Noncommunicable Diseas

Noncommunicable Diseases: A Compendium introduces readers to noncommunicable diseases (NCDs) – what they are, their burden, their determinants and how they can be prevented and controlled.

Focusing on cardiovascular disease, diabetes, cancer and chronic respiratory disease and their five shared main risk factors (tobacco use, harmful use of alcohol, unhealthy diet, physical inactivity and air pollution) as defined by the United Nations, this book provides a synopsis of one of the world's biggest challenges of the 21st century. NCDs prematurely claim the lives of millions of people across the world every year, with untold suffering to hundreds of millions more, trapping many people in poverty and curtailing economic growth and sustainable development. While resources between and within countries largely differ, the key principles of surveillance, prevention and management apply to all countries, as does the need to focus resources on the most cost-effective and affordable interventions and the need for strong political will, sufficient resources, and sustained and broad partnerships. This compendium consists of 59 short and accessible chapters in six sections: (i) describing and measuring the burden and impact of NCDs; (ii) the burden, epidemiology and priority interventions for individual NCDs; (iii) social determinants and risk factors for NCDs and priority interventions; (iv) global policy; (v) cross-cutting issues; and (vi) stakeholder action.

Drawing on the expertise of a large and diverse team of internationally renowned policy and academic experts, the book describes the key epidemiologic features of NCDs and evidence-based interventions in a concise manner that will be useful for policymakers across all parts of society, as well as for public health and clinical practitioners.

Nick Banatvala is the head of the Secretariat of the United Nations Inter-Agency Task Force on the Prevention and Control of Non-communicable Diseases, in WHO, Geneva, that was established to bring the United Nations system and other inter-governmental organizations together to support governments in meeting the NCD-related Sustainable Development Goal targets. Nick is also an honorary professor at the University of Manchester, United Kingdom and honorary Senior Lecturer at Imperial College London.

Pascal Bovet is a senior consultant and former professor of public health at the University Centre for Primary Care and Public Health (Unisanté) in Lausanne, Switzerland, and former head of the NCD Section and co-director of the WHO Collaborating Centre on Cardiovascular Diseases in Populations in Transition. Pascal has for many years advised governments across the world on preventing and controlling NCDs.

Noncommunicable Diseases
A Compendium

Edited by Nick Banatvala and
Pascal Bovet

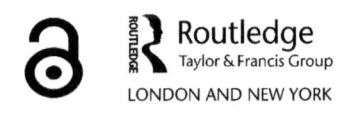

Routledge
Taylor & Francis Group
LONDON AND NEW YORK

The editors and authors alone are responsible for the views expressed in this book and they do not necessarily represent the views, decisions or policies of the institutions or governing bodies with which they are affiliated.

Designed cover image: ajijchan, adapted by Zsuzsanna Schreck.

First published 2023
by Routledge
4 Park Square, Milton Park, Abingdon, Oxon OX14 4RN.

and by Routledge
605 Third Avenue, New York, NY 10158.

Routledge is an imprint of the Taylor & Francis Group, an informa business.

© 2023 selection and editorial matter, Nick Banatvala and Pascal Bovet; individual chapters, the contributors.

The right of Nick Banatvala and Pascal Bovet to be identified as the authors of the editorial material, and of the authors for their individual chapters, has been asserted in accordance with sections 77 and 78 of the Copyright, Designs and Patents Act 1988.

The Open Access version of this book, available at www.taylorfrancis.com, has been made available under a Creative Commons Attribution-Non Commercial-No Derivatives 4.0 license.

Trademark notice: Product or corporate names may be trademarks or registered trademarks, and are used only for identification and explanation without intent to infringe.

British Library Cataloguing-in-Publication Data
A catalogue record for this book is available from the British Library.

Library of Congress Cataloging-in-Publication Data
Names: Banatvala, Nick, editor. | Bovet, Pascal, editor.
Title: Noncommunicable diseases: a compendium/edited by Nick Banatvala and Pascal Bovet.
Other titles: Noncommunicable diseases (Banatvala)
Description: Abingdon, Oxon: New York: Routledge, 2023. | Includes bibliographical references and index.
Identifiers: LCCN 2022041912 (print) | LCCN 2022041913 (ebook) | ISBN 9781032307930 (hardback) | ISBN 9781032307923 (paperback) | ISBN 9781003306689 (ebook)
Subjects: MESH: Noncommunicable Diseases | Chronic Disease | Risk Factors | Social Determinants of Health | Global Health
Classification: LCC RA566 (print) | LCC RA566 (ebook) | NLM QZ 185 | DDC 616.9/8–dc23/eng/20221110
LC record available at https://lccn.loc.gov/2022041912
LC ebook record available at https://lccn.loc.gov/2022041913

ISBN: 978-1-032-30793-0 (hbk)
ISBN: 978-1-032-30792-3 (pbk)
ISBN: 978-1-003-30668-9 (ebk)

DOI: 10.4324/9781003306689

Typeset in Bembo
by Deanta Global Publishing Services, Chennai, India.

Access the Support Material: www.routledge.com/9781032307923

Contents

List of tables xii
List of figures xv
Contributors xvi
Preface xxiv
Foreword xxvi
Credits xxviii
Editors' biographies xxix
Abbreviations xxxi
Editors' note xxxii

PART 1
Describing and measuring the burden and impact of NCDs 1

1 Global burden of NCDs 3
PASCAL BOVET, COLIN MATHERS, NICK BANATVALA, MAJID EZZATI

2 Epidemiologic and demographic transition as drivers of NCDs 14
PASCAL BOVET, FRED PACCAUD, SYLVIE STACHENKO

3 NCDs and sustainable development 21
NICK BANATVALA, AIDAH NAKANJAKO, DOUGLAS WEBB

4 Surveillance of NCDs and their risk factors: Principles 28
PASCAL BOVET, NICK BANATVALA, RICHARD COOPER, LEANNE RILEY

5 Surveillance of NCDs and their risk factors: Selected tools 34
LEANNE RILEY, PASCAL BOVET, NICK BANATVALA, MELANIE COWAN

PART 2
Burden, epidemiology and priority interventions for individual NCDs — 43

6 **Cardiovascular disease: Burden, epidemiology and risk factors** — 45
PASCAL BOVET, NICK BANATVALA, KAY-TEE KHAW, K SRINATH REDDY

7 **Cardiovascular disease: Priority interventions** — 52
PASCAL BOVET, NICK BANATVALA, K SRINATH REDDY, KAY-TEE KHAW

8 **Hypertension: Burden, epidemiology and priority interventions** — 58
PASCAL BOVET, ALTA E SCHUTTE, NICK BANATVALA, MICHEL BURNIER

9 **Diabetes: Burden, epidemiology and priority interventions** — 66
PASCAL BOVET, ISABELLE HAGON-TRAUB, JEAN CLAUDE N MBANYA, NICHOLAS J WAREHAM

10 **Obesity: Burden, epidemiology and priority interventions** — 74
PASCAL BOVET, NATHALIE FARPOUR-LAMBERT, NICK BANATVALA, LOUISE BAUR

11 **Cancer: Burden, epidemiology and principles for priority interventions** — 83
HESHAM GAAFAR, MAY ABDEL-WAHAB, PASCAL BOVET, ANDRÉ ILBAWI

12 **Breast cancer: Burden, epidemiology and priority interventions** — 91
MIRIAM MUTEBI, KARLA UNGER-SALDAÑA, OPHIRA GINSBURG

13 **Cervical cancer: Burden, epidemiology and priority interventions** — 98
NICK BANATVALA, NEERJA BHATLA, SILVINA ARROSSI AND NATHALIE BROUTET

14 **Colorectal cancer: Burden, epidemiology and priority interventions** — 106
JEAN-LUC BULLIARD, SAMAR ALHOMOUD, DIETER HAHNLOSER

15 **Prostate cancer: Burden, epidemiology and priority interventions** — 112
DARIO TRAPANI, MARIANA SIQUEIRA, MANJU SENGAR, DOROTHY C LOMBE

16	**Chronic respiratory diseases: Burden, epidemiology and priority interventions** NILS E BILLO, NICK BANATVALA, PASCAL BOVET, ASMA EL SONY	118

PART 3
Social determinants and risk factors for NCDs and priority interventions — 125

17	**Social determinants of health and NCDs** RUTH BELL, J JAIME MIRANDA, JEAN WOO, MICHAEL MARMOT	127
18	**Tobacco use: Burden, epidemiology and priority interventions** PASCAL BOVET, NICK BANATVALA, JUDE GEDEON, ARMANDO PERUGA	134
19	**Unhealthy diets: Burden, epidemiology and priority interventions** FRANCESCO BRANCA, PASCAL BOVET, NAMUKOLO COVIC, ELISABETTA RECINE	141
20	**Cholesterol, saturated fats and trans fats: Burden, epidemiology and priority interventions** ROGER DARIOLI, PASCAL BOVET, NICK BANATVALA, KAY-TEE KHAW	149
21	**Dietary salt and NCDs: Burden, epidemiology and priority interventions** PASCAL BOVET, MICHEL BURNIER, NICK BANATVALA, LEO NEDERVEEN	157
22	**Dietary sugars and NCDs: Burden, epidemiology, and priority interventions** PASCAL BOVET, NICK BANATVALA, ERIC RAVUSSIN, LEO NEDERVEEN	164
23	**Food reformulation for NCD prevention and control** CHIZURU NISHIDA, RAIN YAMAMOTO, EDUARDO AF NILSON, ALISON TEDSTONE	171
24	**Nutrition labelling for NCD prevention and control** KATRIN ENGELHARDT, CHIZURU NISHIDA, JENNY REID, BRIDGET KELLY	179
25	**Physical inactivity and NCDs: Burden, epidemiology, and priority interventions** ESTELLE VICTORIA LAMBERT, FIONA BULL	186

26 Harmful use of alcohol and NCDs: Burden, epidemiology
and priority interventions 194
PASCAL BOVET, NICK BANATVALA, NICOLAS BERTHOLET, MARISTELA G MONTEIRO

27 Air pollution and NCDs: Burden, epidemiology and
priority interventions 201
JULIA FUSSELL, SOPHIE GUMY, HUALIANG LIN, MALA RAO

28 Infectious diseases and NCDs 209
NICK BANATVALA, EMILY B WONG, GIUSEPPE TROISI, ANTOINE FLAHAULT

29 Genetics and NCDs 216
MURIELLE BOCHUD, AMBROISE WONKAM, PASCAL BOVET, VINCENT MOOSER

PART 4
Global policy for NCD prevention and control 225

30 The WHO Global Strategy for the Prevention and Control
of NCDs 2000 227
NICK BANATVALA, GEORGE ALLEYNE

31 United Nations high-level meetings on NCD prevention
and control 229
NICK BANATVALA, WERNER OBERMEYER, GEORGE ALLEYNE

32 The WHO Global Action Plan for the Prevention and
Control of NCDs 2013–2030 234
NICK BANATVALA, SVETLANA AKSELROD, PASCAL BOVET, SHANTHI MENDIS

33 The WHO Framework Convention on Tobacco Control
and Protocol to Eliminate Illicit Trade in Tobacco Products 240
DOUGLAS WILLIAM BETTCHER, JULIETTE MCHARDY, PASCAL BOVET,
ADRIANA BLANCO MARQUIZO

34 Best buys and other recommended interventions for NCD
prevention and control 246
NICK BANATVALA, PASCAL BOVET, WANRUDEE ISARANUWATCHAI, MELANIE Y
BERTRAM

35	**Accountability for NCD prevention and control** NICK BANATVALA, MELANIE COWAN, MANJU RANI, LEANNE RILEY	253

PART 5
Cross cutting issues around NCD prevention and control   261

36	**Population and individual approaches for NCD prevention and control** PASCAL BOVET, NICK BANATVALA, KAY-TEE KHAW, K SRINATH REDDY	263
37	**A life-course approach for NCD prevention and control** JULIANNE WILLIAMS, KREMLIN WICKRAMASINGHE, SUMUDU K KASTURIARACHCHI, ARNAUD CHIOLERO	271
38	**Universal health coverage and NCD prevention and control** NICK BANATVALA, KASPAR WYSS, PATRICIA AKWEONGO, AUGUST KUWAWENARUWA, VICTOR G RODWIN	277
39	**Financing and allocating resources for NCD prevention and control** NICK BANATVALA, VICTOR G RODWIN, TSEDAY ZERAYACOB, RACHEL NUGENT	285
40	**Making the economic case for investing in NCD prevention and control** ANNA KONTSEVAYA, RACHEL NUGENT, ALEXEY KULIKOV, NICK BANATVALA	294
41	**Fiscal measures for NCD prevention and control** FRANCO SASSI, RONALD CAFRINE, M ARANTXA COLCHERO, NEENA PRASAD	302
42	**Strengthening health systems and service delivery for NCD prevention and control** CHERIAN VARGHESE, BARIDALYNE NONGKYNRIH, PASCAL BOVET, NICK BANATVALA	308
43	**Screening and health checks for NCD prevention and control** KEVIN SELBY, NICK BANATVALA, PASCAL BOVET, JACQUES CORNUZ	317

44	**Access to medicines for NCD prevention and control** CÉCILE MACÉ, DAVID BERAN, RAFFAELLA RAVINETTO, CHRISTOPHE PERRIN	326
45	**Access to medical technologies for NCD prevention and control** ADRIANA VELAZQUEZ BERUMEN, NICOLÒ BINELLO, SASIKALA THANGAVELU, GABRIELA JIMÉNEZ MOYAO	332
46	**Law and NCD prevention and control** BENN MCGRADY, KRITIKA KHANIJO, SUZANNE ZHOU	340
47	**Changing behaviour at scale to prevent NCDs** THERESA M MARTEAU, GARETH J HOLLANDS, DEVAKI NAMBIAR, MARCUS R MUNAFÒ	347
48	**Promoting health behaviours at the individual level for NCD prevention and control** PAUL AVEYARD, WENDY HARDEMAN, ROBERT HORNE	355
49	**Digital technologies for NCD prevention and control** SURABHI JOSHI, CHEICK OUMAR BAGAYOKO, AWA BABINGTON-ASHAYE, ANTOINE GEISSBUHLER	362
50	**Effective communication for NCD prevention and control** JAIMIE GUERRA, ELORM AMETEPE, PASCAL BOVET, NICK BANATVALA	369
51	**NCD prevention and control in emergencies and humanitarian settings** ÉIMHÍN ANSBRO, NICK BANATVALA, SYLVIA KEHLENBRINK, KIRAN JOBANPUTRA	376
52	**The role of human rights in NCD prevention and control** LYNN GENTILE, MARIA CHIARA CAMPISI, NYASHA CHINGORE	384

PART 6
Stakeholder action for NCD prevention and control   391

53 Whole-of-government response for NCD prevention and control   393
ROY SMALL, TAMU DAVIDSON, CONRAD SHAMLAYE, NICK BANATVALA

54 Whole-of-society response for NCD prevention and control   402
NICK BANATVALA, ROY SMALL, PASCAL BOVET, CRISTINA PARSONS PEREZ

55 The role of people living with NCDs in NCD prevention and control   411
JOHANNA RALSTON, CRISTINA PARSONS PEREZ, CHARITY MUTURI, CATHERINE KAREKEZI

56 The role of the private sector in NCD prevention and control   418
NICK BANATVALA, ALAN M TRAGER, MARY AMUYUNZU-NYAMONGO, TÉA COLLINS

57 The role of public–private partnerships in NCD prevention and control   427
ALAN M TRAGER, ETHAN SIMON, SO YOON SIM, NICK BANATVALA

58 Aid effectiveness and the role of multilateral and bilateral development agencies in NCD prevention and control   434
NICK BANATVALA, ANDREA FEIGL, NNENNA EZEIGWE, DUDLEY TARLTON

59 Leadership for NCD prevention and control   442
PEKKA PUSKA, NIZAL SARRAFZADEGAN, BHARATHI VISWANATHAN, NICK BANATVALA

Index   449

Supplement 1. NCD mortality trends and population attributable fractions. The figures (graphs) in this Supplement illustrate NCD mortality estimates displayed in many tables in the compendium. Available at www.routledge.com/9781032307923

Supplement 2. Declarations of interest from authors and editors. Available at www.routledge.com/9781032307923

Tables

1.1 Total deaths and age-standardized rates (per 100,000) for mortality of the four major NCDs by World Bank country income category for 1990 and 2019 (IHME)   8
1.2 Fractions of the global mortality from the four major NCDs that are attributable to modifiable behavioural, metabolic and environmental risk factors (IHME)   10
3.1 Examples of linkages between NCDs and several non-health SDGs   24
5.1 Surveillance tools to measure progress against the WHO Global NCD Action Plan indicators   38
6.1 Mortality for CVD, IHD and stroke (IHME)   46
8.1 Number and percent of deaths and age-standardized mortality attributable to high BP (IHME)   59
9.1 Mortality attributable to diabetes and high fasting blood glucose (IHME)   68
10.1 WHO cut-off points for waist circumference and waist-to-hip ratio and risk of metabolic complications in adults   75
10.2 Mortality attributable to high BMI (IHME)   76
11.1 Mortality and fractions of mortality attributable to modifiable risk factors for leading cancers   84
12.1 Mortality attributable to breast cancer among females (IHME)   92
13.1 Mortality attributable to cervical cancer (IHME)   99
14.1 Mortality for colorectal cancer (IHME)   107
15.1 Mortality for prostate cancer among men (IHME)   113
16.1 Mortality for CRD, including COPD, asthma and pneumoconiosis (IHME)   119
16.2 Examples of WHO global targets and indicators relevant for CRDs   123
17.1 The six areas for action in the Marmot Review with examples of action for the prevention and control of NCDs   130

18.1	Mortality attributable to tobacco use (IHME)	135
19.1	Mortality attributable to dietary risks (IHME)	142
20.1	Mortality attributable to high blood LDL-cholesterol and diet high in trans fat (IHME)	151
20.2	CVD risk categories associated with abnormal blood lipid levels in mmol/l (mg/dl in parentheses)	154
21.1	Mortality attributable to a diet high in sodium (salt)	158
22.1	Mortality attributable to high dietary intake of sugar-sweetened beverages (IHME)	166
24.1	Examples of conditions for nutrient content claims	182
25.1	WHO recommendations on physical activity for children and adolescents, and adults	188
25.2	Mortality attributable to low physical activity (IHME)	189
26.1	Mortality attributable to alcohol use (IHME)	195
27.1	Mortality attributable to air pollution (IHME)	203
29.1	Examples of public health and clinical implications of genetics in relation to NCDs	220
31.1	Challenges to the implementation of WHO best buys and other recommended interventions for the prevention and control of NCDs	232
32.1	Examples of actions described in the WHO Global NCD Action Plan under Objective 1: raising the priority of NCDs in global, regional and national agendas through international cooperation and advocacy (simplified)	238
33.1	Measures to reduce the demand for and supply of tobacco	241
34.1	WHO best buys (interventions with ACER ≤100 international dollars per DALY averted), recommended interventions (those with CEA estimates available but ACER >100), and other recommended interventions (those without CEA estimates)	247
35.1	WHO NCD Global Monitoring Framework	254
36.1	Main characteristics of population-based and high-risk strategies for the prevention and control of diseases	264
39.1	Composition of health spending by funding source in 2019	289
39.2	Official development assistance (official donors, all channels, gross disbursements, for developing countries) in 2020	290
40.1	Economic burden of NCDs, 2011–2030 (trillions of US$ 2010)	296
40.2	Five-year returns on a set of intervention packages to prevent NCDs based on WHO-UNDP investment case methodology across a selection of countries	299
42.1	The six HEARTS modules to strengthen the management of NCDs in primary care	313

42.2	Fifteen health system challenges and opportunities to improve NCD outcomes	315
43.1	Screening and health checks consistent with the WHO best buys and other interventions for NCD conditions	324
47.1	Population-level interventions to change behaviour at scale to prevent NCDs: WHO best buys and other related interventions	349
50.1	Stakeholder or audience analysis for a single overarching communication outcome/objective (SOCO)	372
54.1	The roles of government, the private sector and the media for prevention and control of NCDs	403
55.1	Examples of how the engagement of people living with NCDs can be translated into concrete actions for NCD prevention and control	414
57.1	Business models of public–private partnerships	430
59.1	Styles of leadership	443

Figures

2.1	Decreasing all-cause mortality and changing broad-cause mortality patterns along the four stages of the epidemiologic transition	16
2.2	Demographic transition over time and associated predominant causes of deaths	19
3.1	Poverty contributes to NCDs and NCDs contribute to poverty	22
6.1	The relationship between risk factors and CVD (and other selected NCDs)	48
13.1	The life-course approach to cervical cancer prevention and control	100
17.1	Conceptual Framework of the WHO Commission on Social Determinants of Health	128
24.1	Integrating nutrient declarations, supplementary nutrition information and health and nutrition claims	183
37.1	Impact of interventions across the life-course to reduce cumulative NCD risk	272
38.1	The three key dimensions of UHC: population coverage, service coverage and proportion of costs covered	277
42.1	Challenges in providing optimal healthcare for NCDs	310
43.1	The benefits and harms associated with a screening programme	319
43.2	Example of a framework for screening, counselling and vaccination for the prevention of NCDs and their risk factors at the primary care level in Switzerland	323
56.1	Industries categorized according to value alignment	419

Contributors

Editors

Nick Banatvala and Pascal Bovet

Contributors

May Abdel-Wahab, Division of Human Health, International Atomic Energy Agency, Vienna, Austria.

Svetlana Akselrod, Office of the Deputy Director-General, World Health Organization, Geneva, Switzerland.

Patricia Akweongo, School of Public Health, University of Ghana, Accra, Ghana.

Samar Alhomoud, Colorectal Surgery Section, King Faisal Specialist Hospital and Research Centre, Riyadh, Saudi Arabia.

George Alleyne, Pan American Health Organization, Washington DC, USA.

Elorm Ametepe, Public Relations, Ministry of Health, Accra, Ghana.

Mary Amuyunzu-Nyamongo, African Institute for Health and Development, Nairobi, Kenya.

Éimhín Ansbro, Centre for Global Chronic Conditions, London School of Hygiene and Tropical Medicine, London, UK.

Silvina Arrossi, Health, Economy and Society, Center for the Study of State and Society (CEDES), Buenos Aires, Argentina.

Paul Aveyard, Nuffield Department of Primary Care Health Sciences, University of Oxford, Oxford, UK.

Awa Babington-Ashaye, Division of eHealth and Telemedicine, Geneva University Hospitals, Geneva, Switzerland.

Cheick Oumar Bagayoko, Digital Health and Innovation Center, University of Sciences, Techniques and Technologies of Bamako, Bamako, Mali.

Nick Banatvala, Secretariat of the UN Inter-Agency Task Force on the Prevention and Control of NCDs, World Health Organization, Geneva, Switzerland.

Louise Baur, Sydney Medical School, The University of Sydney, Sydney, Australia.

Ruth Bell, Institute of Health Equity, University College London, London, UK.

David Beran, Division of Tropical and Humanitarian Medicine, University of Geneva, Geneva, Switzerland.

Nicolas Bertholet, Addiction Medicine, Lausanne University Hospital, Lausanne, Switzerland.

Melanie Y Bertram, Department of Delivery for Impact, World Health Organization, Geneva, Switzerland.

Douglas William Bettcher, Office of the Director-General, World Health Organization, Geneva, Switzerland.

Neerja Bhatla, Department of Obstetrics & Gynaecology, All India Institute of Medical Sciences, New Delhi, India.

Nils E Billo, Independent Consultant, Joensuu, Finland, formerly Management of Noncommunicable Diseases Unit, World Health Organization, Geneva, Switzerland.

Nicolò Binello, Medical Devices and In Vitro Diagnostics Team, World Health Organization, Geneva, Switzerland.

Adriana Blanco Marquizo, Secretariat of the WHO Framework Convention on Tobacco Control (an entity hosted by WHO), Geneva, Switzerland.

Murielle Bochud, Department of Epidemiology and Health Systems, University Centre for Primary Care and Public Health (Unisanté), Lausanne, Switzerland.

Pascal Bovet, Department of Epidemiology and Health Systems, University Centre for Primary Care and Public Health (Unisanté), Lausanne, Switzerland.

Francesco Branca, Department of Nutrition and Food Safety, World Health Organization, Geneva, Switzerland.

Nathalie Broutet, Department of Sexual and Reproductive Health and Research, World Health Organization, Geneva, Switzerland.

Fiona Bull, Physical Activity Unit, World Health Organization, Geneva, Switzerland.

Jean-Luc Bulliard, Department of Epidemiology and Health Systems, University Centre for Primary Care and Public Health (Unisanté), Lausanne, Switzerland.

Michel Burnier, Service of Nephrology and Hypertension, Lausanne University Hospital, Lausanne, Switzerland.

Ronald Cafrine, Trade Department, Ministry for Finance, National Planning & Trade, Victoria, Seychelles.

Maria Chiara Campisi, Health Law Programme, International Development Law Organization, Rome, Italy.

Nyasha Chingore, AIDS and Rights Alliance for Southern Africa, Windhoek, Namibia.

Arnaud Chiolero, Population Health Laboratory, University of Fribourg, Fribourg, Switzerland.

M Arantxa Colchero, Center for Health Systems Research, National Institute of Public Health, Cuernavaca, Mexico.

Téa Collins, Global NCD Platform, World Health Organization, Geneva, Switzerland.

Jacques Cornuz, Department of General Medicine, University Centre for Primary Care and Public Health (Unisanté), Lausanne, Switzerland.

Namukolo Covic, International Livestock Research Institute, Addis Ababa, Ethiopia.

Melanie Cowan, Noncommunicable Diseases Department, World Health Organization, Geneva, Switzerland.

Roger Darioli, Swiss Nutrition & Health Foundation, Epalinges, Switzerland.

Tamu Davidson, Chronic Disease and Injury Department, Caribbean Public Health Agency, Port of Spain, Trinidad and Tobago.

Asma El Sony, Epidemiological Laboratory for Public Health, Research and Development, Khartoum, Sudan.

Katrin Engelhardt, Department of Nutrition and Food Safety, World Health Organization, Geneva, Switzerland.

Nnenna Ezeigwe, Independent Consultant, formerly Department of Noncommunicable Diseases, Federal Ministry of Health of Nigeria, Abuja, Nigeria.

Majid Ezzati, Imperial College London, London, UK and University of Ghana, Accra, Ghana.

Nathalie J Farpour-Lambert, Service of Endocrinology, Diabetology, Nutrition and Therapeutic Patient Education, Geneva University Hospitals (HUG), Geneva, Switzerland.

Andrea Feigl, Health Finance Institute, Washington DC, USA.

Antoine Flahault, Institute of Global Health, University of Geneva, Geneva, Switzerland.

Julia Fussell, School of Public Health, Imperial College London, London, UK.

Hesham Gaafar, Department of Noncommunicable Diseases, World Health Organization, Geneva, Switzerland.

Jude Gedeon, Public Health Authority, Ministry of Health, Victoria, Seychelles.

Antoine Geissbuhler, Division of eHealth and Telemedicine, Geneva University Hospitals (HUG), Geneva, Switzerland.

Lynn Gentile, Development and Economic and Social Issues Branch, Office of the United Nations High Commissioner for Human Rights, Geneva, Switzerland.

Ophira Ginsburg, Center for Global Health, U.S. National Cancer Institute, Rockville, USA.

Jaimie Guerra, Department of Communications, World Health Organization, Geneva, Switzerland.

Sophie Gumy, Department of Environment, Climate Change and Health, World Health Organization, Geneva, Switzerland.

Isabelle Hagon-Traub, Endocrinology and Diabetology Unit, Valais Hospital Centre, Sion, Switzerland.

Dieter Hahnloser, Department of Visceral Surgery, Lausanne University Hospital, Lausanne, Switzerland.

Wendy Hardeman, School of Health Sciences, University of East Anglia, Norwich, UK.

Gareth J Hollands, Evidence for Policy and Practice Information and Co-ordinating Centre (EPPI Centre), University College London, London, UK.

Robert Horne, UCL School of Pharmacy, University College London, London, UK.

Wanrudee Isaranuwatchai, Health Intervention and Technology Assessment Program, Ministry of Public Health, Nonthaburi, Thailand.

Gabriela Jiménez Moyao, Health Implementation Support Team, United Nations Development Programme, Geneva, Switzerland.

Kiran Jobanputra, Médecins sans Frontières, London, UK.

Surabhi Joshi, Digital Health and Innovations Department, World Health Organization, Geneva, Switzerland.

Catherine Karekezi, NCD Alliance Kenya, Nairobi, Kenya.

Sumudu K Kasturiarachchi, Independent Consultant, formerly Office of the Deputy Director General for Public Health Services, Ministry of Health, Colombo, Sri Lanka.

Sylvia Kehlenbrink, Division of Endocrinology, Diabetes and Hypertension, Brigham and Women's Hospital, Boston, USA.

Bridget Kelly, School of Health & Society, University of Wollongong, Wollongong, Australia.

Kritika Khanijo, Public Health Law and Policies, World Health Organization, Geneva, Switzerland.

Kay-Tee Khaw, MRC Epidemiology Unit, University of Cambridge, Cambridge, UK.

Anna Kontsevaya, Department of Public health, National Medical Research Center for Therapy and Preventive Medicine, Moscow, Russian Federation.

Alexey Kulikov, Secretariat of the UN Inter-Agency Task Force on the Prevention and Control of NCDs, World Health Organization, Geneva, Switzerland.

August Kuwawenaruwa, Department of Health Systems, Impact Evaluation, and Policy, Ifakara Health Institute, Dar es Salaam, Tanzania.

Estelle Victoria Lambert, Research Centre for Health through Physical Activity, Lifestyle and Sport, University of Cape Town, Cape Town, South Africa.

Hualiang Lin, School of Public Health, Sun Yat-sen University, Guangzhou, China.

Dorothy C Lombe, Regional Cancer Treatment Services, MidCentral District Health Board, Palmerston North, New Zealand.

Cécile Macé, Independent Consultant, formerly Essential Medicines and Health Products Department, World Health Organization, Geneva, Switzerland.

Michael Marmot, Institute of Health Equity, University College London, London, UK.

Theresa M Marteau, Department of Public Health and Primary Care, University of Cambridge, Cambridge, UK.

Colin Mathers, Independent Consultant, formerly Mortality and Health Analysis Unit, World Health Organization, Geneva, Switzerland.

Jean Claude N Mbanya, Department of Internal Medicine and Specialties, University of Yaounde 1, Yaounde, Cameroon.

Benn McGrady, Public Health Law and Policies Unit, World Health Organization, Geneva, Switzerland.

Juliette McHardy, O'Neill Institute for National and Global Health Law, Georgetown Law, Washington DC, USA.

Shanthi Mendis, Independent Consultant, formerly Department of Noncommunicable Diseases, World Health Organization, Geneva, Switzerland.

J Jaime Miranda, CRONICAS Centre of Excellence in Chronic Diseases, Universidad Peruana Cayetano Heredia, Lima, Peru.

Maristela G Monteiro, Noncommunicable Diseases and Mental Health Department, Pan American Health Organization, Washington DC, USA.

Vincent Mooser, Department of Human Genetics, McGill University, Montreal, Canada.

Marcus R Munafò, School of Psychological Science, University of Bristol, Bristol, UK.

Miriam Mutebi, Department of Surgery, Aga Khan University, Nairobi, Kenya.

Charity Muturi, Our Views, Our Voices Global Advisory Committee, NCD Alliance, Nairobi, Kenya.

Devaki Nambiar, Health Systems Sciences Division, George Institute for Global Health, Delhi, India.

Leo Nederveen, Risk Factors and Nutrition Unit, Pan American Health Organization, Washington DC, USA.

Eduardo AF Nilson, Program of Food and Nutrition, Oswaldo Cruz Foundation (Fiocruz), Brasilia, Brazil.

Chizuru Nishida, Department of Nutrition and Food Safety, World Health Organization, Geneva, Switzerland.

Baridalyne Nongkynrih, Centre for Community Medicine, All India Institute of Medical Sciences, New Delhi, India.

Rachel Nugent, Centre for Global NCDs, RTI International, Seattle, USA.

Werner Obermeyer, Director General's Office, World Health Organization, New York, USA.

Fred Paccaud, Department of Epidemiology and Health Systems, University Centre for Primary Care and Public Health (Unisanté), Lausanne, Switzerland.

Cristina Parsons Perez, Capacity Development Unit, NCD Alliance, London, UK.

Christophe Perrin, Independent Consultant, formerly Médecins Sans Frontières Access Campaign, Paris, France.

Armando Peruga, Catalan Institute of Oncology-Biomedical Research Institute of Bellvitge (IDIBELL) & Centro de Investigación Biomédica en Red de Enfermedades Respiratorias (CIBERES), Spain.

Neena Prasad, Bloomberg Philanthropies, New York, USA.

Pekka Puska, Finnish Institute for Health and Welfare (THL), Helsinki, Finland.

Johanna Ralston, Chief Executive Officer, World Obesity Federation, London, UK.

Manju Rani, Department of Healthier Populations and Noncommunicable Diseases, WHO Regional Office for South-East Asia, Delhi, India.

Mala Rao, Department of Primary Care and Public Health, Imperial College London, London, UK.

Raffaella Ravinetto, Department of Public Health, Institute of Tropical Medicine, Antwerp, Belgium.

Eric Ravussin, Clinical Science, Pennington Biomedical Research Center, Baton Rouge, USA.

Elisabetta Recine, Observatory of Food and Nutrition Security Policies, University of Brasilia, Brasilia, Brazil.

K Srinath Reddy, Public Health Foundation of India, Public Health Foundation of India, Gurugram, India.

Jenny Reid, Policy and Trade, Ministry for Primary Industries, Wellington, New Zealand.

Leanne Riley, Noncommunicable Diseases Department, World Health Organization, Geneva, Switzerland.

Victor G Rodwin, Wagner School of Public Service, New York University, New York, USA.

Nizal Sarrafzadegan, Isfahan Cardiovascular Research Center, Isfahan University of Medical Sciences, Isfahan, Iran.

Franco Sassi, Centre for Health Economics & Policy Innovation, Imperial College London, London, UK.

Aletta E Schutte, University of New South Wales, The George Institute for Global Health, Sydney, Australia.

Kevin Selby, Department of Ambulatory Care, Centre for Primary Care and Public Health (Unisanté), Lausanne, Switzerland.

Manju Sengar, Department of Medical Oncology, Tata Memorial Centre, Mumbai, India.

Conrad Shamlaye, Public Health Authority, Ministry of Health, Victoria, Seychelles.

So Yoon Sim, Department of Immunization, Vaccines and Biologicals, World Health Organization, Geneva, Switzerland.

Ethan Simon, PPP Initiative Ltd., Los Angeles, USA.

Mariana Siqueira, Medical Oncology, D'Or Institute of Research and Teaching, Rio de Janeiro, Brazil.

Roy Small, HIV, Health and Development Group, United Nations Development Programme, New York, USA.

Sylvie Stachenko, Independent Consultant, formerly School of Public Health, University of Alberta, Edmonton, Canada.

Dudley Tarlton, HIV Health and Development Group, United Nations Development Programme, Istanbul, Turkey.

Alison Tedstone, Independent Consultant, formerly Office for Health Improvement and Disparities, Department of Health and Social Care, England, London, UK.

Sasikala Thangavelu, Independent Consultant, formerly, Policy, Code and Standard Division, Medical Device Authority, Cyberjaya, Malaysia.

Alan M Trager, The Bartlett School of Sustainable Construction, University College London, London, UK.

Dario Trapani, New Drug Development for Innovative Therapies, European Institute of Oncology IRCCS, Milan, Italy.

Giuseppe Troisi, Secretariat of the UN Inter-Agency Task Force on the Prevention and Control of NCDs, World Health Organization, Geneva, Switzerland.

Karla Unger-Saldaña, Epidemiology Unit, National Cancer Institute, Mexico City, Mexico.

Cherian Varghese, Department of Noncommunicable Diseases, World Health Organization, Geneva, Switzerland.

Adriana Velazquez Berumen, Medical Devices and In Vitro Diagnostics team, World Health Organization, Geneva, Switzerland.

Bharathi Viswanathan, Unit for Prevention and Control of Cardiovascular Diseases, Ministry of Health, Victoria, Seychelles.

Nicholas J Wareham, MRC Epidemiology Unit, University of Cambridge, Cambridge, UK.

Douglas Webb, HIV Health and Development Group, United Nations Development Programme, New York, USA.

Kremlin Wickramasinghe, WHO European Office for Prevention and Control of Noncommunicable Diseases, WHO Regional Office for Europe, Copenhagen, Denmark.

Julianne Williams, WHO European Office for Prevention and Control of Noncommunicable Diseases, WHO Regional Office for Europe, Copenhagen, Denmark.

Emily B Wong, Department of Basic and Translational Science, Africa Health Research Institute, Durban, South Africa.

Ambroise Wonkam, McKusick-Nathans Institute and the Department of Genetic Medicine, Johns Hopkins University, Baltimore, USA.

Jean Woo, Department of Medicine and Therapeutics, The Chinese University of Hong Kong, Hong Kong SAR, China.

Kaspar Wyss, Swiss Centre for International Health, Swiss Tropical and Public Health Institute, Allschwil, Switzerland.

Rain Yamamoto, Department of Nutrition and Food Safety, World Health Organization, Geneva, Switzerland.

Tseday Zerayacob, Independent Consultant, currently Strategic Purchasing Africa Resource Centre, Addis Ababa, Ethiopia.

Suzanne Zhou, McCabe Centre for Law and Cancer, Melbourne, Australia.

Preface

Cardiovascular disease, diabetes, cancer and chronic respiratory disease, collectively referred to as noncommunicable diseases (NCDs) by the United Nations in 2011, are some of the world's biggest challenges of the 21st century. NCDs have a huge socioeconomic impact on individuals, their families and society at large. Tackling NCDs is about more than preventing and treating diseases; it is an integral part of sustainable development.

The compendium restricts itself to the four NCDs above along with five shared main risk factors – tobacco use, harmful use of alcohol, unhealthy diet, physical inactivity and air pollution. While this approach has many proponents, we recognize that others may find this approach reductive.

We are also framing the compendium around the WHO Global Action Plan for the Prevention and Control of Noncommunicable Diseases 2013–2030, including a set of cost-effective, evidence-based interventions that have been endorsed by the World Health Assembly, which all countries should aspire to implement as a public health priority. These are often referred to as WHO best buys and other recommended interventions.

Throughout the compendium we have used the Institute for Health Metrics and Evaluation (IHME)'s internet-based GBD Compare tool to describe the burden of disease, including crude and age-adjusted estimates and population-attributable fractions. We have decided to use this tool as it provides a source that has data available since 1990 and estimates are internally consistent and can be generated by the reader for all countries – and therefore estimates in the compendium can be reproduced. As with all databases, there are limitations, not least that modelling based on a number of assumptions is often required to take into account missing or poor-quality data.

Our target audience is public health and human development professionals, as well as individuals across government and society that can play an important role in advancing NCD prevention and control. We hope that the compendium will also be accessible and meaningful for people living with NCDs, the media and interested members of the public. Each chapter aims to provide a short, easy-to-digest summary of key issues and priority interventions, with a small number of references to signpost readers to further readings. While we are all too conscious that we have not given authors a large-enough space to give issues the full attention and depth that they deserve, we have tried to ensure that each chapter is sufficiently comprehensive and relevant for readers in the majority of settings. Resources between and within countries largely differ, but common public health principles, such as a set of common main surveillance indicators and main prevention and management interventions, tend to apply to all or most countries, as does the need to focus resources on the most cost-effective and affordable interventions and the need for sustained and broad partnerships to improve NCD outcomes as part of broader development goals.

In writing and editing this compendium, we have tried to keep at the forefront of our minds the needs of people affected by NCDs, including those at risk. We both have children, and we want to see them and their children live and thrive in environments that encourage them to make healthy choices in an easy and affordable way. And if they become unwell, we want them to be able to access effective and affordable quality treatment and care.

The compendium was inspired by over 20 residential seminars on the prevention and control of NCDs that have been jointly run since 2010 by WHO and the University of Lausanne, both in Switzerland and in other parts of the world. Public health policymakers and practitioners from more than 110 countries have participated in one or more of these courses so far. Facilitating these seminars has been hugely rewarding, and we were therefore delighted when Routledge suggested that we develop a compendium based on the approach we have used over the last ten years. The faculty for these seminars has always been a mix of staff from WHO and academic institutions – and this multi-author compendium reflects this.

We are immensely grateful to the policy, programme, clinical and academic experts who have worked together over many months to make this compendium a reality. The multifactorial nature of NCDs means that their prevention and control is one of the most challenging areas of public health and goes far beyond technical solutions in the health sector, requiring complex coordinated action and strong political commitment across all parts of government and society.

The prevention and control of NCDs is rapidly advancing. New evidence is constantly emerging on the causes of NCDs and effective interventions to prevent and treat these conditions. We hope to be able to reflect on these changes in future editions of this compendium.

We are extremely grateful to Routledge and Deanta – in particular Helena Hurd, Rosie Anderson, and Shanmugapriya Rajaram, for all the support that they have provided in helping us conceptualize and subsequently develop and finalize the compendium.

Finally, we are all too aware of the limitations of our editing skills, and we ask for the forbearance of readers as they navigate the book. We would be delighted to hear from readers on how we can improve subsequent editions.

Nick Banatvala and Pascal Bovet

Foreword

The world continues to be affected by the huge health and socioeconomic impact of noncommunicable diseases (NCDs). Around 80% of all premature NCD deaths are caused by cardiovascular disease, cancer, chronic pulmonary disease and diabetes. While the good news is that many of these diseases can be prevented and successfully treated through evidence-based, high-impact interventions that can be implemented in all countries, irrespective of income, the tragedy is that millions of people still die too young from NCDs, or suffer unnecessarily because these interventions are not being made available to most people in the world.

This compendium is an important contribution to the global struggle against NCDs. I am delighted that it has been inspired by the NCD seminars that have been running since 2010 that I, in my capacity as Director and Assistant Director-General in WHO, initiated with the University of Lausanne, a WHO Collaborating Centre for cardiovascular disease in countries in transition. These seminars were established to build capacity among health officials and managers of national NCD programmes, principally from low- and middle-income countries.

In line with the seminars, the compendium is framed around the 2000 WHO Global Strategy, and the global NCD and other related action plans and initiatives, which I, as a WHO director and Assistant Director-General, had the honour and privilege of leading for many years. Together these were instrumental in leading to the high-level meeting of heads of state and government on NCDs at the United Nations General Assembly in 2011. The principles and actions set out in these strategies and the commitments agreed upon by all countries at the General Assembly continue to underpin global and country responses to NCDs.

While good progress has been made to increase awareness of NCDs since 2000, and many countries have put in place policies to reduce the impact of NCDs on health and development, action over the last ten years has been slow and uneven – and as a result, many countries are falling behind on their commitments. In order to scale up action, it will be essential to explore, in an objective and transparent way, the existing gaps behind the slow response and the reasons that limit the translation of declared commitments into sustained investments.

By reviewing the epidemiology and impact of the four major NCDs and their shared modifiable risk factors, and focusing on cost-effective, evidence-based interventions to prevent and control them, this comprehensive and concise compendium is an important resource to support policymakers, public health practitioners, clinicians, civil society and other stakeholders working to reinforce political and technical action on NCDs at global, regional and country levels.

Throughout my time at WHO, I was fortunate to work with a great group of colleagues, international experts and partners, many of whom have contributed to this book – which has made writing this foreword a particular pleasure. I congratulate the editors and express deep appreciation for the many individuals who have shared the wealth of their knowledge and experience to assist everyone involved in translating national and international commitments into sustained investment and action, and thereby turning down the tide on NCDs.

Ala Alwan
Professor of Global Health,
London School of Hygiene and Tropical Medicine.
Emeritus Regional Director,
World Health Organization.

Credits

Figure 2.1. Decreasing all-cause mortality and changing broad-cause mortality patterns along the four stages of the epidemiologic transition. Figure adapted from: Bovet P, Paccaud F. Cardiovascular disease and the changing face of global public health: a focus on low and middle income countries. Public Health Rev 2011;33:397-415, with kind permission of the Swiss School of Public Health.

Figure 13.1. The life-course approach to cervical cancer prevention and control
Figure adapted from: Introducing and scaling up testing for HPV as part of a comprehensive programme for prevention and control of cervical cancer: a step-by-step guide. WHO, 2020 with kind permission of the World Health Organization.

Figure 17.1. Conceptual framework of the WHO Commission on Social Determinants of Health.
Figure reproduced from: Solar O, Irwin A. A conceptual framework for action on the social determinants of health. Social Determinants of Health Discussion Paper 2 (Policy and Practice). WHO, 2010 with kind permission of the World Health Organization.

Figure 38.1. The three key dimensions of UHC: population coverage, service coverage and proportion of costs covered. Figure reproduced from: World Health Report. Health systems financing: the path to universal coverage. WHO 2010 with kind permission of the World Health Organization.

Figure 43.1. The benefits and harms associated with a screening programme. Figure reproduced from: Screening programmes: a short guide. Increase effectiveness, maximize benefits and minimize harm. WHO Regional Office for Europe; Copenhagen, 2020 with kind permission of the European Office of the World Health Organization.

Table 54.1. The role of various sectors in society for prevention and control NCDs. Adapted from: Whole-of-society response to address NCDs—what is the role of various stakeholders in society? with kind permission of the South East Asia Regional Office of the World Health Organization.

Editors' biographies

Nick Banatvala is the head of the Secretariat of the United Nations Inter-Agency Task Force on the Prevention and Control of Non-communicable Diseases, in WHO, Geneva, that was established to bring the United Nations system and other inter-governmental organizations together to support governments meet the NCD-related SDG targets.

Nick was head of Global Affairs at the Department of Health in England, where he led the development and implementation of the UK Government's first-ever global health strategy. Before that, he headed up the UK Department for International Development's work on global health partnerships, scaling up health services and communicable diseases. Prior to this, Nick led DFID's health and education programming in Pakistan, Afghanistan and the Middle East. Nick has experience in the non-governmental sector, having worked with the UK aid agency Merlin on a number of humanitarian and development programmes.

Nick trained in paediatrics and infectious diseases before doing public health and epidemiologic research in the East End of London and at the US Centers for Disease Control and Prevention. Nick has held senior posts in UK public health, where his portfolios included cardiovascular disease, diabetes, breast and cervical cancer screening and clinical governance.

Nick has sat on government, non-government and academic boards, as well as national and international committees. He has undertaken consultancies for a number of agencies including the World Bank.

Nick holds an honorary chair at Manchester University and a senior lectureship at Imperial College, London. In addition to being the lead author of a number of United Nations, WHO and UK government publications, Nick has published widely in a range of peer-reviewed journals.

Pascal Bovet is a senior consultant at the University Centre for Primary Care and Public Health (Unisanté) in Lausanne. Prior to this, he was the head of the NCD Section and professor of public health at this institution. He also was the co-director of the WHO Collaborating Centre on Cardiovascular Diseases in Populations in Transition at this institution. Pascal still regularly teaches public health at the University of Lausanne and at other universities. Earlier Pascal was practicing clinical medicine, including as a chief resident or consultant in several hospitals.

Pascal has been a consultant for NCDs for the Ministry of Health of the Republic of Seychelles since 1988, where he has led several population-based NCD surveys and other NCD-related studies. He has contributed to the development of a number of policies, including national NCD plans and strategies, tobacco control legislation, fiscal measures on tobacco and sugar drinks and guidelines for the management of hypertension and diabetes in primary care.

Pascal is currently collaborating with several partners on research and prevention projects related to NCDs in several countries. Pascal has authored or co-authored over 400 publications. Pascal has also been serving as a technical adviser for WHO and several other agencies around the development and evaluation of national NCD plans of action in a number of countries over the past two decades. He has sat on several public health and research-related boards.

Pascal is board certified in both internal medicine and public health (FMH, Switzerland) and holds an MPH degree from UCLA.

Abbreviations

Cardiovascular disease	CVD
Chronic respiratory disease	CRD
High-income countries	HICs
Institute for Health Metrics and Evaluation	IHME
Low-income countries	LICs
Middle-income countries	MICs
Noncommunicable diseases	NCDs
Social Determinants of Health	SDH
Sustainable Development Goals	SDGs
WHO Global Action Plan for the Prevention and Control of Noncommunicable Diseases 2013–2030	WHO Global NCD Action Plan
WHO Framework on Tobacco Control	WHO FCTC
World Health Assembly	WHA
World Health Organization	WHO
United Nations	UN
Universal health coverage	UHC

Editors' note

If you don't have time to read this compendium …

1. The main types of NCDs are cardiovascular disease (such as heart attack and stroke), cancers, chronic respiratory diseases and diabetes; together they kill 41 million people each year, equivalent to 71% of all deaths globally, with cardiovascular diseases accounting for most of these deaths, followed by cancer, chronic respiratory diseases and diabetes.
2. NCDs are not just diseases of high-income countries, as seen by the fact that 77% of all NCD deaths are in low- and middle-income countries, where around 84% of the world's population lives, and the number of people living with NCDs is likely to increase largely because of the growth and aging of populations across the world unless urgent action is taken.
3. Premature deaths and ill health from NCDs curtail economic growth and trap populations in poverty, and improved NCD outcomes support all three dimensions of sustainable development: economic, social and environmental.
4. Socioeconomically disadvantaged people have a higher risk of acquiring NCDs and dying early from them; in large part they are more exposed to a range of modifiable NCD risk factors and also have less access to preventive care and treatment.
5. There are three types of modifiable risk factors for the main NCDs: behavioural, environmental and metabolic.
6. According to the Institute for Health Metrics and Evaluation, when it comes to behavioural risk factors, 8.7 million deaths in 2019 were attributable to tobacco use, 7.9 to an unhealthy diet, 2.4 to harmful use of alcohol and 0.8 million to physical inactivity in 2019; for environmental risk factors, the figure for air pollution for example was 6.7 million deaths; and for metabolic risk factors the figures were 10.8 for high blood pressure, 6.5 for high blood glucose, 5.0 for high body mass index and 4.4 for high blood cholesterol.
7. Cost-effective and affordable evidence-based interventions are available and can be implemented in almost all settings to prevent, detect, screen,

treat and care for people at risk or with NCDs – and, as a result, age-specific rates of most NCDs are now declining in most countries, although more quickly in high- vs low-income countries.
8. Intervention to prevent NCDs lie for a large part outside the health sector and therefore requires leadership and political commitment to act across the whole of government and this requires policies that prioritize public health in multiple sectors, while health systems need to be able to detect, screen, treat and care for people at risk or with NCDs, with government ensuring that everyone is able to access affordable health services for NCDs, as part of universal health coverage.
9. The responsibility for reducing the burden of NCDs lies not only with the government but also with the society as a whole, for example the private sector, civil society, the media and those carrying out research to develop new and evaluate existing interventions.
10. Data, including the levels of the main modifiable risk factors in the population, are essential to chart progress, advocate for resources for evidence-based interventions and hold everyone accountable for their actions.

It is my ambition to say in ten sentences what others say in a whole book.
Friedrich Nietzsche

Part 1
Describing and measuring the burden and impact of NCDs

1 Global burden of NCDs

Pascal Bovet, Colin Mathers, Nick Banatvala, Majid Ezzati

This chapter describes the disease burden of the four NCDs considered in this book – cardiovascular disease (CVD), cancer, diabetes and chronic respiratory diseases (CRD), and their common set of shared risk factors – tobacco use, harmful use of alcohol, unhealthy diet, physical inactivity and air pollution.

Mortality and morbidity can be expressed as 'incidence' (new cases in a given period) or 'prevalence' (number of cases at one moment in time). Incidence and prevalence can be described in absolute numbers (e.g. total numbers of cases in a population) or as rates, frequently per 100,000 population per year.

Assessment of mortality is not straightforward as data are often not collected/registered systematically and the cause of death is frequently unknown/inaccurately recorded. Overall, a little less than half of deaths in the world are registered with their cause, and in Africa, only four countries have national death registration data. Calculating rates is a challenge when the size and age distribution of the population is not known precisely.

Accurate morbidity data are even less available/reliable. Indicators such as numbers of years of life lost (YLLs) and disability-adjusted life years lost (DALYs) rely on complex diagnostic criteria and usually require modelling of some inputs, as well as a number of methodological choices.[1]

Morbidity data can be collected more easily at the health facility level but are not representative of the whole population.

Examples of measures used to describe NCD mortality and morbidity are shown in Box 1.1.

BOX 1.1 EXAMPLES OF MEASURES USED TO DESCRIBE THE NCD BURDEN

Crude estimates

Total numbers (incidence or prevalence) provide information on the actual burden of a particular disease or risk factor in a population. Crude estimates are important for defining public health and health service needs

DOI: 10.4324/9781003306689-2

for this population (e.g. how many people in a country have hypertension or diabetes, how many die from a heart attack or different cancers). Where a population size is increasing and/or ageing (as is the case in most countries, particularly low- and middle-income countries, numbers (both incidence and prevalence) will inevitably increase over time, particularly for NCDs, given that they tend to occur later in life.

Age-standardized rates

Age-standardized incidence or prevalence is calculated by weighting crude estimates against a 'standard' age distribution.[2] This enables us to directly compare incidence or prevalence estimates across different populations and over time, irrespective of differences in population size and age distribution between populations or over time. Age-standardized rates inform us as to whether a disease (or a risk factor) increases or decreases in the population irrespective of demographic changes (i.e. whether differences occur because of different/changing exposures to risk factors and/or prevention/treatment interventions).

Population attributable fractions (PAF)

PAF is the estimated fraction of a disease (based on mortality or other metrics, e.g. DALYs) that would not have occurred if there had been no exposure to one (or several) risk factor(s) in a population.[3] PAF (or population-attributable risk) provides information on the potential public health impact of reducing risk factors in the population. For example, knowing that in a particular country 16% of all deaths are due to tobacco use or that 21% are due to hypertension provides a strong rationale for the need to prioritize and/or strengthen tobacco and hypertension prevention and control interventions.

Years of life lost (YLL) and disability-standardized years of life lost (DALYs)

These metrics integrate morbidity and mortality. Estimation is more complex and requires additional data and a number of assumptions.

Notes:

- The PAF of a disease attributable to several risk factors may be larger when calculated as the sum of PAFs calculated separately for each risk factor than when measured by taking all risk factors together because risk factors may not be fully independent of each other (e.g. PAF of CVD attributable to raised BMI and low physical activity).

- PAFs differ across populations according to the prevalence of risk factors but the impact also varies according to the absolute risk of a disease in a particular population.[4]

Data can be presented at a global, regional, country, or local level. Data can also be disaggregated by age, gender, socio-economic position and/or other variables.

Databases available for understanding the epidemiology of NCDs

National governments, UN/intergovernmental, academic and other agencies publish data on NCDs at a local, national, regional and global level using reported or published data from multiple sources such as civil registration, health facilities and population surveys at national and local levels. Lack of available/reliable data for the reasons described above, means that statistical models are required to prepare mortality, morbidity and PAF estimates for these and other health indicators so that they be compared across countries and/or over time in a meaningful way. Different sources of data, assumptions and modelling explain why estimates can differ between agencies.[5]

Two important global health databases, that include NCDs, are the WHO Global Health Observatory (GHO) and the Institute for Health Metrics and Evaluation (IHME) Global Disease Burden project (GBD). GHO is the WHO's gateway to health-related statistics for its 194 Member States, while GDB is an independent entity. There are differences between GHO and GBD in terms of data sources, funding and models used.[6] As with all databases, there are limitations. They include:

- Extensive statistical modelling, including a number of assumptions for handling missing and poor-quality data, which are not always easy to understand and/or only partially reported. This is particularly the case for morbidity estimates.
- Modelling is inevitably greater for low- and middle-income countries. However, as these countries strengthen their ability to collect data, these limitations are decreasing over time.

The IHME Global Disease Burden project (GBD)

GBD was established as a collaboration between WHO, the World Bank and Harvard University in the 1980s.[7] The GBD 2010 study was set up as a collaboration between IHME and Harvard University, WHO, Johns

Hopkins University and the University of Queensland, as well as drawing on the expertise of around 40 expert working groups. Subsequent rounds of the GBD study were carried out under the auspices/guidance of the IHME alone with inputs from expert groups. Considerable financial and technical resources are used to obtain and generate up-to-date data. GBD also provides estimates of years of life lost and disability-standardized years of life lost. GBD also provides PAFs for around 80 modifiable behavioural, metabolic and environmental risk factors. Updated GBD estimates are published regularly, along with details on methodology.[8,9] The internet-based GBD Compare tool allows users to interrogate the GBD database, including crude and age-standardized mortality as well as PAFs, at country, regional and global levels, by age, sex and year since 1990.

The WHO Global Health Observatory (GHO) and Global Health Estimates (GHE)

GHO provides health-related statistics for WHO Member States. GHO provides GHE on mortality and burden of disease (including NCDs), prevalence of NCD risk factors, and national capacity to prevent and control NCDs' mortality and burden of disease.[10,11] Estimates are based on data from multiple consolidated sources, including national vital registration data, latest estimates from WHO technical programmes, United Nations partners and inter-agency groups, as well as GBD and other scientific studies. GHE data are used across a large number of WHO publications. Data and methods used for preparing these estimates have been described.[12] GHO is used as the source of data for 'NCD Countdown 2030', a collaborative effort that includes WHO, NCD Alliance, Imperial College and *The Lancet* to provide an independent mechanism for countries to monitor their progress toward the SDG 3.4 (reduction in premature mortality from the four major NCDs).[13]

Why this compendium primarily displays mortality data

GBD's crude and age-standardized mortality data (in 2019 and 1990), and PAFs for 2019 are the predominant data displayed in this chapter, as well as in other chapters in this compendium, with breakdown by World Bank income groups. Estimates of morbidity are not systematically included in this compendium, given the lack of space and because, for the reasons described above, they are based on further, often weaker, assumptions than those for mortality. However, as the four NCDs considered in the compendium tend to occur later in life, morbidity estimates generally correlate fairly well with those for mortality, particularly for those that have a high case fatality, but estimates (e.g. number of years lived with disease) can be proportionately larger for those NCDs that have larger survival such as diabetes, stroke and some cancers, partly due to improving treatments and health care.

Why this book primarily displays GBD estimates

The reasons for using GBD data in this chapter, as well as in other chapters of this book, include:

- Data are internally consistent, i.e. have been adjusted to ensure, among other considerations, that the total number of cases (e.g. deaths) amount to the estimated actual total number for a given year and because the same methods are used for national and global estimations, including the way that missing data are managed.
- Data are collated from a large number of sources, from both government and non-government agencies, including universities.
- Data can be freely and easily generated through the web-based GBD Compare tool. This means that figures used in this compendium can be reproduced by readers.
- PAFs can be generated for approximately 300 diseases and 80 risk factors, using internally consistent methods for all risk factors and diseases. GBD continually reviews the evidence on the associations between these risk factors and diseases.

GBD estimates

Table 1.1 summarizes NCD mortality data by World Bank country income category for 1990 and 2019 using IHME data (GBD Compare). Supplement 1 to this compendium provides a set of graphic illustrations on changes in crude and age-standardized mortality according to World Bank country income categories over this time period. The supplement can be accessed at www.routledge.com/9781032307923. As can be seen from the table, a large proportion (generally >75%) of all CVD deaths are attributable to ischemic heart disease and stroke (and a substantial proportion to hypertensive heart disease [Hyp HD]). A large proportion of all chronic respiratory disease (CRD) deaths is attributable to chronic obstructive pulmonary disease (COPD).

Table 1.2 provides global estimates of PAFs for 2019 using IHME data (GBD Compare). The Supplement described above also includes a set of graphical illustrations that show mortality attributable to risk factors in Table 1.2 between 1990 and 2019 according to World Bank country income categories.

Key messages from the GBD tables

Global burden in 2019

- CVD, cancer, CRD and diabetes caused around 60% of deaths worldwide in 2019.

Table 1.1 Total deaths and age-standardized rates (per 100,000) for mortality of the four major NCDs by World Bank country income category for 1990 and 2019 (IHME)

Country income level	CVD	IHD	Stroke	Hyp HD	Cancer	CRD	COPD	Diabetes	Total
Global (population: 7.7 billion)									
% from all deaths in 2019	32.8	16.2	11.6	2.1	17.8	7.0	5.8	2.7	60.4
# (million) in 2019	18.6	9.1	6.6	1.2	10.1	4.0	3.3	1.6	34.2
# among <70 yrs in 2019	6.4	3.2	2.2	0.3	5.2	1.1	0.8	0.7	13.4
% among <70 yrs	34.5	35.5	33.7	27.8	51.3	28.1	24.1	45.6	39.9
# (million) in 1990	12.1	5.7	4.6	0.7	5.8	3.1	2.5	0.7	21.6
Relative change 2019 vs 1990 (%)	54	60	43	77	75	29	30	134	58
Age-standardized mortality rates in 2019	240	118	85	15	125	51	43	19	436
Age-standardized mortality rates in 1990	354	170	132	19	148	88	73	18	608
Relative change 2019 vs 1990 (%)	-32	-31	-36	-21	-15	-42	-42	9	-28
Low- and middle-income countries (population: 6.5 billion)									
% from all causes in 2019	29.7	14.3	10.3	2.0	17.3	6.2	5.1	2.3	55.6
# (million) in 2019	15.0	7.4	5.6	0.9	6.9	3.3	2.8	1.3	26.6
# among <70 yrs in 2019	3.6	2.9	2.1	0.3	4.1	1.0	0.7	0.6	9.3
HICs (pop: 1.2 B; age 70+: 13%)									
% from all causes in 2019	32.5	16.4	8.4	1.9	28.9	5.8	4.9	2.4	69.6
# (million) in 2019	3.5	1.8	0.9	0.2	3.1	0.6	0.5	0.3	7.5
# among <70 yrs in 2019	0.6	0.4	0.1	0.0	1.1	0.1	0.1	0.1	1.9
# (million) in 1990	3.6	2.1	1.0	0.1	2.1	0.4	0.3	0.2	6.3
Relative change 2019 vs 1990 (%)	-2	-15	-9	107	47	59	69	43	20
Age-standardized mortality rates in 2019	134	68	34	7.7	135	24	53	35	327
Age-standardized mortality rates in 1990	283	164	79	8.1	168	30	65	36	518
Relative change 2019 vs 1990 (%)	-53	-58	-56	-4	-20	-20	-18	-5	-37
Upper MICs (population: 2.6 billion; age 70+: 7%)									
% from all causes in 2019	40.7	18.8	16.6	2.6	22.1	7.5	6.9	2.6	72.9
# (million) in 2019	7.9	3.7	3.2	0.5	4.3	1.5	1.3	0.5	14.2
# among <70 yrs in 2019	0.2	1.1	1.0	0.1	2.3	0.3	0.2	0.2	3.1

	C1	C2	C3	C4	C5	C6	C7	C8	Total
# (million) in 1990	4.8	1.9	2.2	0.3	2.3	1.6	1.4	0.2	8.9
Relative change 2019 vs 1990 (%)	64	93	46	52	88	-7	-7	142	60
Age-standardized mortality rates in 2019	267	124	107	18	131	50	46	16	464
Age-standardized mortality rates in 1990	401	163	180	29	158	132	123	15	706
Relative change 2019 vs 1990 (%)	-33	-24	-41	-39	-17	-62	-62	4	-34
Lower MICs (population: 3.2 billion; age 70+: 4%)									
% from all causes in 2019	29.7	16.0	9.8	1.7	10.7	8.1	6.0	2.8	51.2
# (million) in 2019	6.3	3.4	2.1	0.4	2.3	1.7	1.3	0.7	11.0
# among <70 yrs in 2019	3.0	1.6	1.0	0.1	1.5	0.6	0.4	0.4	5.5
# (million) in 1990	3.2	1.6	1.2	0.2	1.0	1.0	0.7	0.2	5.5
Relative change 2019 vs 1990 (%)	97	117	79	108	118	68	85	208	100
Age-standardized mortality rates in 2019	313	168	104	18	97	89	68	33	532
Age-standardized mortality rates in 1990	384	191	140	22	98	122	87	25	629
Relative change 2019 vs 1990 (%)	-18	-12	-26	-15	-1	-27	-22	33	-15
LICs (population: 0.7 billion; age 70+: 2%)									
% from all causes in 2019	16.1	6.2	6.5	1.7	7.5	3.7	2.5	1.4	28.6
# (million) in 2019	0.79	0.31	0.32	0.09	0.37	0.18	0.13	0.10	1.4
# among <70 yrs in 2019	0.40	0.15	0.16	0.04	0.26	0.08	0.05	0.05	0.8
# (million) in 1990	0.44	0.16	0.19	0.05	0.19	0.12	0.07	0.05	0.8
Relative change 2019 vs 1990 (%)	79	97	72	77	93	56	74	96	80
Age-standardized mortality rates in 2019	304	121	123	35	114	72	53	35	524
Age-standardized mortality rates in 1990	355	132	149	41	120	95	65	36	607
Relative change 2019 vs 1990 (%)	-14	-8	-18	-16	-5	-25	-18	-5	-14

Age-standardized rates are per 100,000 population.

Table 1.2 Fractions of the global mortality from the four major NCDs that are attributable to modifiable behavioural, metabolic and environmental risk factors (IHME)

	CVD	Cancer	CRD	Diabetes
Behavioural risk factors				
Tobacco	17.2	25.8	45.4	
Dietary risks	37.0	6.0		25.2
Low physical activity	3.4	0.7		8.1
Alcohol use	2.3	4.9		
Unsafe sex (e.g. leading to HPV transmission, causing cervical cancer)		2.8		
Drug use		5.2		
Metabolic factors				
High blood pressure	53.8			
High blood LDL-cholesterol	23.7			
High fasting blood glucose	20.3	4.2		
High body mass index	17.4	4.6	1.9	40.7
Environmental factors				
Air pollution	19.1	3.9	33.1	19.3
Other	4.6			
Occupational risks		3.3	14.6	

- A total of 40% of all these deaths were premature (before the age of 70 years), which highlights the significant potential for prevention and control strategies.
- CVD accounted for more than half of all NCD deaths globally.

Trends

- Total mortality due to these four major NCDs (i.e. absolute numbers and proportions of all deaths due to these NCDs) has increased between 1990 and 2019, which is largely driven by increasing and aging populations (demographic transition). As mortality is a marker of disease burden, this indicates that most countries need to scale up NCD prevention, treatment and health care services to meet the needs of their populations.
- Age-standardized mortality rates for the four major NCDs have, with the exception of diabetes, decreased between 1990 and 2019 in most parts of the world. This can be explained by a reduction in the underlying causes (i.e. decreasing age-standardized prevalence of some of the risk factors for NCDs) as well as improved case management in many countries. This demonstrates the benefits of public health and healthcare interventions. This is particularly striking for CVD in high-income countries (HICs) and upper-middle-income countries (upper MICs), but also in low-income countries (LICs) to a lesser extent, which to a large extent reflects a reduction in tobacco use, healthier diet, lower cholesterol levels over time, as well as better treatment for some NCD conditions, such as hypertension and heart disease.

- Irrespective of the changes that arise from demographic transition, a decrease in age-standardized *incidence* (new cases) or *mortality* does not imply a decrease in age-standardized *prevalence* (i.e. number of persons living with a condition), particularly when life expectancy for many living with NCDs is increasing because of improved treatment and care. For example, age-standardized CVD *incidence* and *mortality* decreased by 46% and 33% respectively between 2000 and 2015 in Canada, but the age-standardized *prevalence* increased by 21%;[14] this has large implications for the provision of health care.

Geographic variations

- The large majority of deaths from these four major NCDs are in low- and middle-income countries. This is in line with the large majority of the world's population living in low- and middle-income countries and emphasizes that NCDs are a major problem for all countries, including low- and middle-income countries.
- The crude proportions and total numbers of deaths from these four major NCDs are higher in low- and middle-income countries than in HICs (mainly because the population is largest in the former).
- Age-standardized mortality rates for several of these four NCDs are also higher in low-and middle-income countries. For example, the age-standardized mortality rates of CRDs are several times higher reflecting much higher levels of ambient and household pollution and poorer access to effective healthcare.

Risk factors

- The large PAFs for several of these four major NCDs emphasize the large potential to reduce these diseases through risk factor reduction in the whole population. Benefits are largest for CVD, highlighting that CVD is largely preventable: much of the improved life expectancy in the world, including in low- and middle-income countries, is the result of decreasing age-standardized CVD rates.[15]
- Nearly one-quarter of cancer deaths and one-fifth of CVD deaths would be avoided if exposure to tobacco was eliminated.
- Nearly half of global diabetes deaths would be prevented if none of the world's population was overweight or obese.

GHO estimates

Although specific estimates inevitably differ from those from GBD for the reasons described above, the overall picture is the same.[16] A comparison between data from GHO and GBD and the challenges facing WHO and its Member States in collecting and reporting on global health statistics has been described.[17]

- Globally, 41 million of 55 million (71%) deaths in 2019 were due to NCDs, with 77% of these in low- and middle-income countries.
- More than 15 million people died from one of the four major NCDs between the ages of 30 and 69 years (defined by WHO as premature deaths, corresponding to a global target in the WHO Global NCD Action Plan) and 85% of these were in low- and middle-income countries.
- CVD accounted for most NCD deaths in 2019 (17.9 million people), followed by cancers (9.3 million), respiratory diseases (4.1 million) and diabetes (1.5 million).
- Up to 80% of premature deaths from heart disease and stroke, and a majority of deaths from type-2 diabetes, could be prevented.[18]

Further observations about the burden of these four major NCDs and their implications for prevention and control are provided in other chapters. As highlighted above, country-level estimates from global databases such as IHME and GHE are based on considerable assumptions and extrapolations. For countries where real data are lacking, efforts should be made to develop their surveillance systems to provide robust data on the incidence and prevalence of NCD mortality and morbidity (Chapters 4 and 5 on surveillance).

Notes

1. Murray CJ. Quantifying the burden of disease: the technical basis for disability-adjusted life years. *Bull WHO* 1994;72:429–45.
2. Ahmad OB et al. Age standardization of rates: a new WHO standard. GPE Discussion Paper Series: No.31. WHO, 2001.
3. Mansournia MA, Altman DG. Population attributable fraction. *BMJ* 2018;360:k757.
4. Powles J et al. National cardiovascular prevention should be based on absolute disease risks, not levels of risk factors. *Eur J Public Health* 2010;20:103–06.
5. Boerma T, Mathers CD. The World Health Organization and global health estimates: improving collaboration and capacity. *BMC Med* 2015;13:50.
6. Mahajan M. The IHME in the shifting landscape of global health metrics. *Global Policy* 2019;10(Suppl 1):110–19.
7. Das P, Samarasekera U. The story of GBD 2010: a "super-human" effort. *Lancet* 2012;380:2067–70.
8. GBD 2019 Diseases and Injuries Collaborators. Global burden of 369 diseases and injuries in 204 countries and territories, 1990–2019: a systematic analysis for the Global Burden of Disease Study 2019. *Lancet* 2020;396:1204–22.
9. GBD 2019 Risk Factors Collaborators. Global burden of 87 risk factors in 204 countries and territories, 1990–2019: a systematic analysis for the Global Burden of Disease Study 2019. *Lancet* 2020;396:1223–49.
10. WHO. Global health estimates 2000–2019.
11. WHO. Global health observatory. NCDs. https://www.who.int/data/gho/data/themes/noncommunicable-diseases.
12. WHO methods and data sources for country-level causes of death 2000–2019. Global Health Estimates Technical Paper WHO/DDI/DNA/GHE/2020.2.
13. NCD Countdown 2030 Collaborators. NCD countdown 2030: efficient pathways and strategic investments to accelerate progress towards the sustainable development goal target 3.4 in low-income and middle-income countries. *Lancet* 2022;399:1266–78.

14 Blais J et al. Complex evolution of epidemiology of vascular diseases, including increased disease burden: from 2000 to 2015. *Can J Cardiol* 2020;36:740–46.
15 Foreman KJ et al. Forecasting life expectancy, years of life lost, and all-cause and cause-specific mortality for 250 causes of death: reference and alternative scenarios for 2016–40 for 195 countries and territories. *Lancet* 2018;392:2052–90.
16 WHO. Noncommunicable diseases fact sheet. https://www.who.int/news-room/fact-sheets/detail/noncommunicable-diseases.
17 Mathers CD. History of global burden of disease assessment at the World Health Organization. *Arch Public Health* 2020;78:77.
18 Ford ES et al. Healthy living is the best revenge: findings from the European prospective investigation into cancer (EPIC) and nutrition–potsdam study. *Arch Intern Med* 2009;169:1355–62.

2 Epidemiologic and demographic transition as drivers of NCDs

Pascal Bovet, Fred Paccaud, Sylvie Stachenko

Epidemiologic and demographic transition refers to changing disease and demographic patterns in populations along socio-economic development. The magnitude and speed of these changes over time are modulated by the changing exposures to risk factors and public health responses in populations.[1]

In brief, the following sequence is observed in populations: (i) a first phase where overall mortality is very high, the population is predominantly young (life expectancy [LE_0] ~30–40 years), and infectious diseases are the predominant cause of mortality; (ii) a later phase with larger proportions of older persons, LE_0 increases (~50–70 years) and the disease burden shifts from infectious diseases (largely owing to the public health response) to the four NCDs that are the topic of this compendium (e.g. cardiovascular disease [CVD] and cancer, as the prevalence of risk factors such as tobacco use and a diet high in saturated fats increases); and (iii) a final phase with a large proportion of older persons, longer LE_0 (~80+ years), and the disease burden shifting away from the four main NCDs (e.g. owing to tobacco control, healthier diet, treatment of hypertension) to lesser preventable/treatable NCDs (e.g. neurodegenerative conditions such as Alzheimer's disease).[2]

Trends in epidemiologic and demographic patterns explain why, for example, total numbers of deaths from NCDs such as CVD or lung cancer can markedly increase in a population (because of population growth and aging) while the age-standardized mortality rates (which express a risk irrespective of population growth and age structure) decrease, as is observed in high-income countries (HICs) and in an increasing number of low- and middle-income countries. Trends between 1990 and 2019 for both crude (total deaths) and age-standardized (risk) NCD mortality are shown in Table 1.1 in the chapter on the global burden of NCDs.

Demographic, epidemiologic and public health transition are described separately in this chapter, but they are strongly interrelated and also referred to as the 'health transition'.

Epidemiologic transition

Risks of diseases in populations change as exposures to risk factors and the public health response evolve. For example, the risk of infectious diseases is higher

DOI: 10.4324/9781003306689-3

when sanitary conditions are poor and vaccines are unavailable, while the risk of some cancers and CVD increases when cigarettes become widely available, and the risk of CVD and lung cancer decreases when exposure to cigarettes is reduced as a result of tobacco control measures.

The paradigm of the epidemiologic transition has been widely described[3,4] and posits four stages (Box 2.1).

BOX 2.1 THE FOUR STAGES OF THE EPIDEMIOLOGIC TRANSITION

1. *Pre-transition.* The 'age of pestilence' dominated by famine, malnutrition, infectious diseases and high levels of infant and child mortality. Life expectancy at birth (LE_0) is typically <30 years.
2. *Early transition.* The 'age of receding epidemics', with urbanization and industrialization resulting in improved public health (more diverse diet, clean water and sewage systems, as well as interventions including immunization). Death rates begin to fall. As birth rates remain high, the population grows rapidly. LE_0 is typically 30–50 years.
3. *Late transition.* The 'age of degenerative or man-made diseases', with the four NCDs (CVD, cancer, chronic respiratory diseases, diabetes) and their risk factors becoming predominant. Birth rates decline and the rate of population growth decelerates. LE_0 is typically 50–70 years.
4. *Post-transition.* The 'age of delayed degenerative diseases', with a decline in some of the NCDs such as CVD as a consequence of reduced exposure to NCD risk factors (owing to prevention and treatment), but less preventable conditions (e.g. dementia, arthrosis) increase. Post-transitional populations are characterized by both low birth rates and low death rates. Population growth is negligible or declining. LE_0 is typically >70–80 years.

More recently a fifth phase of the epidemiologic transition has been suggested, the 'age of obesity and inactivity', which is associated with several cardiometabolic diseases and threatens progress in postponing illness and death to later years in adult life spans.[5]

Figure 2.1 depicts mortality trends according to broad disease groups. Two main observations can be made. First, all-cause mortality declines markedly over time, largely owing to decreasing mortality from infectious diseases at young ages. Second, there is no uniform decline in mortality by cause of death but, rather, a sequence of causes of death that 'rise and fall'. The course of the sequence depends on exposures to risk/protective factors in the population at a certain

16 Pascal Bovet et al.

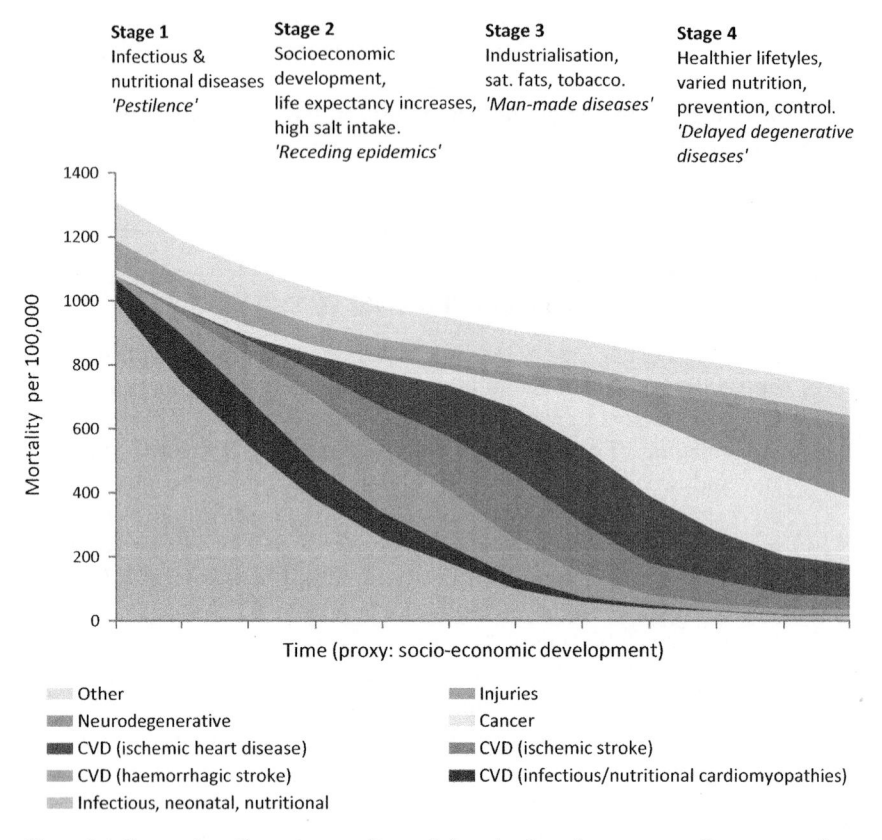

Stage 1	Stage 2	Stage 3	Stage 4
Infectious & nutritional diseases 'Pestilence'	Socioeconomic development, life expectancy increases, high salt intake. 'Receding epidemics'	Industrialisation, sat. fats, tobacco. 'Man-made diseases'	Healthier lifetyles, varied nutrition, prevention, control. 'Delayed degenerative diseases'

Figure 2.1 Decreasing all-cause mortality and changing broad-cause mortality patterns along the four stages of the epidemiologic transition. (adapted from Bovet P, Paccaud F. Cardiovascular disease and the changing face of global public health: a focus on low and middle income countries. *Public Health Rev* 2011;33:397–415).

period and the public health response. The 'rise and fall of diseases' may perhaps better be described as 'sequentially falling diseases'.[6]

A bell-shaped relationship between socio-economic development and CVD risk factors has been observed in many populations.[7] For example, mean blood cholesterol, blood pressure and (to a lesser extent) body mass index increase, plateau and then decrease along a country's socio-economic development as a consequence of the changing levels of their determinants in populations and the public health efforts to prevent and control them.[8] These changing levels of risk factors over time determine the 'rise and fall' (or 'sequential falls') of diseases. For example, the risk (age-standardized rate) of coronary heart disease peaked in HICs in the late 1960–1980s when the prevalence of several main modifiable CVD risk factors was highest (e.g. tobacco use and intake of saturated fats) but then declined over the next three decades by nearly 80%

owing to prevention and treatment, yet remaining a leading cause of death. This sequence is also increasingly observed in low- and middle-income countries along socio-economic development.[9] The epidemiologic transition model also predicts that the predominant disease burden will shift away from some NCDs (when they are prevented and controlled) to other lesser preventable and treatable NCDs, such as neurodegenerative diseases and diseases of the musculoskeletal system.

Demographic transition

Demographic transition is defined as the changes in population size and age structure over time that result from changes in mortality and birth rates. The population typically increases in size (growth) and age (with increasing LE_0) as a consequence of a time gap between the decline in all-cause mortality and the decline (decades later) in birth rates. The demographic transition is complete when both the mortality and birth rates reach low levels (as is already the case in a minority of high-income countries) and, at this stage, the population no longer increases in size and can even decline when birth rates fall below the population replacement ratio (e.g. fertility ratio of <2.1 children per woman). The causes of the decreasing birth rates and fertility rates are not fully understood but can be associated with societal changes in disease patterns, education, economic models (e.g. more women joining the workforce), societal values (e.g. a large number of children no longer considered as a necessary goal for families), and access to contraceptive means.

According to the UN, the global birth rate in 2019 was more than two times higher than mortality (1.85% vs 0.76%), meaning that the demographic transition was ongoing, with the world population size increasing by 1.1% per year.[10] The UN predicts that the world's population will stop growing in around 2100. According to IHME, the world population would peak in the 2060s at 10 billion and then decrease to 8.8 billion by 2100 (with 2.4 billion individuals aged >65 years).[11] Fertility rates would fall below the population replacement ratio in 151 countries by 2050, and in 183 by 2100. More than 20 countries (e.g. Japan, Thailand and Spain) are forecasted to have population declines greater than 50% between 2017 and 2100 (and a 48% decline from 1.4 billion to 768 million in China). Yet, fertility rates are expected to remain high in some countries, and sub-Saharan Africa is expected to become the most populated continent, with 3.0 billion individuals in 2100 and Nigeria would be the most populated country in the world with 790 million people (from 207 million in 2017).

UN estimates indicate that the percent of the world population aged >65 years (when most NCDs occur) was 9.3% in 2019 but is expected to reach 16% in 2050 (1.5 billion) – and some consider this figure may be an underestimate if different assumptions are made around maximal LE_0[12] and mortality compression during the few last years of life (the so-called 'rectangularization' of the survival curve).[13,14] Given that NCDs predominantly develop in middle-aged and older individuals, these demographic predictions have important implications in terms of the expected numbers of persons with NCDs and the need for health care in the coming decades (including sufficient numbers of health workers and home carers).

Figure 2.2 illustrates how demographic and epidemiological previsions can be used to identify future public health needs.

Public health transition

The health transition is the set of interventions developed and implemented in response to demographic and epidemiological changes. This includes efforts for primary prevention through reducing the modifiable determinants in the whole population (to decrease the incidence of diseases) and for strengthening the healthcare system (to curb disease progression and reduce case fatality at the individual level).

Implications of demographic and epidemiologic transition for NCD policy and planning include:

- The need for robust health information systems, including surveillance to chart changes in levels of NCDs (as well as other diseases) over time (Chapters 4 and 5 on surveillance) to plan for health and healthcare services. NCD estimates should be presented using both age-standardized rates (to assess trends in NCD risk independently of size and age of populations, hence to evaluate the impact of prevention and treatment strategies) and total numbers (which largely depend, for NCDs, on changes in population size and age, and are useful to inform health care needs).
- Developing public health responses to meet the needs of people with NCDs, including the financing and delivery of preventive, treatment and care services, as well as other conditions such as neurodegenerative and musculoskeletal diseases, which are beyond the scope of this compendium.
- Recognition that the linkages and associations between infectious diseases and NCDs, and the ongoing double burden of disease (communicable diseases and NCDs) in many low- and middle-income countries, means that health systems need to have the capacity to address the full range of public health challenges in an integrated manner (Chapter 28 on infectious diseases and NCDs). As trends in the burden of different diseases can be partly predicted, health systems should anticipate and plan for future needs associated with these changes.
- Understanding that demographic transition will continue to evolve in the years ahead with direct and indirect impacts on incidence, health care and financing of NCDs. The *increasing* population size in many countries will also exert a significant impact on climate change and the environment as well as economic and geopolitical consequences, including food supply (which all have an impact on NCDs). Where populations are or will be, *declining*, future welfare will be increasingly threatened, including a

Epidemiologic and demographic transition   19

Demographic characteristics & predominant causes of deaths				
Population size	++	+++	+++	+(−)
% young vs older	>>>	>	<	=
Mortality	+++	++	++	low
Birth rate	+++	++	+	low
Neurodegenerative diseases	−	(+)	+	+++
Cancers (less preventable*)	(+)	+	++	+++
Cancers (more preventable*)	(+)	+	++	+
Ischaemic heart disease	(+)	++	+++	+
Haemorrhagic stroke	+	++	+	(+)
Infectious diseases	+++	++	+	(+)

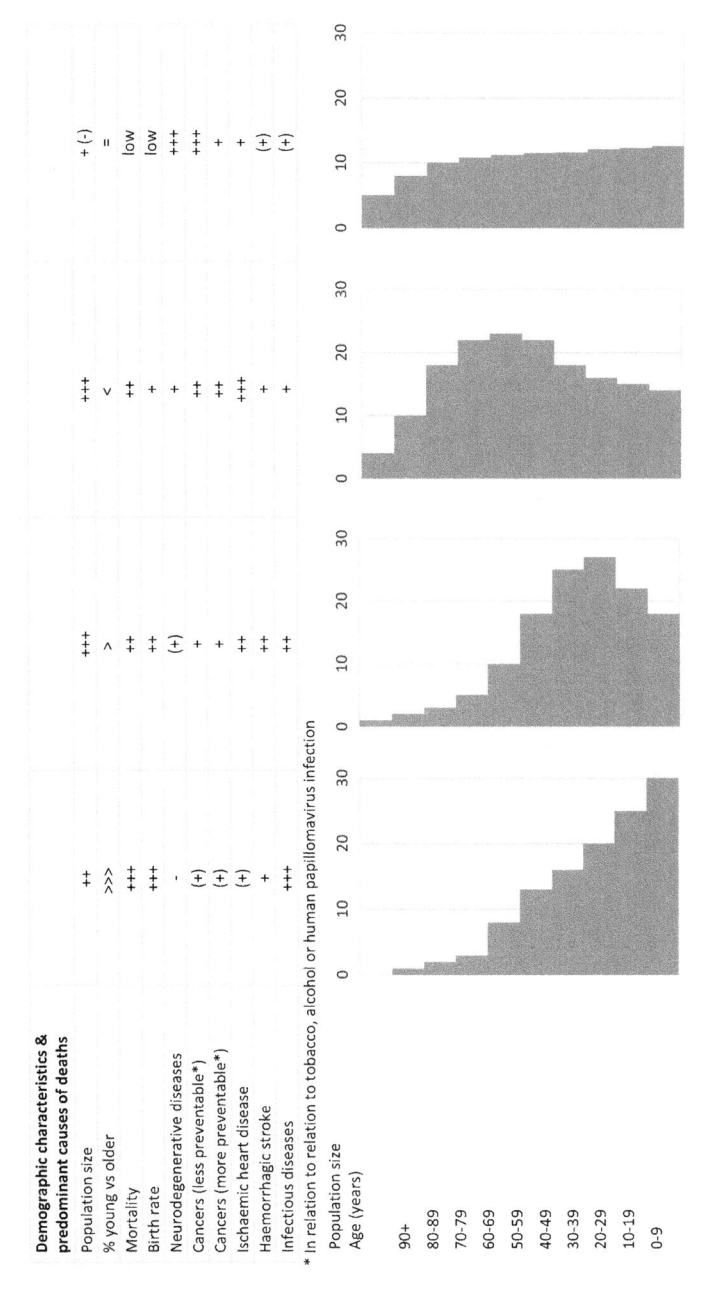

* In relation to tobacco, alcohol or human papillomavirus infection

Population size				
Age (years)				
90+				
80-89				
70-79				
60-69				
50-59				
40-49				
30-39				
20-29				
10-19				
0-9				

Figure 2.2 Demographic transition over time and associated predominant causes of deaths.

decreasing workforce able to respond to the increasing demand for health care for aging populations and individuals living with an NCD.[15] Planners therefore need to consider public health responses based on different scenarios.

Notes

1 Egger G. Health, "illth", and economic growth: medicine, environment, and economics at the crossroads. *Am J Prev Med* 2009;37:78–83.
2 Miranda JJ et al. Major review: on-communicable diseases in low- and middle-income countries: context, determinants and health policy. *Trop Med Int Health* 2008;13:125–34.
3 Omran AR. The epidemiologic transition: a theory of the epidemiology of population. *Milbank Q* 1971;49:509–538, 57.
4 Olshansky SJ et al. The fourth stage of the epidemiologic transition: the age of delayed degenerative diseases. *Milbank Q* 1986;64:355–91.
5 Gaziano JM. Fifth phase of the epidemiologic transition: the age of obesity and inactivity. *JAMA* 2010;303:275–76.
6 Mackenbach JP. The rise and fall if diseases: reflections on the history of population health in Europe since ca. 1700. *Eur J Epidemiol* 2021;36:1119–205.
7 Danaei G et al. The global cardiovascular risk transition: associations of four metabolic risk factors with national income, urbanization, and Western diet in 1980 and 2008. *Circulation* 2013;127:1493–502.
8 Ezzati E et al. Rethinking the 'diseases of affluence' paradigm: global patterns of nutritional risks in relation to economic development. *PLoS* 2005;2:e133.
9 Stringhini S et al. Declining stroke and myocardial infarction mortality between 1989 and 2010 in a country of the African region. *Stroke* 2012;43:2283–88.
10 https://population.un.org/wpp/Graphs/1_Demographic%20Profiles/World.pdf.
11 Vollset SE et al. Fertility, mortality, migration, and population scenarios for 195 countries and territories from 2017 to 2100: a forecasting analysis for the Global Burden of Disease Study. *Lancet* 2020;396:1285–306.
12 Oeppen J, Vaupel J. Broken limits to life expectancy. *Science* 2002;296:1029–31.
13 Anson J. The second dimension: a proposed measure of the rectangularity of mortality curves. *Genus* 1992;48:1–17.
14 Rousson V, Paccaud F. A set of indicators for decomposing the secular increase of life expectancy. *Pop Health Metrics* 2010;8:18.
15 Ezeh AC et al. Family planning 1: Global population trends and policy options. *Lancet* 2012;380:142–48.

3 NCDs and sustainable development

Nick Banatvala, Aidah Nakanjako, Douglas Webb

Globally, 41 million (71%) of the 55.4 million deaths in 2019 were due to noncommunicable diseases, with 77% of these in low- and middle-income countries.[1] More than 15 million people died from an NCD between the ages of 30 and 69 years and 85% of these were in low- and middle-income countries. And yet, large proportions of premature deaths from heart attack, stroke, diabetes and selected cancers can be prevented (see chapters on these diseases).

Premature deaths from NCDs curtail economic growth and trap populations in poverty. Poverty disproportionately exposes people to both behavioural and environmental risk factors for NCDs, and, in turn, the resulting NCDs may become an important driver to the downward spiral that leads families towards poverty and the maintenance of overall economic and health inequities (Figure 3.1). In many countries, treatment for NCDs can quickly drain household resources. NCDs exacerbate social inequity because in many countries significant payments for healthcare are private and out-of-pocket (e.g. long-term treatment for diabetes or hypertension, rehabilitation after stroke, cancer treatment, etc.); such costs weigh more heavily on those least able to afford them.[2] The chronic nature of NCDs, and the projected increase in the absolute number of people living with NCDs (Chapter 2 on health transition), means that the economic impact of NCDs will continue to grow over many years.

The differential prevalence of NCDs within and across populations in developing countries constitutes one of the major challenges for development in the 21st century, which undermines social and economic development throughout the world and threatens the achievement of the Sustainable Development Goals. The rise of NCDs among younger populations in developing countries now jeopardizes the 'demographic dividend' – the economic benefits expected when a relatively large proportion of the population is of working age.

In addition to the costs of healthcare, NCDs often require family members, usually girls or women, to care for the sick, which means less time for them to learn and earn. Many of the costs of NCDs are thus absorbed by the informal economy (e.g. those working in domestic settings, local markets and the black market), which is not usually included in calculations comprising economic indicators such as GDP. At a macro level, less sickness leads to higher

DOI: 10.4324/9781003306689-4

POVERTY AT HOUSEHOLD LEVEL ➡ **POPULATIONS IN LOW- AND MIDDLE-INCOME COUNTRIES**

GLOBALIZATION
URBANIZATION
POPULATION AGEING

Increased exposure to common modifiable risk factors:
-Unhealthy diets
-Physical inactivity
-Tobacco use
-Harmful use of alcohol

Loss of household income from unhealthy behaviours

Noncommunicable diseases:
-Cardiovascular diseases
-Cancers
-Diabetes
-Chronic respiratory diseases

Loss of household income from poor health and premature death

Limited access to effective and equitable health-care services which respond to the needs of people with noncommunicable diseases

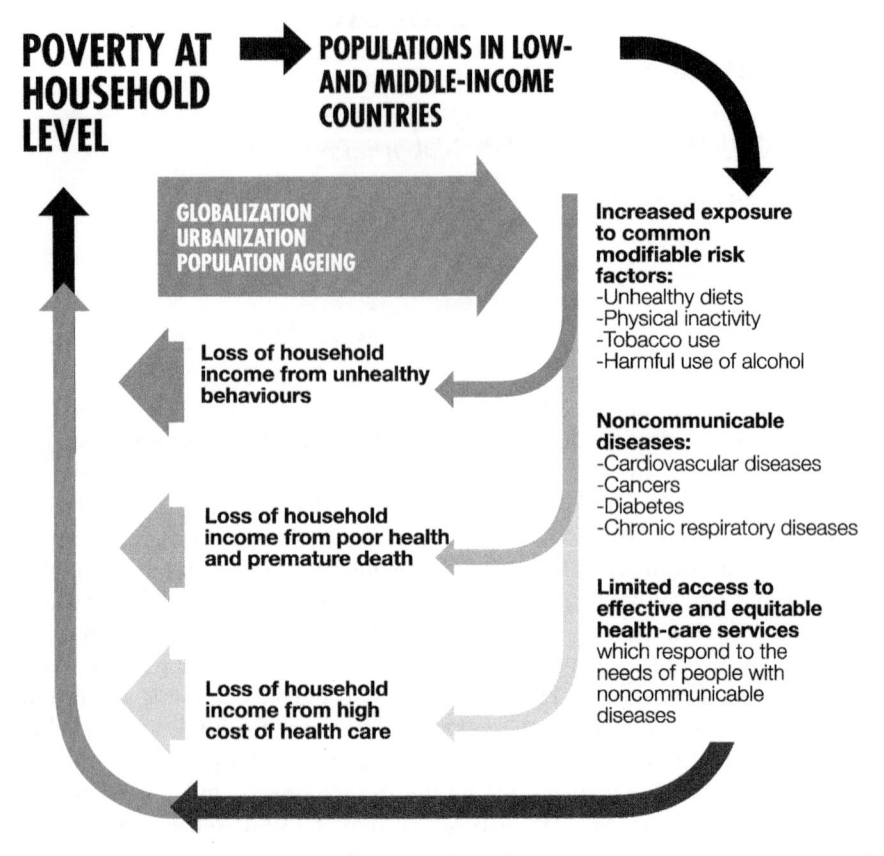

Loss of household income from high cost of health care

Figure 3.1 Poverty contributes to NCDs and NCDs contribute to poverty. (WHO and UNDP. Guidance note on the integration of noncommunicable diseases into the United Nations development assistance framework. 2015).

productivity and regional and national economic growth. The costs of NCDs are not confined to the health sector – they impact productivity and GDP (Chapter 40 on the economic case for investing in NCDs). NCDs are therefore a powerful driver of poverty and inequalities through their direct impact on families, health systems and the economy at large.[3]

Improved NCD outcomes support all three dimensions of sustainable development: economic, social and environmental – and the integration of NCDs into the global development architecture in the form of Agenda 2030 is absolute. Better health of individuals drives socio-economic development (e.g. productivity, consumption of goods, active participation in society), while socio-economic development enables individuals to enjoy better health. This overall improvement in health status is driven by determinants such as lower exposure to air pollution, greater access to food that make up a healthy diet, and better levels of education and income that allow individuals and their families to live healthier lifestyles and to be able to access better healthcare.

Numerous global and international declarations, resolutions and agreements underscore these interconnections across NCDs, health and sustainable development, including the 2030 Agenda for Sustainable Development.[4] Sustainable Development Goal (SDG) 3 is to ensure healthy lives and promote well-being for all at all ages. Targets that are most relevant to NCDs are shown in Box 3.1.

BOX 3.1   NCD AND NCD-RELATED SDG TARGETS

3.4   By 2030, reduce by one-third premature mortality from NCDs through prevention and treatment and promote mental health and well-being.
3.5   Strengthen the prevention and treatment of substance abuse, including narcotic drug abuse and harmful use of alcohol.
3.8   Achieve universal health coverage, including financial risk protection, access to quality essential healthcare services and access to safe, effective, quality and affordable essential medicines and vaccines for all.
3.9   By 2030, substantially reduce the number of deaths and illnesses from hazardous chemicals and air, water and soil pollution and contamination.
3.a   Strengthen the implementation of the WHO Framework Convention on Tobacco Control.
3.b   Support the research and development of vaccines and medicines for the communicable diseases and NCDs that primarily affect developing countries; provide access to affordable essential medicines and vaccines, in accordance with the Doha Declaration on the TRIPS Agreement and Public Health, which affirms the right of developing countries to use to the full the provisions in the Agreement on Trade-Related Aspects of Intellectual Property Rights (an international legal agreement between all the member nations of the World Trade Organization), regarding flexibilities to protect public health, and, in particular, provide access to medicines for all.
3.c   Substantially increase health financing and the recruitment, development, training and retention of the health workforce in developing countries, especially in the least developed countries and small island developing States.

There are important and powerful linkages between NCDs and a number of the non-health SDGs (Table 3.1).

The implications of the interconnectedness of NCDs, health and broader development are that there are large win–wins across sectors that can result. For example, sound environmental policies (e.g. efforts to reduce air pollution or tobacco control measures to reduce tobacco use) can improve NCD

Table 3.1 Examples of linkages between NCDs and several non-health SDGs

SDG	Linkage with SDGs
SDG 1. No poverty.	Individuals and households that are burdened with out-of-pocket and catastrophic payments of NCDs are pushed into poverty (Chapter 38 on universal health coverage and NCDs). Those living with NCDs may not be able to continue to be economically productive. In addition to the costs to the health system, NCDs cause a loss to the economy and reduce economic growth through premature mortality, absenteeism and presenteeism. (Chapter 40 on the economic case for investing in NCD prevention and control).
SDG 2. Zero hunger.	Children who are undernourished in their early years and who put on weight rapidly later in childhood and adolescence are at high risk of NCDs.[a] (Chapter 37 on life-course approach to NCDs).
SDG 4. Quality education.	Quality education includes encouraging healthy behaviours and improving health literacy around NCDs (Chapter 48 on behaviour change on NCDs).[b] Children with obesity have lower life satisfaction and are more prone to being bullied by schoolmates. This can lead to lower class participation and reduced educational performance.[c]
SDG 5. Gender equality.	Gender influences the development and course of NCDs and their risk factors as well as their capacity to access health services.[d]
SDG 7. Affordable and clean energy.	Premature deaths due to air pollution cost the global economy more than US$ 5 trillion in 2013,[e] equating to over 7% of GDP in some countries. Co-benefit interventions range from divesting from fossil fuels, enabling active transport and promoting sustainable food systems. (Chapter 27 on air pollution and NCDs).
SDG 8. Decent work and economic growth.	NCDs reduce the productivity of the workforce and are a drain on business productivity. NCDs are often responsible for preventing people from finding and/or sustaining employment. A healthy workplace can make an important contribution to the prevention of NCDs and the care of people living with NCDs.[f] (Chapter 17 on social determinants).
SDG 10. Reduced inequalities.	Prioritizing action to prevent and treat NCDs (including tackling their underlying social determinants) that have the greatest impact on disadvantaged populations is a way of reducing health and broader inequalities, e.g. health taxes, and increasing healthcare facilities in marginalized communities. (Chapter 17).
SDG 11. Sustainable cities and communities.	Sustainable and well-designed cities provide win-win opportunities for reducing the NCD risk burden. Healthy people are important for prosperous cities and communities. Urban areas should be designed to promote public transport and safe walking and cycling, thus reducing air pollution and increasing physical activity. (Chapters 10 and 25).

(Continued)

Table 3.1 (Continued)

SDG	Linkage with SDGs
SDG 12. Responsible consumption and production.	Reduction in the use of fossil fuels (e.g. through increasing public transport), increase in the use of low-emissions fuels (including in healthcare centres), and more sustainable food and agriculture systems (e.g. promoting local, seasonal, plant-based diets) has an impact on levels of NCDs and levels of air pollution. (Chapter 20).
SDG 13. Climate action.	Well-designed climate change policies in sectors such as energy, transportation, agriculture, land and forestry, and construction provide win-win opportunities for climate change mitigation, improving air quality and reducing NCDs.[g,h] Heat waves are associated with increased rates of cardiovascular disease mortality. (Chapter 27).

a Victora CG. Maternal and child undernutrition: consequences for adult health and human capital. *Lancet* 2008;371:340–57.
b Heine M et al. Health education interventions to promote health literacy in adults with selected non-communicable diseases living in low-to-middle income countries: a systematic review and meta-analysis. *J Eval Clin Pract* 2021;27:1417–28.
c OECD. The heavy burden of obesity: The economics of prevention. OECD Health Policy Studies, 2019.
d PAHO and International Diabetes Federation. Non-communicable diseases and gender. Success in NCD prevention and control depends on attention to gender roles.
e World Bank and Institute for Health Metrics and Evaluation. The cost of air pollution: strengthening the economic case for action, 2016.
f Tackling noncommunicable diseases in workplace settings in low- and middle-income countries. A call to action and practical guidance. NCD Alliance and Novartis Foundation, 2017.
g Human health, global environmental change and transformative action: the case for health co-benefits. Institute for Advanced Sustainability Studies, 2018.
h Air pollution and climate change – links between greenhouse gases climate change and air quality. Institute for Advanced Sustainability Studies, 2022.

outcomes. Similarly, improved access to healthcare and the advancement of health technology worldwide not only leads to improved health of people but also stirs technological innovation and economic development. Furthermore, interventions with primary objectives beyond health (e.g. education, housing, urban design, public transport, agriculture) often also have a favourable impact on health (and NCDs in particular), once again emphasizing the interconnectedness of different SDGs and the co- and multi-benefits of addressing them. The linkages between NCD prevention and control and broader development is described in more detail in other chapters, e.g. Chapter 17 (social determinants), Chapter 54 (whole-of-government), and Chapter 56 (private sector).

Tackling NCDs as a development issue must mean the integration of the prevention and control of NCDs and their risk factors into development strategies and plans of action at a national level. The severity of the economic impacts of NCDs warrants their attention in legal, economic and cross-sector planning frameworks. For example, health taxes that aim to reduce the consumption of tobacco, alcohol and sugar-sweetened beverages, while both raising domestic revenues and reducing health inequities, should be consistent features of fiscal tools and cross-sector budgeting processes such as integrated national financial frameworks (Chapter 41). Similarly combatting air pollution through reducing carbon emissions is an important goal of fossil fuel subsidy reform and an important development financing process (in addition to benefiting health).[5] Because of their widespread benefits and constraints, these issues highlight that prevention and control of NCDs should not be left to the discretion and responsibility of the ministry of health alone.

NCDs and gender

NCD risk factor behaviours are influenced by gender norms, roles and relations, which affect exposure to risk factors (e.g. social customs related to physical mobility may reduce women's opportunities for physical activity and many societies view tobacco smoking as a desired masculine norm), health-seeking behaviour and thus the development of NCDs. Interactions with the health system, including treatment adherence and outcomes, also vary based on gender. The majority of the world's poor are women, who are least able to allocate funds for NCD treatment. In many settings, households with limited funds see these resources predominantly spent on the health needs of men, with women having less say than men in decisions regarding health expenditures. In other settings, the behaviour of men may mean that they are less likely to seek preventive healthcare, as well as less readily referring themselves for early diagnosis and treatment. In addition, women and girls are often the main providers of care to those with NCDs, with the result that women may have to stop working or girls may drop out of school. NCD prevention and care can be a useful entry point for strengthening gender equality. Policies that reduce or eliminate healthcare user fees are important in encouraging men and women to access healthcare.

NCDs, COVID-19 and sustainable development

The pandemic has made the achievement of the SDGs even more challenging.[6] NCDs and their risk factors are associated with greater susceptibility to COVID-19 infection and increased risks of severe disease and death from COVID-19[7] – with smokers for example facing a 40–50% higher risk of severe disease and death from COVID-19.[8] The COVID-19 pandemic has also exacerbated inequality, including in NCDs.[9] In many disadvantaged communities, COVID-19 and NCDs have been experienced as a 'syndemic', a co-occurring, synergistic pandemic that is interacting with and increasing social and economic inequalities. Poverty, discrimination, and gender and cultural norms have shaped health-seeking behaviour for both NCDs and COVID-19 and also access to health and other basic services, health decision-making, exposure to risks and caretaking burdens. In addition, the pandemic has highlighted the risk to those with NCDs for marginalized communities including people living in fragile and humanitarian settings with chronically weak health systems. Building back better to achieve the 2030 Agenda for Sustainable Development means that NCDs must be an integral part of whole-of-government COVID-19 response and recovery efforts, as well as pandemic preparedness, with a systemic focus on protecting those furthest behind.[10]

Notes

1. WHO. Noncommunicable diseases. Key facts. https://www.who.int/news-room/fact-sheets/detail/noncommunicable-diseases. April 2021.
2. Lancet NCDI Poverty Commission. National commission reports. http://www.ncdipoverty.org/national-commission-reports.
3. Bukhman G et al. Reframing NCDs and injuries for the poorest billion: a Lancet Commission. *Lancet* 2015;386:1221–22.
4. Transforming our world: the 2030 Agenda for Sustainable Development. United Nations, A/RES/70/1, 2015.
5. UNDP. Future investment: a toolkit for a fair energy pricing reform. https://dontchooseextinction.com/en/policies/.
6. *The Sustainable Development Goals Report 2020*. New York: United Nations, 2020.
7. Nikoloski Z et al. Covid-19 and non-communicable diseases: evidence from a systematic literature review. *BMC Public Health* 2021;21:1068.
8. WHO supports people quitting tobacco to reduce their risk of severe COVID-19, 2021. https://www.who.int/news/item/28-05-2021-who-supports-people-quitting-tobacco-to-reduce-their-risk-of-severe-covid-19.
9. Economist Intelligence Unit. Examining the intersection between NCDs and COVID-19: lessons and opportunities from emerging data. Defeat-NCD Partnership, 2021.
10. Responding to non-communicable diseases during and beyond the COVID-19 pandemic. WHO and UNDP, 2020.

4 Surveillance of NCDs and their risk factors

Principles

Pascal Bovet, Nick Banatvala, Richard Cooper, Leanne Riley

Noncommunicable disease surveillance is the ongoing systematic collection, analysis, interpretation and dissemination of data to provide appropriate information regarding a country's NCD disease burden, including the main causes of NCD mortality, the population groups at risk, morbidity, risk factors and determinants, coupled with the ability to track NCD-related health outcomes and risk factor trends over time. NCD surveillance is essential to support the planning, implementation and evaluation of NCD prevention and control efforts, particularly when it is closely integrated with the timely dissemination of these data to those who need to know and act.

Surveillance and monitoring of NCDs enables patterns of health and disease to be monitored in populations over time, which ensures the most relevant public health and healthcare interventions can be prioritized, and then the impact of these interventions to be measured. Surveillance therefore empowers decision-makers to act more effectively by providing timely and useful evidence ('data for action', 'what gets measured gets done') and to advocate for the necessary resource for action.

Despite the importance of surveillance and monitoring, these activities are often not prioritized and sufficiently resourced. Accurate data from countries is vital to reverse the global rise in death and disability from NCDs. Currently, many countries have little useable mortality data and weak NCD surveillance. Surveillance is a core component of the health system, and it needs to be prioritized as such. Data on NCDs need to be well integrated into national health information systems, including routine capture of patient health information status as part of patient management systems. Improving country-level surveillance and monitoring continues to be a top priority in the fight against NCDs.

A surveillance framework that comprehensively monitors exposures (risk factors and determinants), outcomes (morbidity and mortality) and health system responses (interventions and capacity) is essential. Ideally, surveillance should work towards capturing an agreed set of standardized indicators on these components, using methods that are as practical, uniform and simple to implement as possible, yet valid and accurate.

This chapter focuses on the principles of surveillance for NCDs, including mortality, morbidity and the prevalence of risk factors. Many of the principles

DOI: 10.4324/9781003306689-5

are also relevant for generating information on the public health response to NCDs over time (e.g. national policies, plans of action, guidelines, health system responses).

Surveillance enables policymakers to know the frequency and distribution of NCDs, risk factors and associated characteristics in their population in order to monitor and inform prevention and control programmes and policy. Information on current levels of NCD risk factors in the population also enables a prediction to be made on the NCD burden in the future and is important for planning services and interventions given the often long interval between current levels of risk factors and the occurrence of ill health (e.g. heart attack, stroke, cancer).

WHO recommends that their Member States have systems in place for generating reliable cause-specific mortality data on a routine basis, a comprehensive set of measures of NCD service quality and availability and for tracking clinical health outcomes for the facility-based patient and programme monitoring of NCDs and that a suitable survey to assess NCD risk factors is done every five years.[1] The results of these population-based surveys are essential for countries to report against the WHO Global NCD Accountability Framework (Chapter 35).

Key issues

Engage stakeholders. To ensure that the results from surveillance activities are used to support the development of policy and programming, it is important that key stakeholders (including community leaders) are involved in the full process, from design to the dissemination of results. It is better to collect small amounts of valid and useful data than collect larger amounts of information that may be less reliable or of limited use.

Ensure robust governance. It is imperative that when data are being collected, systems are in place to ensure participant confidentiality and information governance, with agreement on how aggregated and disaggregated data will be used.

Ensure enumerators (data collectors) are well-trained. Investing in the training of those conducting surveys or those recording patient status is critical to ensure that they understand the importance of collecting high-quality data.[2]

Collect only those data that will be used. Ensuring clarity on the purpose of each data item that is being collected is important in order not to waste resources associated with the collection, storage, analysis and dissemination. Data obtained must be properly summarized and aggregated, along with a description of the main findings and the implications for relevant authorities, in a timely manner.

Ensure a high level of participation. Nonresponse (both through the inability to make contact with survey participants or individuals that refuse to participate) has the effect of reducing the sample size from that required to draw meaningful results and increases the risk of bias as nonrespondents (e.g. those with illness or marginalized groups) may differ from respondents in terms of characteristics measured.

Collect sufficient data to allow for disaggregation. Accurate prevalence surveys based on random sampling require a relatively small number of participants, often as little as a few thousands, even in large countries. Nevertheless, it is important that data obtained from such surveys can allow for disaggregation by socio-demographic variables when this is important for understanding the epidemiology and designing NCD prevention and control programmes and policy. These variables include age, gender, urban-rural divide, occupation and socioeconomic status.[3]

Disseminate findings. Publishing the results of population-based surveys and aggregated data from patient and facility-based monitoring and civil and vital registration systems in the peer-review literature is an important way of increasing access to the work and provides a further layer of quality control.

- *Total numbers* for overall incidence (including mortality) and overall prevalence (i.e. the total number of people with certain risk factors) inform on the needs in terms of use of health services (e.g. numbers needed to be treated and volume of services needed to treat them). The total numbers of people with NCDs or with risk factors inevitably (which are generally strongly associated with age) significantly increase over time in most populations as the mean age and the size of most populations increase over time (i.e. demographic transition), even if the risk of a NCD or the age-standardized prevalence of a risk factor is decreasing over time.

- *Rates* provide a measure of the frequency with which an event occurs in a defined population either over a specified period or at one point in time. Rates can be used to describe either new cases of (or deaths from) a particular NCD (incidence) or existing cases of a particular NCD or risk factor (prevalence). Given that NCDs and most risk factors are strongly associated with age: age-standardized rates (i.e. rates that have been weighted to a same standard age distribution)[4] are particularly useful as they can be directly compared over time in the same population or between populations and inform about disease risk in the population irrespective of age and size of the population.

Assessing NCD mortality and morbidity in the population

Assessing NCD mortality requires accurate information on the number and distribution of deaths – including causes of death, usually obtained from well-functioning civil and vital registration systems where the entire population is covered and the system generates reliable, continuous and timely data on age- and-cause-specific mortality. Monitoring NCD mortality can only be achieved with reliable vital registration systems that count all deaths and reliably certify their causes. National initiatives to strengthen vital registration systems and cause-specific mortality are a key priority for many countries. Physicians must be trained on the importance of completing death certificates. In settings where many deaths are not attended by a physician, alternate methods, such as verbal autopsy, may be used to complement data collected from death certificates. The global goal of high-quality mortality data will require long-term investment in civil registration.

Assessing NCD morbidity also requires robust health information systems capable of tracking the number and characteristics of those who are screened, diagnosed and treated for an NCD. Good systems should routinely collect, aggregate, analyze and report data on key NCDs including cancer, diabetes, cardiovascular disease and chronic respiratory diseases, among others. The use of a set of standardized indicators capable of tracking the cascade of screening, diagnosis, treatment and control is important for improving NCD programme responsiveness and effectiveness and for planning future service capacity. This helps health care providers, facility managers, Ministry of Health staff and their partners to better plan, target, tailor and scale interventions; assess whether programmes are being implemented with quality; respond effectively when they are not implemented as planned; and report on standardized global indicators. The challenges for completeness and accuracy of data from these systems include the need for the use of standardized criteria for diagnosis and standardized indicator aggregation and reporting, along with the inclusion of data from across all health facilities (including private sector providers). Such data may not be representative of the entire population — with bias against those not accessing health services, such as the poor, those in rural areas or those attending private health or other services that are not routinely included. Further, generating and using morbidity data requires strict robust governance procedures to be in place to protect the confidentiality and misuse of data.

Another source of morbidity metrics for the whole or part of the population may be from population-based registries for specific conditions and diseases, such as those for cancer and diabetes. Some morbidities will also need to be derived from population-based surveys, e.g. hypertension and diabetes prevalence, due to challenges in capturing these metrics completely from patient and program monitoring systems.

Assessing the levels of NCD risk factors in the population

Assessing levels of NCDs risk factors in the entire population is impractical, and therefore surveys that sample a scientifically selected sample of the population of interest are used. It is crucial that eligible participants are scientifically selected from the whole population in order to provide data that can be extrapolated to the whole population concerned. School-based surveys can provide population-based estimates among children and adolescents where there is a high level of school attendance. Assessing risk factors based on those accessing health care services is unlikely to provide accurate estimates across the whole population.

There are several types of surveys to assess risk factors in the population. They include:

Health examination surveys where eligible participants are requested to attend survey centres. Levels of participation are variable and can be as low as 30% in some settings (e.g. high-income countries). Low attendance can result in biased estimates, but this can be partly compensated (e.g. by weighing crude results to the expected distribution of the population in relation to some variables, such as education or income).

Household-based surveys require household visits and therefore need significant resources (e.g. travel to people's homes, availability of portable equipment, access to a secluded place to conduct the survey).

Phone- and internet-based surveys are increasingly used as they can require fewer resources. Challenges include obtaining contact details for eligible participants, bias towards those who have access to fixed and mobile phones and computers, and low response rates. Physical measurements (e.g. height, weight and blood pressure) rely on participants providing accurate information. In addition, participants may not respond to unsolicited calls, although participation can be substantially improved if incentives are provided.

Surveys based on electronic health records enable the rapid, up-to-date, inexpensive and ongoing collection of large amounts of information (risk factors, clinical and laboratory, etc.). If information is available at the entire (or nearly entire) population level ('whole of population surveillance'), prevalence estimates can be inferred to the entire population, e.g. national health systems in the UK, Spain, Denmark, Korea[5] or from health care providers (e.g. health and medical insurance companies). As electronic health records are increasingly used in many countries, surveillance of NCD risk factors based on electronic records is likely to be used more widely in the future. Health data can also be linked with other electronic databases (e.g. medical prescriptions, social services, etc.), which can provide useful information on NCD control rates and health services use and efficiency and, possibly, assist with effective real-time prevention and control measures at the population and health care levels. Challenges include information only from those accessing health services, which may not be representative of the whole population.

Surveys of the capacity of health systems to perform NCD surveillance and of the health response to NCD prevention and control

A variety of surveys and/or tools exist for assessing issues that do not directly assess NCD outcomes in the population but are indirectly linked with surveillance. This includes surveys of the capacity of the health system to perform surveillance tasks, funding available for surveillance tasks, the existence of units/

sections for performing surveillance tasks, etc. Surveys of the public health response to NCDs assess governance, implementation of policies and strategies in a country to address NCDs and their risk factors in the population, the health care response for NCD service delivery and the management of NCDs.[6]

Notes

1. Noncommunicable Diseases Progress Monitor. WHO, 2020.
2. Croome A, Mager F. *Doing research with enumerators*. Nairobi: Oxfam, 2018.
3. GBD 2017 Causes of Death Collaborators. Global, regional, and national age-sex-specific mortality for 282 causes of death in 195 countries and territories, 1980–2017: a systematic analysis for the Global Burden of Disease Study 2017. *Lancet* 2018;392:1736–88.
4. Ahmad OB et al. Age standardization of rates: a new WHO standard. GPE Discussion Paper Series: No.31. WHO, 2001.
5. Carstensen B et al. Components of diabetes prevalence in Denmark 1996–2016 and future trends until 2030. *BMJ Open Diabetes Res Care* 2020;8:e001064.
6. Assessing national capacity for the prevention and control of NCDs: report of the 2019 global survey. WHO, 2020.

5 Surveillance of NCDs and their risk factors
Selected tools

Leanne Riley, Pascal Bovet, Nick Banatvala, Melanie Cowan

Chapter 4 describes the purpose of NCD surveillance and its underlying principles. This chapter describes examples of tools that are commonly used including those developed by WHO.[1]

Assessing the prevalence of risk factors

These instruments require eligible participants to be scientifically selected from the population so that the results are generalizable. Data are obtained from standardized questionnaires and, in some cases, include a physical examination and/or biochemical measurements. Findings may be reported as crude or age-standardized estimates (see chapter 1 on the global burden of NCDs) and can be presented according to age, sex, income, education or other categories. There is a range of ethical considerations when collecting data through surveys[2] and they should be reviewed and approved by the relevant ethics committee/institutional review board, which will address, among other issues, that data management systems are in place to protect participants' privacy and that participation includes informed consent. It is imperative that those involved in surveys received adequate training and that support is on hand for those conducting the survey.

The WHO STEPwise Approach to NCD Risk Factor Surveillance (STEPS) has been developed to collect, analyze and disseminate responses to a set of questions on the key behavioural risk factors including alcohol and tobacco use, physical inactivity, unhealthy diet, along with the history of selected NCD conditions (Step 1); physical measures to assess the main biological risk factors such as overweight and obesity and raised blood pressure (Step 2); and biochemical measures of blood glucose, cholesterol and urinary sodium and creatinine (Step 3) among those aged 18–69 years. Where resources are available, an expanded set of measurements are available for each step. STEPS can be expanded to cover other public health priorities with additional add-on modules, including cervical cancer, objective measurement of physical activity, tobacco policy, oral health, mental health, sexual health, eye and ear health, and violence and injury. Countries can choose to add variables of local relevance. Scientific sampling of eligible participants is typically by clusters, e.g.

DOI: 10.4324/9781003306689-6

across regional, district and household levels. STEPS requires data collectors to visit the homes of participants for conducting Steps 1 and 2, and Step 3 (the latter being usually conducted in health centres or special study sites). All the tools required for STEPS are readily accessible, including those for electronic data entry on mobile devices, which allows rapid data analysis and generation of reports. Surveys should be repeated at regular intervals (e.g. every 5–10 years). While STEPS requires resources, the information it provides means it is important that these are seen as a priority. STEPS surveys have been conducted in many countries for more than 20 years, with many countries having undertaken repeat surveys to determine trends over time and to enable comparisons with other countries. Data from these surveys are included in the WHO NCD microdata repository.[3] Results are often disseminated widely through WHO publications, peer-reviewed journals, and data are included in a range of global public health databases.

The *Global School-based Student Health Survey (GSHS)* is a collaborative surveillance approach led by WHO that allows countries to assess behavioural risk and protective factors in ten core areas (alcohol, drugs, dietary behaviour, hygiene, mental health, physical inactivity, sexual and reproductive health, tobacco, violence, bullying and injury) among school-going adolescents aged 13 to 17 years.[4] Because the survey is based on a scientifically selected sample of schools and classes in the whole country or a country sub-region, the GSHS is a relatively low-cost survey, which uses a self-administered anonymous questionnaire. Physical measurements of height and weight are also included in calculating students' body mass index (BMI). Expanded sets of questions are available for each module, and additional country-specific questions about other topics of unique importance or interest can be added. Answer sheets can be rapidly scanned, with an automated analysis of results. GSHS can be conducted over a few days or weeks (after a preparation period). As with STEPS, GSHSs have been conducted once or several times in many countries, reports are widely available and data are included in a range of global public health databases. Data from these surveys are included in the WHO NCD microdata repository.

The *Global Youth Tobacco Survey (GYTS)*, developed by WHO and the US Centers for Disease Control and Prevention, is a self-administered school-based survey of those aged 13 to 15 years. It is designed to monitor tobacco use among youth and to guide the implementation and evaluation of tobacco prevention and control programmes.[5] GYTS is based on a scientifically selected sample of schools and classes. GYTS is an important tool to assist countries design, implement and evaluate tobacco control demand reduction measures.

The *Health Behaviour in School-aged Children Survey (HBSC)* is a cross-national study led by the WHO Regional Office for Europe. It is a collaborative cross-national study, initiated in 1982, which is conducted every four years in more than 40 (mostly European) countries. The study aims to gain insight into the well-being, health behaviours and social of 11–15-year-old adolescents.[6] Summary and raw data are available on NCD risk factors. Reports are widely available.

Many countries have developed national surveillance tools that focus on or include NCD risk factors. These surveys may include a physical examination (e.g. the US National Health and Nutrition Examination Survey [NHANES]),[7] the Korea National Health and Nutrition Examination Survey), done by telephone (e.g. Switzerland Health Survey) or through the internet (e.g. Constance in France). As for all surveys, it is essential that samples of the eligible participants accurately represent the whole population. Population-based cohort studies are an alternative way to obtain information data, but the results can be difficult to extrapolate to the whole population for reasons that include selection and other biases. In some countries (e.g. Spain, Denmark), health and medical data (including on NCDs and their risk factors) are collated electronically from all healthcare providers, which provides a form of 'whole population surveillance', given that the majority of the population attend health care centres at some point in time.

Measuring NCD events

Tracking NCD events in the population is complex and resource-demanding and requires the ability to identify and report all (or nearly all) deaths and new events of NCDs. This requires access to deaths in public and private health services as well as those outside health centres across all parts of the country and that the causes of disease/death are assessed in a standardized manner (e.g. the WHO International Classification of Diseases) with a reliable knowledge of the main cause of illness/death among possibly several comorbidities (e.g. whether the death was due to a stroke or to a pulmonary infection). Clearly, there are some events that are likely to be described more accurately than others.

National civil registration and vital statistics. Data capable of reporting cause-specific mortality in the population rely on death certificates in which the primary, secondary and associated causes of death are systematically recorded and are, ideally, completed by healthcare professionals that either attended the death or knew the medical history of the deceased. Overall, less than half of all deaths in the world are registered with their cause and even when death certificates are available, the cause of death is often unreliable. It is important that those certifying deaths received training on completing meaningful returns.[8] Calculating mortality rates also requires the size and age distribution of the entire population to be known.

Demographic surveys assess incidence (mortality and, to some extent, morbidity), typically in definite geographical areas populated by a few thousand or hundreds of thousands of people. Health officers visit each household at regular intervals (e.g. every six months), with the cause of death determined by *verbal autopsies* that enable the likely cause of death to be established.

Disease registries are available in some countries where resources are available. They can be either population-based or hospital-based. Population-based cancer registries are used to determine cancer patterns among various populations or sub-populations, monitor trends and improve patient care. Registries also exist for other chronic diseases (e.g. stroke, heart diseases, kidney disease, hypertension, diabetes, inheritable conditions) and are generally established at hospital and/or primary health care levels: their main focus is to improve patient care.

Patient record systems are used to collect, store and report clinical information important to the delivery of NCD-related patient care and are an important source of data for those accessing health services regarding NCD diagnosis, management and care. A comprehensive set of reliable measures of service quality, service availability and clinical health outcomes for the facility-based patients and programme monitoring for NCDs, as well as practical and simple digital reporting tools, can address gaps in monitoring. WHO has developed a set of indicators to support standards-based data recording and reporting in health facilities at the primary care level in low-resource settings, and related tools to integrate these indicators are currently being piloted for inclusion, such as DHIS2 (District Health Information Software, developed by the Health Information Service Provider [HISP] global network, led by the University of Oslo)[9] and other health information management system/electronic patient record platforms.[10] A key challenge is that these data are often not fully representative of population health (as they only reflect people who access health services) and may be incomplete or of uneven quality.

Assessing services for NCDs

The Service Availability and Readiness Assessment (SARA) tool was developed by WHO and the US Agency for International Development (USAID).[11] It is designed to assess and monitor health services availability and readiness and provides information to support the planning and managing of a health system. Data collected include information on the availability of key human and infrastructure resources and the availability of basic equipment, basic amenities, essential medicines and diagnostic capacities (around NCDs and other health issues). Countries have also developed their service assessment instruments.[12]

Surveillance tools for measuring progress against the WHO Global NCD Action Plan indicators

Examples of tools that countries can use to measure indicators in the WHO Global NCD Action Plan are shown in Table 5.1.

Challenges when it comes to obtaining high-quality data from NCD risk factor surveillance include: (i) governments and their partners not prioritizing this area of work sufficiently with inadequate integration of NCD risk factor surveillance into national health information systems; (ii) the often high turnover of personnel involved in surveillance; (iii) the lack of resources available at the country level to support surveillance activities with weak infrastructure

Table 5.1 Surveillance tools to measure progress against the WHO Global NCD Action Plan indicators[a]

Element	Target	Indicator	Examples of surveillance tools
Mortality and morbidity			
Premature mortality from NCDs.	1. A 25% relative reduction in mortality from CVD, cancer, diabetes or chronic respiratory diseases.	1. Unconditional probability of dying between the ages of 30 and 70 from CVD, cancer, diabetes or chronic respiratory diseases. 2. Cancer incidence, by type of cancer, per 100,000 population.	National civil registration and vital statistics capable of reporting cause of death, verbal autopsy tools, DHS, etc. Population censuses are also needed.
Behavioural risk factors			
Harmful use of alcohol.	2. At least a 10% relative reduction in the harmful use of alcohol, as appropriate within the national context.	3. Total alcohol per capita (aged 15+ years old) per year (litres of pure alcohol). 4. Prevalence★ of heavy episodic drinking in adolescents and adults. 5. Alcohol-related morbidity and mortality in adolescents and adults.	STEPS, NHS, GSHS, DHS and similar surveys (with or without examination).
Physical inactivity.	3. A 10% relative reduction in the prevalence of insufficient physical activity.	6. Prevalence of insufficiently physically active adolescents (<60 minutes of moderate to vigorous intensity activity daily). 7. Prevalence★ of insufficiently physically active adults (<150 minutes of moderate-intensity activity per week, or equivalent).	Idem (as for alcohol). Surveys must include physical activity at work, at home, for transport and during leisure time.
Salt/sodium intake.	4. A 30% relative reduction in mean population intake of salt/sodium.	8. Mean★ population intake of salt per day in adults.	Idem. Biological samples are needed if spot or 24-hour urine samples are taken.

(*Continued*)

Table 5.1 (Continued)

Element	Target	Indicator	Examples of surveillance tools
Tobacco use.	5. A 30% relative reduction in the prevalence of current tobacco use in adults.	9. Prevalence of current tobacco use in adolescents. 10. Prevalence★ of current tobacco use in adults.	Idem.
Biological risk factors			
Raised BP.	6. A 25% relative reduction in the prevalence of raised BP or contain the prevalence of raised BP, according to national circumstances.	11. Prevalence★ of raised BP in adults (≥140/90 or treatment) and mean systolic BP.	Idem. Physical measurements of BP are needed (self-reported values are not accepted).
Diabetes and obesity.	7. Halt the rise in diabetes and obesity.	12. Prevalence★ of raised BP/diabetes in adults (glucose ≥7.0 mmol/l (126 mg/dl) or treatment). 13. Prevalence of overweight and obesity in adolescents (WHO growth reference). 14. Prevalence★ of overweight and obesity in adults (BMI ≥25 kg/m² and ≥ 30 kg/m²).	Idem. Biological measurements of blood glucose and physical measurements of height and weight are needed. (self-reported values are not accepted).
		15. Proportion★ of total energy intake from saturated fatty acids in adults. 16. Prevalence★ of adults consuming <5 servings (400 g) of fruit and vegetables per day. 17. Prevalence★ of raised cholesterol in adults (≥5.0 mmol/l or 190 mg/dl); and mean★ total cholesterol concentration.	Idem.

(Continued)

Table 5.1 (Continued)

Element	Target	Indicator	Examples of surveillance tools
National systems response			
Drug therapy to prevent heart attacks and strokes.	8. At least 50% of eligible people receive drug therapy and counselling to prevent heart attacks and strokes.	18. Proportion of persons aged ≥40 years with 10-year CVD risk ≥30% receiving drug therapy and counselling for hypertension or diabetes.	Idem. Patient record systems.
Essential NCD medicines and basic technologies to treat major NCDs.	9. An 80% availability of affordable basic technologies and essential medicines to treat major NCDs in both public and private facilities.	19. Availability and affordability of quality, safe and efficacious essential NCD medicines, including generics, and basic technologies in both public and private facilities.	SARA, other facility-based surveys.

*Age-standardized.
CVD: cardiovascular disease; BP: blood pressure, BMI: body mass index, adults: persons aged 18+ years. DHS: demographic health survey.
a Noncommunicable diseases global monitoring framework: indicator definitions and specifications. WHO, 2014.

(e.g. travel and transport systems) that make household surveys difficult, weak country capacity in data management, analysis and report writing; and (iv) out-of-date sampling frames and lack of geographical accessibility of some areas in some countries.[13]

Notes

1 Surveillance systems & tools. www.who.int/teams/noncommunicable-diseases/surveillance/systems-tools/.
2 Hammer MJ. Ethical considerations for data collection using surveys. *Oncol Nurs Forum* 2017;44:157–59.
3 WHO NCD microdata repository. https://extranet.who.int/ncdsmicrodata/.
4 Global school-based student health survey. WHO. www.who.int/teams/noncommunicable-diseases/surveillance/systems-tools/global-school-based-student-health-survey.
5 Global youth tobacco survey. WHO. www.who.int/teams/noncommunicable-diseases/surveillance/systems-tools/global-youth-tobacco-survey.
6 Health behaviour in school-aged children. WHO collaborative cross-national survey. www.hbsc.org/about/index.html.
7 National Health and Nutrition Examination Survey. US Centre for Disease Control and Prevention. https://www.cdc.gov/nchs/nhanes/index.htm.

8 Brooks EG, Reed KD. Principles and pitfalls: a guide to death certification. *Clin Med Res* 2015;13:74–84.
9 What is DHIS2? https://docs.dhis2.org/en/use/what-is-dhis2.html.
10 Webster P. The rise of open-source electronic health records. *Lancet* 2011;377:1641–42.
11 Service availability and readiness assessment (SARA). WHO. www.who.int/data/data-collection-tools/service-availability-and-readiness-assessment-(sara)?ua=1.
12 Hoa NT et al. Development and validation of the Vietnamese primary care assessment tool – provider version. *Prim Health Care Res Dev* 2019;20:e86.
13 Riley L et al. The World Health Organization STEPwise approach to noncommunicable disease risk-factor surveillance: methods, challenges, and opportunities. *Am J Public Health* 2016;106:74–78.

Part 2
Burden, epidemiology and priority interventions for individual NCDs

Part 2

6 Cardiovascular disease
Burden, epidemiology and risk factors

*Pascal Bovet, Nick Banatvala, Kay-Tee Khaw,
K Srinath Reddy*

This is one of two chapters on cardiovascular disease (CVD). Chapter 7 focuses on priority interventions for CVD and monitoring and evaluation.

Definitions

CVD is a term for conditions affecting the heart and blood vessels. The two main sites for CVD are ischaemic heart disease (IHD) and cerebrovascular disease (such as ischaemic or haemorrhagic stroke). Common manifestations of IHD include angina pectoris (chest pain due to insufficient oxygen supply in the coronary arteries), heart attack (also called myocardial infarction, which causes the loss of a part of the heart muscle) and heart failure (impairment of the heart pumping function due to weakened heart muscle). Cerebrovascular disease can result in lasting neurological damage, including hemiplegia and severe brain cognitive alterations. Transient ischaemic attacks (TIAs) are similar to a stroke but last only a few minutes or hours and cause no lasting disability, but a third of persons with a TIA can subsequently develop a full stroke.

Common to IHD and ischaemic stroke is atherosclerosis (an intravascular build-up of cholesterol, calcium, fibrous tissue and platelets) that progressively over many decades results in narrowed and inelastic arteries, which results in decreased blood flow and oxygen supply (hence the word 'ischaemic') and ultimately total vessel block (causing heart attack or stroke). Haemorrhagic stroke is particularly strongly associated with hypertension.

Other cardiovascular diseases include congenital heart disease malformations, heart valves defects (including rheumatic heart disease), cardiomyopathies (diseases of the heart muscle that are not directly related to ischaemia), arterial aneurysm, peripheral arterial disease, deep vein thrombosis and pulmonary embolism.

This chapter focuses on IHD and stroke because they cause around 80% of the global CVD mortality (IHME, 2019), and they share (along with some other CVDs such as peripheral arterial disease) a common set of modifiable risk factors and therefore similar prevention and management strategies. For these reasons, the focus on CVD in the WHO Global NCD Action Plan is on IHD and stroke and their main risk factors.

DOI: 10.4324/9781003306689-8

Disease burden and trends

The three most important elements of the epidemiology of CVD are: (i) the increasing total CVD burden owing to the increasing and aging populations in the world, i.e. demographic transition; (ii) the decreasing age-standardized CVD mortality rates in most countries because progress is being made in tackling risk factors and improving treatment; and (iii) large differences in age-standardized CVD mortality between countries as a result of markedly different risk factor levels across populations and large differences in implementation of population-wide prevention and control programmes, including effective health care.

Based on data from IHME, there were 523 million people living with a CVD in 2019 of which 197 were IHD and 101 were stroke. CVD accounted for 18.6 million deaths in 2019, while IHD accounted for 9.1 million deaths.[1]

Table 6.1 shows that CVD (including IHD and stroke) in 2019 accounted for 32.8% (18.6 million) of all deaths globally, IHD for 16.2% (9.1 million) and stroke for 11.2% (6.6 million) (data from IHME).

However, there are large differences between countries from different World Bank income categories. The proportion – from all deaths – of CVD deaths for CVD, IHD and stroke were high in 2019 in high-income countries (HICs) but had decreased compared to 1990; were highest in upper-middle-income countries (MICs) in 2019 (an increase from 1990); and were lowest in lower-MICs and low-income countries (LICs), but a twofold increase from 1990. These differences in regions partly reflect changing age distributions of populations.

Although IHD and stroke deaths are more common above the age of 70, they also cause substantial premature mortality. For example, nearly 30% of all deaths worldwide between 50 and 69 years in 2019 were from IHD and stroke.

Decreasing age-standardized mortality

Table 6.1 also shows that the age-standardized mortality rates from CVD, IHD and stroke (which are not influenced by the age distribution of the populations

Table 6.1 Mortality for CVD, IHD and stroke (IHME)

	Global		HICs		Upper-MICs		Lower-MICs		LICs	
	1990	2019	1990	2019	1990	2019	1990	2019	1990	2019
Proportion of all deaths (%)										
All CVD	25.9	32.8	42.2	32.5	32.3	40.7	17.4	29.7	9.1	16
IHD	12.2	16.2	24.4	16.4	12.7	18.8	8.5	16	3.2	6.2
Stroke	9.8	11.6	11.8	8.4	14.8	16.6	6.4	9.8	3.9	6.5
Age-standardized mortality rates (per 100,000)										
All CVD	345	240	283	134	401	267	384	313	355	304
IHD	170	118	164	68	163	124	191	169	131	121
Stroke	132	84	79	34	180	107	141	104	149	123

compared) were higher in low- and middle-income countries than in HICs. However, the rates *decreased* over time in all income groups, with a large two-fold decrease in HICs, and a marked decrease in upper-MICs, but only a small decrease in lower-MICs and LICs.

Decreasing CVD mortality is due to a decrease in both incidences (of new cases) and case fatality (among cases) over time.[2] The decreasing incidence reflects a downward shift in several CVD risk factors in the population due to prevention and treatment (e.g. tobacco use, BP and blood cholesterol),[3] while increasing survival reflects improving case management.[4] Large gains in life expectancy at birth observed over the past few decades worldwide largely resulted from the decrease in age-standardized CVD mortality but, in several regions, including Africa, also largely resulted from reductions in maternal and child mortality.[5]

However, the downward trend in age-standardized CVD mortality has been slowing in many countries over recent years, including in HICs, particularly among younger adults, which has been in part attributed to the increasing prevalence of obesity and diabetes.

Variations across countries

Age-standardized CVD rates vary by more than ten-fold between countries, for example <30/100,000 population in 2019 (and still decreasing) in Japan and France compared to >700/100,000 population (but decreasing) in Uzbekistan for IHD, with a similar magnitude of variation for stroke (IHME).

Proportions of IHD/stroke mortality that are attributable to modifiable risk factors (population-attributable fractions)

These fractions express the estimated proportions (or percentages) of the total IHD/stroke burden that could be prevented if a risk factor was eliminated in the *whole* population (i.e. if all individuals in the population had this risk factor at the optimal level range).[6] At a global level, in 2019, these fractions were as follows:[7]

- *Environmental*: particulate matter (e.g. pollution, indoor smoke) 21%; non-optimal temperature 7%.
- *Physiologic/metabolic*: high blood pressure 51%; high blood cholesterol 28%; high blood glucose 23%; kidney dysfunction 11%.
- *Behaviours*: unhealthy diet 41%★; tobacco use 19%; physical inactivity 4%; harmful use of alcohol 1%.

    ★This includes: high sodium (salt) and low whole grains (10% each); low vegetables and fruit (7% and 5% respectively); high red meat, high trans fat, low nuts and seeds low fibre (4% each); low vegetables, alcohol (3% each), low polyunsaturated fats and low omega-3 fatty acids (2% each); processed meat and sugar-sweetened beverages (1% each).

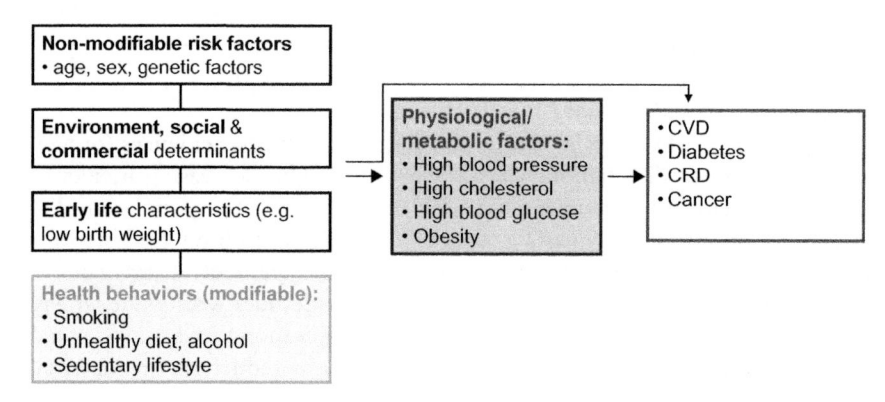

Figure 6.1 The relationship between risk factors and CVD (and other selected NCDs).

These large attributable fractions across a wide range of risk factors emphasize the need to prevent IHD and stroke through a large number of interventions, and these are addressed in the following chapter and other chapters.

Risk factors

The relationships between modifiable and non-modifiable risk factors, as well as broader determinants of health with physiological and metabolic risk factors and with IHD and stroke, are shown in Figure 6.1. Peripheral vascular disease, as well as cancer and chronic respiratory disease, are included to highlight the relationship between these risk factors and NCDs more broadly. The relationship between risk factors and CVD outcomes is graded (i.e. dose-dependent). This explains why the majority of CVD outcomes arise in individuals with moderate rather than high levels of risk factors (i.e. the majority of the population) rather than from those (a minority of the population) at high risk. This underscores the need to reduce risk factors in the whole population, not only among those at the highest risk. Chapter 36 on population and high-risk strategies provides a description of this 'prevention paradox'.

Main modifiable risk factors

The main modifiable CVD risk factors were identified in the late 1940s and 1950s when the CVD epidemic was rapidly progressing in high-income countries. The pioneering Framingham cohort study (started in the late 1940s) showed that both the 10- and 30-year risk of CVD risk was <5% among individuals who were non-smokers, with low BP, low blood cholesterol and no diabetes, but the 10- and 30-year risks were as high as around 40% and 80%, respectively, among individuals with elevated levels of these four risk factors, emphasizing the importance of interventions to reduce exposure to these risk factors.[8]

Other studies have shown that individuals with healthy behaviours, including not smoking, being physically active, with a healthy diet, and being lean (which can be interpreted as having healthy nutrition and regular physical activity), had a very low incidence of heart attacks and stroke (as well as diabetes and cancer),[9] emphasizing the critical role of this small number of healthy behaviours. Consistent with this, many studies have shown large protection for CVD among individuals with low levels of these main risk factors, described by the American Heart Association as 'Life Simple 7', which includes three 'ideal health factors' (BP <120/80 mmHg, total cholesterol <5.2 mmol/L, blood glucose <5.6 mmol/L) and four 'ideal health behaviours' (not smoking, regular physical activity, healthy diet, and body mass index <25 kg/m^2).[10] While there is some evidence that low alcohol consumption (e.g. ≤1 drink per day) may reduce the risk of IHD, anything more is associated with increased risk. Hundreds of clinical trials have shown an approximately 20–30% lower relative risk of CVD when reducing one risk factor with therapy (behavioural or medication), and much more when reducing several risk factors at the same time.[11] A list of main modifiable CVD risk factors, and their potential contribution to the CVD incidence (e.g. as assessed by population-attributable fractions), is described in the previous section; a more detailed description of related interventions appears in other chapters in the book (hypertension, diabetes, fats and cholesterol, tobacco, salt, diet, physical activity, alcohol, etc.).

Age, genetics and other risk factors

Chronological age is by far the most important CVD risk factor, independent of the risk factors above. However, biological or physiological age (how old a person seems) is even more important and is a combination of an individual's chronological age, phenotype (e.g. blood pressure, blood sugar level or extent of vascular atherosclerosis), and genetic makeup and alterations over time (e.g. detrimental chromosomal telomere changes with age).[12]

Genetic makeup plays a significant role in CVD.[13] Single gene alterations are rare but important causes of CVD, e.g. familial hypercholesterolemia that causes heart attack at an early age. In contrast, polygenic alterations (i.e. abnormal single nucleotide polymorphisms) are common (e.g. a prevalence of up to 30% for the presence of one particular isolated abnormal SNP associated with CVD), but the effect on CVD is generally small in the presence of one or a few such alterations but can be substantial when many abnormal SNPs are present. However, while a high polygenic risk score (i.e. a score based on many SNPs associated with CVD) can raise CVD risk by as much as two-fold, the impact is reduced among those with healthy lifestyles and diets.[14] In addition, epigenetic factors associated with CVD (i.e. alterations in gene expression, how the body 'reads' DNA rather than alterations of the genetic code itself) can also increase the risk of CVD. These alterations are, for example, enhanced by exposure to risk factors such as tobacco smoke.[15] The above suggests that polygenic risk scores are likely to play an important role in personalized CVD prevention and treatment in the future[16] (Chapter 29 on genetics).

Psycho-social factors (e.g. stress, depression) and socio-economic variables such as income, education, employment status, and neighbourhood characteristics are associated with CVD, either directly or indirectly (e.g. depression, stress or other unfavourable psycho-social conditions can lead people to smoke more, have a poorer diet, consume more alcohol, do less physical activity, and seek less frequent care for their health).[17] Low birth weight is associated with an increased risk of several cardiometabolic disorders (e.g. obesity, diabetes, CVD) in adulthood,[18] which has significant public health implications in low-income countries. Further details are provided in Chapter 17 on social determinants of health and chapter 37 on a life-course approach to NCDs.

The role of economic development, globalization and urbanization

The relationship between a society's economic development and the development of CVD is complex. Early in the health transition (Chapter 2), individuals of higher socio-economic status (SES) have the highest levels of risk factors, with the correspondingly greatest incidence of CVD events. Individuals of higher SES are, however, the first to acquire an understanding of CVD risks and they modify their behaviour accordingly (e.g. they reduce tobacco consumption and adopt a healthier diet), resulting in a decrease in CVD incidence. In the meantime, those in the lower socio-economic groups are more exposed to risk factors, with a high incidence of disease.

As a result, the relationship between socio-economic development and CVD risk factors generally follows a bell shape curve, with levels of mean blood cholesterol, blood pressure and (to a lesser extent) body mass index rapidly increasing, plateauing and then decreasing as a country's socio-economic development increases over time.[19] These trends partly reflect a transition from (healthy) unrefined traditional foods, to inexpensive (unhealthy) energy-dense processed foods, until a later stage where a broader variety of foods is available (both healthy and unhealthy). In summary, economic development (and by extension globalization) presents both challenges and opportunities with regard to CVD – ones that need to be tackled respectively through policies that impact CVD and health more broadly.[20] There is also emerging evidence that the argument that urbanization is invariably detrimental to cardiovascular health is not always the case. For example, the prevalence of obesity is now increasing faster in rural rather than urban settings in low- and middle-income countries.[21] These issues are also described further in Chapter 2 on the health transition.

Notes

1 Roth GA et al. Global burden of cardiovascular diseases and risk factors, 1990–2019: update from the GBD 2019 study. *J Am Coll Cardiol* 2020;76:2982–3021.

2 Camacho X et al. Relative contribution of trends in myocardial infarction event rates and case fatality to declines in mortality: an international comparative study of 1·95 million events in 80·4 million people in four countries. *Lancet Public Health* 2022;7:e229–39.
3 Shah ASV et al. Clinical burden, risk factor impact and outcomes following myocardial infarction and stroke: a 25-year individual patient level linkage study. *Lancet Reg Health Eur* 2021;7:100141.
4 Ezzati M et al. Contributions of risk factors and medical care to cardiovascular mortality trends. *Nat Rev Cardiol* 2015;12:508–30.
5 Foreman KJ et al. Forecasting life expectancy, years of life lost, and all-cause and cause-specific mortality for 250 causes of death: reference and alternative scenarios for 2016–40 for 195 countries and territories. *Lancet* 2018;392:2052–90.
6 Fractions are not independent of each other (e.g. salt & hypertension) and vary in relation to the prevalence of the risk factors in the population. Source of data: IHME.
7 https://vizhub.healthdata.org/gbd-compare.
8 Pencina MJ et al. Predicting the 30-year risk of CVD: The Framingham heart study. *Circulation* 2009;11:3078–84.
9 Ford ES et al. Healthy living is the best revenge: findings from the European prospective investigation into cancer (EPIC) and nutrition–potsdam study. *Arch Intern Med* 2009;169:1355–62.
10 Han L et al. National trends in American Heart Association revised life's simple 7 metrics associated with risk of mortality among US adults. *JAMA Netw Open* 2019;2:e1913131.
11 Arnett DK et al. 2019 ACC/AHA guideline on the primary prevention of cardiovascular disease. *Circulation* 2019;140:e563–95.
12 Arsenis NC et al. Physical activity and telomere length: impact of aging and potential mechanisms of action. *Oncotarget* 2017;8:45008–19.
13 Vrablik M et al. Review: genetics of cardiovascular disease: how far are we from personalized CVD risk prediction and management? *Int J Mol Sci* 2021;22:4182.
14 Khera AV et al. Genetic risk, adherence to a healthy lifestyle, and coronary disease. *NEJM* 2016;375:2349–58.
15 Maas Clin SCE et al. Smoking-related changes in DNA methylation and gene expression are associated with cardio-metabolic traits. *Epigenetics* 2020;12:157.
16 Sun L et al. Polygenic risk scores in cardiovascular risk prediction: a cohort study and modelling analyses. *PLoS Med* 2021;18:e1003498.
17 Schultz WM et al. Socioeconomic status and cardiovascular outcomes: challenges and interventions. *Circulation* 2018;137:2166–17.
18 Arima Y et al. Developmental origins of health and disease theory in cardiology. *J Cardiol* 2020;76:14–17.
19 Ezzati E et al. Rethinking the "diseases of affluence" paradigm: global patterns of nutritional risks in relation to economic development. *PLoS* 2005;2:e133.
20 Stuckler D et al. Manufacturing epidemics: the role of global producers in increased consumption of unhealthy commodities including processed foods, alcohol, and tobacco. *PLoS Med* 2012;9:e1001235.
21 NCD Risk Factor Collaboration. Rising rural body-mass index is the main driver of the global obesity epidemic in adults. *Nature* 2019;569:260–64.

7 Cardiovascular disease
Priority interventions

Pascal Bovet, Nick Banatvala, K Srinath Reddy, Kay-Tee Khaw

This is one of two chapters on cardiovascular disease (CVD). Chapter 6 focuses on CVD burden, epidemiology and risk factors.

Rationale

Around 50–60% of the decline in age-standardized ischaemic heart disease (IHD) mortality in the last few decades (at least in high-income countries) can be attributed to a multiple risk factor reduction through population-level interventions while around 40–50% is from treatment.[1] This means that improving CVD public health requires both interventions in multiple sectors aimed at reducing risk factors in the entire population and health care interventions among individuals with NCD or at high risk.

Since atherosclerosis starts at a young age (fatty streaks and increasing arterial thickness – the precursors to atheroma are already present in coronary arteries of a significant proportion of children and adolescents), it is important to aim at reducing risk factors from early life for both physiological reasons (atherosclerosis accumulates in arteries over time and is largely not reversible) and behavioural reasons (many behaviours are acquired early in life; they tend to track over age and it is challenging for individuals to modify them when they become internally ingrained). The large proportion of sudden deaths (which are largely due to IHD),[2] i.e. before a person can receive care, further emphasizes the importance of primary prevention.

Hence, CVD (and indeed NCD) public health programmes must therefore act across the full range of modifiable risk factors and start from an early age if CVD risk factors levels are to be maintained at low levels throughout the life-course or, when elevated, managed effectively (Chapter 37 on the life-course approach). The majority of the WHO best buys and effective interventions have an impact on CVD or their risk factors (as well as on several other NCDs).

Interventions at the population level

These interventions aim at reducing the exposure to modifiable CVD risk factors in the whole population and require action across multiple sectors.

DOI: 10.4324/9781003306689-9

A list of the main modifiable CVD risk factors and their potential importance in contributing to CVD incidence (i.e. population-attributable fractions) is described in the previous chapter. A number of interventions are described in more detail in chapters on specific CVD risk factors (e.g. hypertension, blood lipids, tobacco, diet and physical inactivity). The examples below are adapted from Disease Control Priorities 2.[3] It is important to note that the WHO Global NCD Action Plan, in addition to highlighting specific cost-effective interventions to reduce CVD risk, also draws attention to the broader upstream actions on environmental and socio-economic factors ('the causes of the causes'). These are described in more detail in Chapter 17 on social determinants and in other chapters (whole-of-government response, fiscal measures, law, etc.).

- *Policy to increase/decrease access, availability or exposure to healthy/unhealthy foods or products*
  - Alter the content of foods and beverages (e.g. salt, trans-fats, saturated fats and sugar in selected foods).
  - Limit marketing, supply and availability of unhealthy foods.
  - Ban smoking or alcohol use in selected premises.
- *Policies around transportation to improve active mobility*
  - Limit the role of private vehicles and develop the use of public transport to promote active mobility (e.g. walking/cycling).
  - Promote healthy cities, e.g. structures that promote physical activity for all such as green spaces.
- *Economic/fiscal policies to increase/reduce the demand/supply of healthy/unhealthy items*
  - Differential tax rates/subsidies on healthy foods vs unhealthy energy-dense ones.
  - Excise taxes on tobacco, alcohol, sugar drinks.
- *Initiatives at the community level*
  - Most effective when multifaceted, involving the community and culturally acceptable.
  - Dose and duration of interventions should be large enough and sustained over time.
- *Educational programmes*
  - Increasing population awareness of NCDs and their risk factors through the media and in different settings (e.g. schools, workplaces).

Several WHO technical packages have been developed to support countries reduce CVD risk factors at the population level, and these are described in relevant chapters in this book.

Interventions at the individual level

A number of WHO best buys and other recommended interventions are available to identify, diagnose and treat individuals at risk of CVD or with established CVD, including at the primary health care level.

1. *WHO best buys for CVD*
    - Drug therapy (including glycaemic control for diabetes and control of hypertension) using a total CVD risk approach and counselling to individuals who have had a heart attack or stroke and to persons with high risk ($\geq 30\%$) or moderate to high risk ($\geq 20\%$) of a fatal or non-fatal CVD event in the next ten years. This intervention is feasible, to different extents, in all resource settings, including by non-physician health workers. This should also include treatment to lower blood cholesterol, in line with the WHO HEARTS package and recommendations from a number of heart societies. The threshold for defining CVD risk can be set at lower levels to enable greater numbers of people to receive treatment where resources allow (see the section below on the total risk approach and CVD risk scoring). Other chapters describe interventions to reduce individual CVD risk factors, e.g. hypertension (Chapter 8), diabetes (Chapter 9), and dyslipidaemia (Chapter 20).
2. *WHO effective interventions for CVD*
    - Treatment of new cases of acute heart attack with antiplatelet therapy (low dose aspirin and/or clopidogrel), thrombolysis, or primary percutaneous coronary interventions – the approach taken will be dependent on the capacity of the health system.
    - Treatment of acute ischemic stroke with intravenous thrombolytic therapy where capacity exists to diagnose ischemic stroke. A number of specialized centres use mechanical thrombectomy to remove the obstructing blood clot.
3. *Other WHO-recommended interventions*
    - Treatment of congestive cardiac failure with angiotensin-converting-enzyme inhibitor, beta-blocker and diuretic.
    - Cardiac rehabilitation post-myocardial infarction.
    - Antiplatelet therapy (e.g. low-dose aspirin) for ischemic stroke.
    - Care of acute stroke and rehabilitation in stroke units.

Detailed guidance for implementing the above interventions has been developed by WHO and authoritative professional bodies.

Key issues that policymakers and programme managers need to be aware of are given below.

Total absolute risk approach and CVD risk scoring

The total risk approach is an important principle when it comes to the management of CVD as it recognizes that the risk of developing CVD is determined by the combined effect of cardiovascular risk factors, which often commonly coexist and act multiplicatively. An individual with several mildly raised risk factors may be at a higher total risk of CVD than someone with just one elevated risk factor. Conversely, CVD total risk can be reduced equivalently by reducing any of the modifiable risk factors, irrespective of their baseline values. A number of CVD risk stratification charts (risk calculators) are available to determine the ten-year risk of a cardiovascular event (e.g. Framingham, SCORE, QRISK, AHA/ACC and WHO).[4,5] Important considerations with regard to CVD risk charts are:

- Risk calculators should aim to obtain the optimal ratio of the size of the population needing treatment for the greatest impact on reducing subsequent CVD events, and minimize the number of eligible patients that need to be treated (NNT) to prevent one CVD event given the limited resources available in a particular country (i.e. identify those individuals who will benefit most from therapy in terms of absolute CVD risk reduction).[6]
- Age alone contributes up to 80% of the predictive value of any given CVD risk score.[7] Risk scores over periods longer than ten years, for example 30 years, can be useful to assess more accurately long-term or lifetime CVD risk in younger individuals (e.g. aged <40 years).[8,9]
- CVD risk scores perform accurately to predict the average underlying CVD risk in the population, but they perform less well at the individual level because not all risk factors are included in a given risk prediction score, the associations between risk factors and CVD are relatively weak, and risk scores results are simplified into only two categories ('at risk' vs 'not at risk') while the relation between risk factors and CVD is graded. This highlights the need for an ever more accurate assessment of CVD risk at an individual level, where relevant and possible, that takes into account other risk factors, health conditions and measurements (e.g. family history, psychosocial wellbeing, kidney function, coronary artery calcium).
- As total CVD risk varies significantly between populations and over time (often as much as a 3% annual decrease in some countries), risk prediction scores need to be developed or validated, and regularly recalibrated, to the relevant population.

Individuals with a previous CVD hard outcome ('secondary prevention')

Individuals who have established IHD or stroke are at very high risk of subsequent CVD events and death. These people are the top priority for receiving treatment and lifestyle advice to reduce their risk: risk stratification charts are not required. However, despite their risk, many studies, including in high-income countries, have shown that these individuals are not receiving adequate treatment, including antiplatelet therapy, beta-blockers, and blood pressure/blood cholesterol-lowering medications, despite their high efficacy to reduce recurrent CVD and the possibility of prescribing these fairly simple and safe therapies in primary care.[10]

Fixed-dose medication combination (polypill). There has been significant interest in simple treatments that can be widely used to reduce the risk of

CVD events among individuals at high risk.[11] Fixed-dose combination drug regimens, also known as polypills, are options that along with non-pharmacological approaches can be used for both primary and secondary prevention.[12] Polypills generally contain three to five different medications combined in one daily pill (e.g. two to three different blood pressure lowering drugs, a statin and – in some cases – aspirin, at full or half dose). Clinical trials in several countries have shown that polypills improve adherence to treatment, lower risk factor levels and decrease CVD mortality.[13] Polypills are also a cost-effective way of delivering treatment and are more straightforward for the prescriber, especially in primary health care and among non-physician health professionals.

Health care packages for CVD

WHO has developed the HEARTS[14] package to support countries to strengthen primary health CVD management. HEARTS includes six modules: (i) healthy-lifestyle counselling; (ii) evidence-based treatment protocols; (iii) access to essential medicines and technology; (iv) risk-based CVD management; (v) team-based care; and (vi) systems for monitoring. The HEARTS technical package is part of the broader Global Hearts Initiative, which includes the MPOWER package for tobacco control in line with the WHO Framework Convention on Tobacco Control, the ACTIVE package for increasing physical activity, the SHAKE package for salt reduction, and the REPLACE package to eliminate industrially produced trans fat from the global food supply. A WHO package of essential noncommunicable (PEN) disease interventions aimed at low- and middle-income countries has also been developed to support countries improve the coverage of appropriate services for people with NCDs in primary care settings.[15]

Detailed guidelines on CVD prevention and management are also regularly issued by other well-recognized public health bodies (e.g. the American Heart Association, the European Society of Cardiology as well as by many national health authorities).

Monitoring

Achieving all nine targets in the WHO Global NCD Action Plan will have an impact on CVD. The majority of the 25 indicators of the WHO Global Monitoring Framework (Chapter 35 on accountability) are therefore key in monitoring and evaluating processes towards a reduction in CVD. Population-based surveys of risk factors among adults (e.g. STEPS) and children (e.g. GSHS) are central to the surveillance of CVD risk factors (i.e. their prevalence and awareness/treatment/control levels). Regular assessment of health care services, including how patients with CVD are managed, is also important using tools such as SARA. These are described in more detail in Chapter 5 on surveillance tools. Vital statistics are important in assessing CVD deaths at a population level but are resource-intensive.

Notes

1 Ford ES et al. Explaining the decrease in U.S. deaths from coronary disease, 1980–2000. *NEJM* 2007;356:2388–98.
2 Camacho X et al. Relative contribution of trends in myocardial infarction event rates and case fatality to declines in mortality: an international comparative study of 1·95 million events in 80·4 million people in four countries. *Lancet Public Health* 2022;7:e229–39.
3 Jamison D et al. *Disease control priorities in developing countries.* Washington, DC: World Bank and Oxford University Press, 2006. https://openknowledge.worldbank.org/handle/10986/7242.
4 The WHO CVD Risk Chart Working Group. WHO cardiovascular disease risk charts: revised models to estimate risk in 21 global regions. *Lancet Global Health* 2019;7:e1332–45.
5 Damen JAAG et al. Prediction models for cardiovascular disease risk in the general population: systematic review. *BMJ* 2016;353:i2416.
6 Ndindjock R et al. Potential impact of single-risk-factor versus total risk management for the prevention of cardiovascular events in Seychelles. *Bull WHO* 2011;89:286–95.
7 Pencina MJ et al. Quantifying importance of major risk factors for coronary heart disease. *Circulation* 2019;139:1603–11.
8 Pencina MJ et al. The expected 30-year benefits of early versus delayed primary prevention of cardiovascular disease by lipid lowering. *Circulation* 2020;142:827–37.
9 Leening MJ et al. Lifetime perspectives on primary prevention of atherosclerotic cardiovascular disease. *JAMA* 2016;315:1449.
10 Yusuf S et al. Use of secondary prevention drugs for cardiovascular disease in the community in high-income, middle-income, and low-income countries (the PURE Study): a prospective epidemiological survey. *Lancet* 2011;378:1231–43.
11 Wald NJ, Law MR. A strategy to reduce cardiovascular disease by more than 80%. *BMJ* 2003;326:1419.
12 Selak V et al. Reaching cardiovascular prevention guideline targets with a polypill-based approach: a meta-analysis of randomised clinical trials. *Heart* 2019;105:42–8.
13 Joseph P et al. Fixed-dose combination therapies with and without aspirin for primary prevention of cardiovascular disease: an individual participant data meta-analysis. *Lancet* 2021;398:1133–46.
14 https://www.who.int/publications/i/item/hearts-technical-package.
15 https://www.who.int/publications/i/item/who-package-of-essential-noncommunicable-(pen)-disease-interventions-for-primary-health-care.

8 Hypertension

Burden, epidemiology and priority interventions

Pascal Bovet, Alta E Schutte, Nick Banatvala, Michel Burnier

Raised blood pressure (BP) is the leading cause of mortality worldwide and the main risk factor for cardiovascular disease (CVD). Most people with raised BP have no symptoms and are only diagnosed through screening, through a health check or when they have a CVD event, such as a stroke, a heart attack or heart failure. Reducing the prevalence of raised BP is one of the nine targets of the WHO Global NCD Action Plan. A number of cost-effective interventions at the population and individual levels are available to prevent and control raised BP. Diagnosis and treatment of hypertension should be a priority public health intervention in all countries as well as the main component of any programme aiming to reduce CVD.

Definitions

'Optimal' BP is most often defined as <120/80 mmHg. Hypertension is usually defined as BP ≥140 and/or 90 mmHg[1,2] but reduced to ≥130/80 mmHg for example in guidelines in the USA.[3] As BP increases, so does the risk of CVD. Accurate measuring of BP is critically important because once a patient is started on the treatment they often should remain on it for life. Therefore to confirm the diagnosis of hypertension, multiple readings of high BP need to be obtained over a period of time. The increase in BP that transiently results from the normal physiological response to stress or during physical activity is not hypertension.

Prevalence and disease burden

Prevalence of high BP

The global number of persons with high BP has doubled over the past 30 years, affecting around 1.3 billion people in 2019,[4] and numbers will continue to increase because of growing and aging populations. Prevalence of hypertension in most countries ranges from 2–10% at 5–30 years of age to 15–40% (30–60 years) and 30–60% (60+ years). It is therefore important to standardize for age when comparing the prevalence of high BP across different populations or over time. The age-standardized mean BP seems to have decreased between

DOI: 10.4324/9781003306689-10

Table 8.1 Number and percent of deaths and age-standardized mortality attributable to high BP (IHME)

	Global		HICs		Upper-MICs		Lower-MICs		LICs	
	2019	*1990*	*2019*	*1990*	*2019*	*1990*	*2019*	*1990*	*2019*	*1990*
Number of deaths (million)	10.9	6.8	1.9	2.1	4.6	2.6	3.8	1.8	0.5	0.3
% of all deaths	19.2	14.5	17.5	24.9	23.8	17.4	18.1	9.8	9.8	5.2
Age-standardized mortality rates (per 100,000)	139	198	73	166	153	214	187	215	183	203

1975 and 2015 in high-income countries (HIC), but with varying trends in other countries, reflecting differences in prevention, treatment and progression of the obesity epidemic across countries.[5]

Disease burden attributable to high BP

High BP caused 10.9 million deaths worldwide (19.2% of all deaths) in 2019 (Table 8.1), of which 92% were attributable to CVD (mainly heart attack, heart failure, and stroke) and 8% were attributable to kidney disease (IHME). The overall disease burden attributable to high BP increased between 1990 and 2019 in most regions (except in HICs), largely because of growing and aging populations. However, age-standardized mortality rates attributable to high BP decreased in most countries between 1990 and 2019, more markedly in HICs than in low- and middle-income countries again, partly reflecting better prevention and control in the former than the latter.

Risk factors

The main modifiable risk factors of hypertension are overweight/obesity, unhealthy diet (high in salt and low in vegetables and fruit), harmful use of alcohol and physical inactivity. Being overweight/obese alone can account for up to 20–50% of cases of hypertension,[6] especially among children. The majority of obese people with high BP will reduce their BP to normal if they return to normal weight. Diets rich in fruit and vegetables, which are high in potassium (which can include substituting sodium chloride for potassium chloride), reduce BP and thus CVD risk.[7] Similarly, hypertension is less common among populations that are lean and physically active.

Interventions at the population level

Population-based interventions to reduce the exposure to the risk factors described above can have a large impact on the hypertension-related burden because they lower BP in the entire population – and even if this is by a small amount it can have a significant impact on the population level (see Chapter 36).[8] These interventions (which include several WHO best buys) are described in detail in other chapters of the compendium.

Interventions at the individual level

Diagnosis of hypertension

Measuring BP should be considered at any face-to-face consultation with a healthcare professional and health checks provide an opportunity to do this (Chapter 43 on health checks). For young adults, measurement of BP every 3–5 years is reasonable. For older adults, this should be more frequent.[9]

Where an initial reading is elevated, at least one or two additional readings should be taken on the same visit, and readings repeated on at least two additional visits at several day or week intervals. In up to 20% of patients, BP can be systematically higher (and sometimes substantially higher) when assessed in a healthcare setting compared to being measured at home. BP self-measurement at home using a personal BP device should therefore be encouraged to support measurements done in the clinic.[10] Guidelines are available on how to measure BP accurately (e.g. cuff width in relation to arm circumference, rest duration before a reading is made, time intervals between BP readings).

Where BP is dangerously high (≥180/120 mmHg), or there has been an acute CVD event, or damage is identified to the heart, kidney or other organs as a result of raised BP, immediate treatment should be provided.

Management of hypertension

Reducing behavioural risk factors

Before initiating medical treatment, individuals should be encouraged to develop a healthier lifestyle, including a healthy diet (reducing salt intake to <5 g daily, eating more fruit and vegetables and limiting the intake of foods high in saturated fats and reducing/eliminating trans fats), being physically active, controlling their body weight and reducing alcohol consumption. Together, these interventions can reduce BP by around 5–10 mmHg on average in standard clinical settings. All patients should also be strongly encouraged to quit smoking to reduce their CVD risk.

Medication

Drug treatment should be started if BP remains high after a few weeks or months of lifestyle changes – the time depends on the level of BP and risk of CVD risk. A number of national and international authorities have published guidelines on when to start treatment, including by WHO. The criteria below are those from WHO:

- Systolic BP is ≥140 mmHg and/or diastolic BP is ≥90 mmHg.
- Systolic BP is ≥130 mmHg in individuals with existing CVD and individuals without CVD but with high CVD risk, diabetes or chronic kidney disease.

Generic antihypertensive drugs are commonly available and are generally inexpensive. Most have relatively few side effects. It is now well recognized that a larger benefit can result from combining several drugs in single-pill combinations.[11,12]

A number of authorities have issued guidance on treatment regimens. Those from WHO are that initial treatment should be with a single-pill combination (to improve adherence and persistence), consisting of ≥2 drugs from the following classes: diuretics (thiazide or thiazide-like), angiotensin-converting enzyme inhibitors or angiotensin-receptor blockers and calcium channel blockers. The aim should be to reduce BP to <140/90 mmHg (<130 for those with a history of CVD, diabetes or chronic kidney disease). Beta-blockers are recommended for patients with hypertension and cardiac diseases.

Other classes of medications can be useful in particular situations (e.g. labetalol [a beta blocker] or methyldopa for hypertension in pregnancy or resistant hypertension). Antihypertensive treatment typically reduces office BP by ~10–30 mmHg on average, which translates into a 20–60% relative reduction in the risk of CVD. Medication will normally be required for life, yet a major challenge is to ensure that patients continue to take treatment over the long term to maintain BP control.

After the start of treatment or when changing treatment, patients should be reviewed monthly until the target BP is reached, and then at 3-6 months intervals afterwards. A CVD risk assessment (see below) and screening for comorbidities should be undertaken where feasible and provided this does not delay treatment.

As high BP is asymptomatic, and in many settings the costs are significant and/or the availability of drugs is limited, adherence to treatment decreases rapidly over time and does not exceed 50% globally.[13,14] In LICs, less than 10–20% of those with hypertension have their BP effectively controlled.[15] There is therefore continued interest in tools and interventions that can support treatment adherence, e.g. using polypills, pill organizers or the use of mobile technologies.[16]

Resistant hypertension and secondary hypertension

Where BP is not decreasing with treatment and it is not believed to be due to lack of adherence to medication (which is the most common cause, albeit often difficult to ascertain), an underlying cause ('secondary hypertension') can be investigated (such as a renal or endocrine conditions, such as primary aldosteronism)[17], with hypertension responding sometimes to appropriate treatment.

Surgery

Where individuals are morbidly obese, gastric surgery is performed in some settings. This procedure often reduces BP significantly and, in many cases, to levels that no longer require treatment.[18]

Ongoing care

This is required to monitor BP, ensure optimal treatment and assess risk or emergence of CVD, renal and/or other diseases and manage them appropriately. This can all be managed at a primary care level, in partnership between local healthcare workers and the patient. Low-cost electronic BP monitors are now widely available for patients to use and can improve adherence to treatment and a healthy lifestyle. It is important to ensure this equipment is reliable and accurate.[19,20]

Hypertension as part of total CVD risk assessment and treatment

Screening and treatment of hypertension should be part of a broader assessment of CVD risk and management programme. CVD risk assessment takes into account additional risk factors such as age, BMI, blood lipids, glucose levels, tobacco use, alcohol consumption and history of CVD. A range of charts and calculators are available to assess an individual's risk of CVD.[21,22] Ideally, risk scores should be underpinned by data obtained from the local population and updated regularly to take account of changing risk (as CVD risk is decreasing in most populations). Where this is not possible, risk scores are available, for example WHO region-specific risk scores.[23]

The importance of strong health services and systems

The very large numbers of people who need individual-based management for their hypertension, which is often lifelong, emphasize the importance of effective and efficient health services and systems (Chapter 42). This includes:

- Patient-centred services that reduce barriers to use and access, including low-cost or free medical visits and medications, convenient times for consultations and repeat (and in stable patients multi-month) prescriptions, once-daily/single-pill combination treatment regimens, ready access to free BP monitoring (including devices for self-measurement), and the opportunities to increase health literacy around BP control and CVD.
- Community-based multidisciplinary teams, with task sharing so the healthcare workers who are most accessible to patients can provide care,

including adjusting regimens. Pharmacological treatment of hypertension may be provided by non-physician professionals such as pharmacists and nurses, provided the following are in place: proper training, prescribing authority, specific management protocols and physician oversight.
- Uninterrupted supply of quality-assured medications.
- Patient registers for easy retrieval of risk factors measurements and treatment over time. Electronic medical files are particularly helpful.
- Regular training of healthcare staff on the diagnosis and management of hypertension and NCDs.
- Treatment protocols. These need to be simple and practical, yet provide sufficient detail on diagnosis and management, including treatment regimens, as well as criteria for referral.

The WHO HEARTS technical package provides an example of a strategic approach to improving cardiovascular health through a set of six modules (**h**ealthy-lifestyle counselling, **e**vidence-based treatment protocols, **a**ccess to essential medicines and technology, **r**isk-based CVD management, **t**eam-based care, **s**ystems for monitoring).[24]

Relevant WHO Global NCD Action Plan targets for raised BP

A 25% relative reduction in the prevalence of raised BP, or contain the prevalence of raised BP, according to national circumstances.	Age-standardized prevalence of raised BP among persons aged 18+ years (defined as systolic/diastolic BP ≥140/90 mmHg) and mean systolic BP.
At least 50% of eligible people receive drug therapy and counselling (including glycaemic control) to prevent heart attacks and strokes.	Proportion of eligible persons (defined as age 40+ years with a ten-year CVD risk ≥30%, including those with existing CVD) receiving drug therapy and counselling (including glycaemic control) to prevent heart attacks and strokes.
An 80% availability of affordable basic technologies and essential medicines, including generics, required to treat major NCDs in both public and private facilities.	Availability and affordability of quality, safe and efficacious essential NCD medicines, including generics, and basic technologies in both public and private facilities.

Global targets on reducing: (i) harmful use of alcohol; (ii) salt/sodium intake; and (iii) physical inactivity, as well as the target to halt the rise in diabetes and obesity are important related targets.

Monitoring

Population-based surveys such as STEPS (Chapter 5) are required to estimate the prevalence of raised BP, as well as trends in the proportions receiving treatment/counselling and being controlled. Ideally, surveys should allow BP to be measured in individuals who have raised BP on more than one occasion as surveys based on measurements on a single day tend to overestimate the actual prevalence of hypertension.[25] The availability of equipment, medicines and protocols for treating raised BP can be assessed through surveys such as the Health Service Availability and Readiness Assessment (SARA) which are used to monitor the delivery of NCD services.

Notes

1 Unger T et al. 2020 International Society of Hypertension global hypertension practice. *J Hypertens* 2020;38:982–1004.
2 Guideline for the pharmacological treatment of hypertension in adults. WHO, 2021.
3 Whelton PK et al. Guideline for the prevention, detection, evaluation, and management of high blood pressure in adults: a report of the ACA/ AHA Task Force on clinical practice guidelines. *Hypertension* 2018;71:e13–115.
4 NCD Risk Factor Collaboration (NCD-RisC). Worldwide trends in hypertension prevalence and progress in treatment and control from 1990 to 2019: a pooled analysis of 1201 population-representative studies with 104 million participants. *Lancet* 2021;398:957–80.
5 Zhou B et al. Global epidemiology, health burden and effective interventions for elevated blood pressure and hypertension. *Nat Rev Cardiol* 2021;18:785–802.
6 Mills KT et al. The global epidemiology of hypertension. *Nat Rev Nephrol* 2020;16:223–37.
7 Neal B et al. Effect of salt substitution on cardiovascular events and death. *NEJM* 2021;385:1067–77.
8 Olsen MH et al. A call to action and a lifecourse strategy to address the global burden of raised blood pressure on current and future generations: the Lancet Commission on hypertension. *Lancet* 2016;388:2665–712.
9 Krist AH et al. Screening for hypertension in adults: US Preventive Services Task Force reaffirmation recommendation statement. *JAMA* 2021;325:1650–56.
10 Stergiou GS et al. 2021 European Society of Hypertension practice guidelines for office and out-of-office blood pressure measurement. *J Hypertens* 2021;39:1293–302.
11 Chow CK et al. Initial treatment with a single pill containing quadruple combination of quarter doses of blood pressure medicines versus standard dose monotherapy in patients with hypertension (QUARTET). *Lancet* 2021;398:1043–52.
12 Webster R et al. Fixed low-dose triple combination antihypertensive medication vs usual care for blood pressure control in patients with mild to moderate hypertension in Sri Lanka: a randomized clinical trial. *JAMA* 2018;320:566–79.
13 Bovet P et al. Monitoring one-year compliance to antihypertension medication in the Seychelles. *Bull WHO* 2002;80:33–9.
14 Burnier M et al. Adherence in hypertension. *Circ Res* 2019;124:1124–40.
15 Geldsetzer P et al. The state of hypertension care in 44 low-income and middle-income countries: a cross-sectional study of nationally representative individual-level data from 1.1 million adults. *Lancet* 2019;394:652–62.
16 Gazit T et al. Assessment of hypertension control among adults participating in a mobile technology blood pressure self-management program. *JAMA Network Open* 2021;4:e2127008.
17 Funder JW, Carey RM. Primary aldosteronism: where are we now? Where to from here? *Hypertension* 2022;79:726–35.
18 Reynolds K et al. Comparative effectiveness of gastric bypass and vertical sleeve gastrectomy for hypertension remission and relapse: the ENGAGE CVD Study. *Hypertension* 2021;78:1116–25.

19 Picone DS et al. How to check whether a blood pressure monitor has been properly validated for accuracy. *Clin Hypertens* 2020;22:2167–74.
20 Stride BP. https://www.stridebp.org/.
21 Examples include: WHO CVD Risk Charts, Framingham Risk Score, Atherosclerotic Cardiovascular Disease Risk Algorithm (AHA/ACC-ASCVD), European Systematic Coronary Risk Evaluation (SCORE), etc.
22 Sudharsanan N et al. Variation in the proportion of adults in need of BP-lowering medications by hypertension care guideline in low- and middle-income countries: A cross-sectional study of 1,037,215 individuals from 50 nationally representative surveys. *Circulation* 2021;143:991–1001.
23 WHO package of essential noncommunicable (PEN) disease interventions for primary health care. WHO, 2020.
24 HEARTS Technical Package. WHO, 2018.
25 Bovet P et al. Assessing the prevalence of hypertension in populations: are we doing it right? *J Hypertens* 2003;21:509–17.

9 Diabetes

Burden, epidemiology and priority interventions

Pascal Bovet, Isabelle Hagon-Traub, Jean Claude N Mbanya, Nicholas J Wareham

Diabetes is one of the biggest challenges facing society in the 21st century. In the past three decades the prevalence of type-2 diabetes (T2D), which is closely related to obesity, has risen dramatically in almost all countries.[1] A number of interventions are available to control all forms of diabetes and for the prevention of T2D.

Definitions

Diabetes mellitus is a chronic, metabolic disease characterized by elevated levels of blood glucose. Over time the high glucose levels and the associated metabolic disorders can lead to serious damage to the heart, blood vessels, eyes, kidneys and nerves. The different types of diabetes and their characteristics are shown in Box 9.1. Around 95% of all cases are T2D.

BOX 9.1 TYPES OF DIABETES (ADAPTED AND SIMPLIFIED FROM THE WHO CLASSIFICATION)[2]

Type-1 diabetes (T1D). The immune system attacks and destroys the cells in the pancreas that produces insulin. Persons with T1D must take insulin every day to stay alive. Although T1D often develops at an early age, T1D can appear at any age. There are no known measures to prevent this form of diabetes. Without prompt diagnosis and treatment, T1D is rapidly fatal. The incidence of T1D may be underestimated in areas with deficient health services where deaths from T1D may go unrecognized.

Type-2 diabetes (T2D). The body does not produce enough insulin to maintain normal glucose levels. In nearly all cases of T2D, there is 'insulin resistance', meaning that the pancreas must produce increasingly higher amounts of insulin to 'force' blood glucose to enter into body cells. T2D and insulin resistance largely occur in response to

---

DOI: 10.4324/9781003306689-11

increased adipose tissue. T2D develops most often in middle-aged and older people but also increasingly in young adults and adolescents who are overweight or obese.

Gestational diabetes. This form of diabetes develops during pregnancy and disappears after giving birth. It appears in the second or third trimester and is more common in women with a high body mass index (BMI). Gestational diabetes can affect the pregnancy for both the foetus and the mother. Women with gestational diabetes have a greater risk of developing T2D later in life. T1D and T2D can also be diagnosed during pregnancy.

Other causes of diabetes. Less common causes of diabetes include inherited monogenic diabetes and disease of the pancreas (cystic fibrosis-related diabetes, pancreatitis). Elevated levels of blood glucose can also be seen in acute or chronic diseases.

Diagnosis of diabetes is based on one of the following:

- Fasting plasma glucose ≥7.0 mmol/l.
- Two-hour post-glucose-load plasma glucose ≥11.1 mmol/l after a 75 g oral glucose tolerance test (variations are often used for gestational diabetes).
- HbA1c ≥48 mmol/mol (≥6.5%).
- A random blood glucose ≥11.1 mmol/l in the presence of signs and symptoms.

Pre-diabetes is a term often used to describe moderately elevated levels of blood glucose (but blood insulin level is generally already substantially increased), which is associated with metabolic complications and a higher risk of progression to T2D. Its prevalence in the population can be two or three times higher than that of diabetes. There is no universally accepted definition of 'pre-diabetes' since the attribution of the diagnostic label has different implications for preventive action in different countries. Generally, it is based on one of the following criteria:

- Fasting plasma glucose ≥6.1 to <7.0 mmol/l according to WHO or ≥5.5 to <7.0 mmol/l according to the American Diabetic Association (ADA).
- Two-hour post-load plasma glucose ≥7.8 to <11.1 mmol/l after a 75 g oral glucose tolerance test.
- HbA1c ≥42 to <48 mmol/mol (6.0–<6.5%) in most countries or 5.7–6.4% according to ADA.

Disease burden

More than 500 million adults have diabetes, of whom 80% live in low- and middle-income countries, in line with the larger proportion of people living in these countries.[3]

68 *Pascal Bovet et al.*

Table 9.1 Mortality attributable to diabetes and high fasting blood glucose (IHME)

	Global		HICs		Upper-MICs		Lower-MICs		LICs	
	1990	2019	1990	2019	1990	2019	1990	2019	1990	2019
Diabetes as a direct cause of death										
Proportion of all deaths (%)	1.4	2.7	2.1	2.3	1.4	2.6	1.2	3.3	1.0	1.9
Age-standardized mortality rates (per 100,000)	18	20	14	10	15	16	36	34	24	33
High blood glucose as a risk for other diseases										
Proportion of all deaths (%)	6.2	11.5	11.3	12.8	6.7	11.9	4.3	11.8	2.6	5.7
Age-standardized mortality rates (per 100,000)	84	83	75	54	83	76	93	123	101	107

Diabetes was the direct (immediate) cause (e.g. diabetic renal disease, diabetic coma) of 0.7 million deaths (1.4%) in 1990 and 1.5 million, globally, in 2019 (2.7%) (Table 9.1, estimates from IHME). As a risk factor (e.g. high blood glucose increases the risk of CVD by two to four times[4]), high blood glucose (including moderately elevated glucose defining 'pre-diabetes') accounted for 6.5 million deaths (11.5% of all deaths in 2019 globally), an increase from 2.9 million in 1990. The percentage of deaths attributable to high blood glucose increased in all regions between 1990 and 2019, with a steeper increase in low- and middle-income countries, a twofold increase, than in high-income countries (HICs), partly owing to aging populations. The age-standardized mortality rates attributable to high blood glucose (which are not influenced by the age distribution of the populations compared) were lower in HICs and upper-middle-income countries (where rates decreased over time) than in low- and middle-income countries (where rates increased), partly reflecting a steeper increase in the prevalence of T2D and poorer blood glucose control in low- and middle-income countries than HICs.[5]

According to IHME, the following proportions of T2D mortality were attributable to modifiable risk factors globally in 2019: increased body mass index 42%, dietary risks (low fruit, high red/processed meat, low whole grain, high sugar-sweetened drinks) 26%, ambient and household air pollution 20%, tobacco use 16%, low physical activity 8%.

Consequences of diabetes

Very high blood glucose concentration results in acute symptoms of polyuria (excessive urination), thirst, loss of weight, hunger and tiredness, the classic way that those with T1D first present. If T1D is untreated, diabetic ketoacidosis, coma and death follow.

Over many years, elevated blood glucose in T1D and T2D affects the inner linings of both large (macrovascular damage) and small arteries (microvascular damage). Microvascular damage can result in blindness and kidney failure and destroys the sensory nerves, particularly in the lower limbs, which makes injury a major risk. Healing of injuries and wounds is less effective in patients with diabetes, and this, coupled with vascular impairment, can lead to ulceration and persistent infection which may require amputation. Macrovascular complications of diabetes include ischaemic heart disease (IHD), stroke and peripheral arterial disease. Diabetes is also associated with increased susceptibility to infections and more serious complications from infections.[6]

Diabetogenic environment

This concept of a diabetogenic environment is essentially the same as that for the obesogenic environment described in Chapter 10 on obesity. This has resulted in the current high and increasing levels in nearly all countries of 'diabesity', the combined 'epidemic' of obesity and T2D.

Interventions at the population level

Tackling the diabetogenic environment requires the same sorts of macro-policy interventions across multiple sectors as described for the obesogenic environment (Chapter 10, Box 3). Tackling the diabetogenic environment also requires behaviour change at scale as well as whole-of-government (e.g. legal, fiscal and regulatory policies to address the commercial determinants of NCDs) and whole-of-society (e.g. civil society and the private sector) actions. These issues are considered in more detail in other chapters.

Screening

Although it is unclear if systematic testing of blood glucose in the entire population is cost-effective,[7] opportunistic testing of high-risk individuals has been shown to be cost-effective in some settings for detecting diabetes and pre-diabetes and reducing their associated disease burden,[8] and, for example, the US Preventive Services Task Force recommends that overweight or obese adults aged 35–70 years are screened for diabetes and pre-diabetes.[9]

Interventions at the individual level

Risk factor reduction. Weight control is central to the management of T2D and pre-diabetes.[10] For diabetic patients who are overweight or obese, intensive weight management (e.g. loss of >10 kg) markedly improves blood glucose and associated metabolic risk factors[11] and can even result in remission to a non-diabetic state in a significant proportion of patients.[12] Interventions targeting weight control at the individual level are described in Chapter 10 on obesity, including the extreme but highly effective 'bariatric surgery'.[13] Encouraging physical activity, quitting smoking and reducing alcohol consumption are also important. WHO best buys include advice on healthy lifestyles and medical treatment of risk factors among individuals with high CVD risk.

Pharmacologic treatment for T1D. Insulin is the cornerstone of treatment. However, insulin is not sufficiently available or affordable in many settings, resulting in an increased risk of death. Good glycaemic control can be achieved with fastidious attention to insulin dosing and tight monitoring of blood glucose (including self-monitoring). Newer biosimilar products (insulin analogues, such as glargine which is included in the WHO Essential Medicines List) may help achieve tighter glycaemic control but at a much higher cost.[14,15] Newer devices, ranging from fairly inexpensive pens that make injections easier, to complex and very expensive automated insulin delivery systems, are increasingly available to support patients in strengthening their ability to monitor and control blood glucose levels more effectively.[16]

Pharmacologic treatment for T2D. Metformin is inexpensive and is the drug of first-choice. Sulphonylureas, at least first generations, are no longer recommended as a first–line agent since they may cause weight gain. Insulin is often required when oral hypoglycaemic medications cannot reduce blood glucose sufficiently. However, insulin often increases body weight, which further increases insulin resistance. This highlights the opportunity that comes from newer treatments which, like metformin, reduce blood glucose but also impact favourably on body weight and prevent diabetes complications. GLP-1 analogues (glucagon-like peptide-1 receptor agonists, e.g. semaglutide, exenatide) reduce satiety (and thus lower body weight) and also reduce CVD risk. SGLT-2 inhibitors (sodium-glucose cotransporter-2 inhibitor, e.g. gliflozins) slow chronic kidney disease progression and reduce heart failure and CVD risk.[17,18] These treatments can be even more effective than insulin, and some of them also have the advantage of requiring less frequent administration.[19] Although expensive, their costs are decreasing, making them increasingly cost-effective, even in low- and middle-income countries.[20] As many patients with T2D have comorbidities, and given that diabetes is a strong risk factor for developing CVD, additional drugs, for example, to control BP and lower blood cholesterol, are most often also required[21] (see Chapters 6 on CVD, 36 on high-risk approaches and 20 on cholesterol). Guidelines and protocols for the management of T2D are widely available.[22,23,24]

Follow-up

Patients with diabetes need to be able to access care to prevent and manage acute and long-term complications. Hypoglycaemia (often a result of treatment) and hyperglycaemia (which can result from insufficient treatment, changes in diet or levels of physical activity or acute infection) can be life-threatening, so patients and those around them should be able to recognize hypo- or hyperglycaemic emergencies and how to manage these situations should be managed.

Patients should be supported to be assiduous in monitoring their blood glucose (including self-monitoring), regularly examining and examining their skin and feet, and using suitable footwear and bedding. Follow-up also involves diligent and rigorous long-term monitoring for: (i) eye disease (retinopathy, cataract and glaucoma), which should be done every two years at a minimum; (ii) kidney disease (through annual assessment, including measurement of serum creatinine and albuminuria); (iii) diabetic neuropathy (through annual assessment); and (iv) long-term macrovascular complications (IHD, cerebrovascular disease and peripheral vascular disease), which includes regular assessment and treatment of BP, blood lipids, smoking cessation and daily acetylsalicylic acid for patients who have had a CVD event and no history of major bleeding. Patient support groups are an important source of advice and support.

The importance of strong health services and systems

Effective long-term care requires partnerships between patients and multiple healthcare professionals, with both taking responsibility for managing the disease. As with all NCDs, optimal long-term care for patients with diabetes requires strong health services and systems (Chapter 42). However, evidence-based care for people with diabetes is sub-optimal in all countries, even the most well-off countries.[25] In addition, half of all adults across the world with T2D are undiagnosed, and large proportions of those diagnosed are untreated or insufficiently treated,[26] and these proportions are much higher in low- and middle-income countries.[27] Continuing lack of access to effective care, particularly access to insulin, highlights a range of deep systemic issues, including that: (i) three multinational companies control over 95% of the global insulin supply, although the inclusion of insulin in the WHO Prequalification of Medicines Programme is an opportunity to facilitate entry of new companies into the market; (ii) many governments lack policies on the selection, procurement, supply, pricing and reimbursement of insulin; (iii) mark-ups in the supply chain affect the final price to the consumer; (iv) expenses related to diabetes often require out of pocket payments; and (v) the organization of diabetes management within the healthcare system often affects patient access to insulin.[28]

Targets and indicators in the WHO Global NCD Action Plan

Target	To halt the rise in diabetes and obesity between 2010 and 2025. (Combining diabetes and obesity into one target emphasizes the strong relationship between the two).
Indicators	Age-standardized prevalence of overweight and obesity in persons aged 18+ years (respectively BMI ≥25 kg and ≥30 kg/m^2).
	Prevalence of overweight and obesity in adolescents (defined according to the WHO growth reference for children and adolescents).

Monitoring

Examination population surveys are useful to estimate the proportion of the population with diabetes/pre-diabetes and the proportion of those who are treated and adequately controlled. Indicators at health care level are also useful, including the proportion of patients treated/controlled for blood glucose, BP and blood lipids, frequency of exams to assess complications (e.g. eye, kidney or foot), and broader indicators, such as the presence and use of diabetes protocols, monitoring systems and availability of medicines.

In 2021, WHO launched the Global Diabetes Compact,[29] an initiative to bring partners together to improve access to equitable, comprehensive, affordable and quality treatment and care, as well as to support the prevention of T2D. The initiative also sets priority metrics and targets to serve as diabetes-related health objectives for all countries of the world to achieve by 2030.[30]

Notes

1 Zimmet P et al. Global and societal implications of the diabetes epidemic. *Nature* 2001;414:782–87.
2 Classification of diabetes mellitus. WHO, 2019.
3 NCD-RisC. Worldwide trends in diabetes since 1980: a pooled analysis of 751 population-based studies with 4.4 million participants. *Lancet* 2016;387:1513–30.
4 Dal Canto E et al. Diabetes as a cardiovascular risk factor: an overview of global trends of macro and micro vascular complications. *Eur J Prev Cardiol* 2019;26(Suppl 2):25–32.
5 Magliano DJ et al. Trends in all-cause mortality among people with diagnosed diabetes in high-income settings: a multicountry analysis of aggregate data. *Lancet Diabetes Endocrinol* 2022;10:112–19.
6 Casqueiro J et al. Infections in patients with diabetes mellitus: a review of pathogenesis. *Indian J Endocrinol Metab* 2012;16:S27–S36.
7 Herman WH et al. Early detection and treatment of type 2 diabetes reduce cardiovascular morbidity and mortality: a simulation of the results of the Anglo-Danish-Dutch study of intensive treatment in people with screen-detected diabetes in primary care (ADDITION-Europe). *Diabetes Care* 2015;38:1449–55.
8 Zhou X et al. Cost-effectiveness of diabetes prevention interventions targeting high-risk individuals and whole populations: a systematic review. *Diabetes Care* 2020;43:1593–16.
9 Screening for prediabetes and type 2 diabetes: US Preventive Services Task Force recommendation statement. *JAMA* 2021;326:736–43.
10 Lingvay I et al. Obesity management as a primary treatment goal for type 2 diabetes: time to reframe the conversation. *Lancet* 2022;399:394–405.
11 The Look AHEAD Research Group. Cardiovascular effects of intensive lifestyle intervention in type 2 diabetes. *NEJM* 2013;369:145–54.
12 Lean MEJ et al. Durability of a primary care-led weight-management intervention for remission of type 2 diabetes: 2-year results of the DiRECT open-label, cluster-randomised trial. *Lancet Diabetes Endocrinol* 2019;7:344–55.
13 Kirwan JP et al. Diabetes remission in the alliance of randomized trials of medicine versus metabolic surgery in type 2 diabetes (ARMMS-T2D). *Diabetes Care*;45:1574–83).
14 Unnikrishnan R et al. Newer antidiabetic agents: at what price will they be cost effective? *Lancet Diabetes Endocrinol* 2021;9:801–03.
15 Dafny LS. Radical treatment for insulin pricing. *NEJM* 2022;386:2157–59.

16. Braune K et al. Open-source automated insulin delivery: international consensus statement and practical guidance for health-care professionals. *Lancet Diabetes Endocrinol* 2022;10:58–74.
17. Drucker DJ et al. The incretin system: glucagon-like peptide-1 receptor agonists and dipeptidyl peptidase-4 inhibitors in type 2 diabetes. *Lancet* 2006;368:1696–705.
18. Marx N et al. Guideline recommendations and the positioning of newer drugs in type 2 diabetes care. *Lancet Diabetes Endocrinol* 2021;9:46–52.
19. Battelino T et al. Efficacy of once-weekly tirzepatide versus once-daily insulin degludec on glycaemic control measured by continuous glucose monitoring in adults with type 2 diabetes (SURPASS-3 CGM): a substudy of the randomised, open-label, parallel-group, phase 3 SURPASS-3 trial. *Lancet Diabetes Endocrinol* 2022;10:407–17.
20. Global Health & Population Project on Access to Care for Cardiometabolic Diseases (HPACC). Expanding access to newer medicines for people with type 2 diabetes in low-income and middle-income countries: a cost-effectiveness and price target analysis. *Lancet Diabetes Endocrinol* 2021;9:825–36.
21. Joseph JJ et al. Comprehensive management of cardiovascular risk factors for adults with type 2 diabetes: a scientific statement from the American Heart Association. *Circulation* 2022;145:e722–59.
22. Chatterjee S et al. Type 2 diabetes. *Lancet* 2017;389:2239–51.
23. American Diabetes Association. Standards of medical care in diabetes – 2021. *Diabetes Care* 2021;44(Suppl 1):1–225.
24. Diagnosis and management of type 2 diabetes (HEARTS-D). WHO, 2020.
25. Fang M et al. Trends in diabetes treatment and control in U.S. adults, 1999–2018. *NEJM* 2021;384:2219–28.
26. Manne-Goehler J et al. Health system performance for people with diabetes in 28 low- and middle-income countries: a cross-sectional study of nationally representative surveys. *PLoS Med* 2019;16:e1002751.
27. Basu S et al. Estimation of global insulin use for type 2 diabetes, 2018–30: a microsimulation analysis. *Lancet Diabetes Endocrinol* 2018;7:25–33.
28. Beran D et al. A global perspective on the issue of access to insulin. *Diabetologia* 2021;64:954–62.
29. The Global Diabetes Compact. WHO, 2021.
30. Reducing the burden of noncommunicable diseases through strengthen in prevention and control of diabetes. WHO, 2021.

10 Obesity

Burden, epidemiology and priority interventions

Pascal Bovet, Nathalie Farpour-Lambert, Nick Banatvala, Louise Baur

The obesity epidemic is one of the biggest challenges facing society in the 21st century. In addition to multiple physical and mental health effects, obesity has considerable socio-economic impacts, as well as broader development implications, across a nexus that includes health and education, agriculture and industry, and climate action and the environment.[1] The fact that there is no chance of reaching the WHO Global NCD Action Plan target of a zero increase in rates of obesity and diabetes between 2010 and 2025 emphasizes that new bold approaches are required if the world is to tackle the issue of overweight and obesity.

Definition of overweight and obesity

Being overweight is a condition characterized by excessive adiposity, and obesity is defined as a chronic complex disease defined by excessive adiposity that can impair health. Obesity is in most cases a multifactorial disease due to obesogenic environments, psycho-social factors and genetic variants. In a subgroup of patients, single major etiological factors can be identified (diseases, immobilization, iatrogenic procedures, monogenic disease/genetic syndrome). Body mass index (BMI) is a surrogate marker of adiposity calculated as weight divided by height squared (kg/m^2). In adults, there are three levels of obesity severity in recognition of different management options, and the BMI categories for defining obesity vary by age and gender in infants, children and adolescents (Box 10.1).

BOX 10.1 DEFINITION OF OVERWEIGHT AND OBESITY IN ADULTS AND CHILDREN[2]

Adults

- Overweight: BMI ≥25
- Obesity: BMI ≥30
    - Obesity Class I: BMI 30.0–34.9
    - Obesity Class II: BMI 35.0–39.9
    - Obesity Class III: BMI ≥40

> **Children aged between 5 and 19 years**
>
> - Overweight: BMI-for-age >1 standard deviation (SD) above the WHO growth reference median.
> - Obesity: BMI-for-age >2 SD above the WHO growth reference median.
>
> **Children under 5 years**
>
> - Overweight: weight-for-height or BMI-for-age >2 SD above the WHO child growth standards median.
> - Obesity: weight-for-height or BMI-for-age >3 SD above the WHO child growth standards median.
>
> International charts/tables for children aged 5–19 years and those <5 years are available from WHO and elsewhere.[3] Some countries have developed charts/tables for their populations.

While BMI provides the most useful population-level measure of overweight and obesity as thresholds that do not depend on the sex and age in adults, it remains a fairly rough marker of adiposity in different individuals.[4] BMI does not distinguish well between muscle and fat mass, and some individuals with a normal BMI can have increased adipose tissue and cardiometabolic risk, while some muscular individuals may have a high BMI with normal adipose tissue and no increased risk.

Waist circumference (or waist circumference ratio, Table 10.1) is also a useful measure of adiposity, particularly abdominal adipose tissue. Similar to BMI, it is a fairly good predictor of cardiometabolic risk (e.g. increased blood glucose, triglycerides, insulin resistance, and reduced HDL-cholesterol) and can be used on its own or in conjunction with BMI.[5]

Overall, both BMI and waist circumference (or waist-to-hip ratio) fall short of gold standards (such as dual-energy x-ray absorptiometry, MRI, or isotope dilution methods), with a correlation of around 0.8 for predicting adipose

Table 10.1 WHO cut-off points for waist circumference and waist-to-hip ratio and risk of metabolic complications in adults

Indicator	Cut-off points (men/women)	Risk of metabolic complications
Waist circumference	>94/80 cm	Increased
	>102/88 cm	Substantially increased
Waist-to-hip ratio	≥0.90/0.85	Substantially increased

Table 10.2 Mortality attributable to high BMI (IHME)

	Global 1990	Global 2019	HICs 1990	HICs 2019	UMICs 1990	UMICs 2019	UMICs 1990	UMICs 2019	LICs 1990	LICs 2019
Number of deaths (million)	2.2	5.0	0.8	1.1	0.9	2.0	0.5	1.7	0.06	0.2
Proportion of all deaths (%)	4.7	8.9	9.5	10.4	5.9	10.4	2.5	7.9	1.4	3.8
Age-standardized mortality (per 100,000)	60	63	64	47	63	63	47	72	44	60

tissue but are adequate as screening tools for clinical and population use. Gold standards are clinically impractical and too costly for routine use.[6]

Disease burden

According to IHME, increased high BMI (≥25 kg/m^2) accounted for 8.9% of all deaths (5 million) in 2019 globally, as compared to 2.2 million in 1990, as a result of a combination of the increasing prevalence of obesity and growth and aging of populations over time (Table 10.2). Mortality attributable to high BMI, in percent of all deaths, increased in all regions. Age-standardized mortality rates attributable to high BMI increased in most regions but decreased in high-income countries (HICs), possibly owing to better control of complications of obesity in HICs than in low- and middle-income countries. Mortality attributable to high BMI was as follows globally in 2019 (IHME): 64% was attributable to CVD, 20% to diabetes and 9% to cancer. Increased BMI accounted globally for 4.9% of years lived with an obesity-related disease, mainly attributable to diabetes (64%).

Prevalence of overweight and obesity[7,8,9]

Around 2 billion adults were overweight in 2016, and 650 million of them had obesity (i.e. 39% and 13% of the world's population respectively). In 2016, over 340 million children and adolescents aged 5–19 were overweight or had obesity, and in 2020, 39 million children under the age of five years were overweight or had obesity. The worldwide prevalence of obesity nearly tripled between 1975 and 2016 in both adults and children.

Levels of overweight and/or obesity among adults are highest (up to 50–70%) in the Pacific and Caribbean islands, the Middle East, Mexico and the USA. In Africa, the number of overweight children under five years has increased by nearly 24% percent since 2000. While the prevalence of overweight/obesity was typically higher among wealthier vs poorer populations until a few decades ago (in part because food was less accessible to poorer vs wealthier people), this has reversed in many countries (in part because of the increased availability of inexpensive energy-dense foods).

Health consequences of overweight and obesity

Increased BMI is associated with impairment of blood glucose and lipids levels, increased blood pressure, cardiovascular disease (CVD), many types of cancer (e.g. endometrial, oesophageal, stomach, liver and kidney, breast and colorectal) and premature mortality.[10,11,12] Obesity is also associated with other conditions, including respiratory (e.g. obstructive sleep apnoea), gastrointestinal (e.g. non-alcoholic fatty liver disease, reflux oesophagitis), musculoskeletal (e.g. lower extremity malalignment, lower back pain, osteoarthritis), soft tissue (e.g. cellulitis), reproductive (e.g. early puberty, polycystic ovary syndrome) and greater likelihood of postoperative complications. No less are the psycho-social consequences, including weight stigma, discrimination, lower wages, lower quality of life and a likely susceptibility to depression. The combination of several cardio-metabolic indicators (increased BMI and/or waist circumference, blood glucose, triglycerides and blood pressure, and decreased HDL-cholesterol) is referred to as metabolic syndrome and is associated with an increased risk of CVD risk.[13]

Obesogenic environments

Most world populations now live in environments which promote weight gain and increased rates of obesity. Commercial, societal and cultural factors contribute to the development of obesogenic environments. Commercial factors include massive advertising and promotion of ultra-processed foods and sugar-sweetened beverages and the ubiquitous supply of and access to low cost high-energy processed foods that have high shelf durability and large profit margins.[14] The loss of recreation spaces and walkable environments, as well as the ever-increasing use of motorized transport, and electric or electronic appliances have reduced opportunities for physical activity at work and home. In some societies, being overweight is perceived as a sign of wealth, good health and fertility. Home and work pressures also contribute to the obesogenic environment, with compensatory calorie intake, including through 'convenient', rapid and easy-to-prepare energy-dense meals largely based on processed foods.

The importance of neuroendocrine systems and genetics

Satiety and hunger are regulated through complex, tight regulatory loops that involve hormones and peptides released by the adipose tissue (leptin, etc.), stomach and intestine (ghrelin, glucagon-like peptide 1, etc.), pancreas (insulin, glucagon etc) and brain/hypothalamus (melanocortin system, dopamine, etc.) in response to energy balance. This complex neuroendocrine system tends to defend adipose accumulation by stimulating energy intake (hunger) over energy expenditure (including through adjusting resting basal metabolic rate).[15]

These effects are enhanced by processed, and particularly ultra-processed foods (that require little in the way of chewing before swallowing and then being rapidly absorbed by the intestine), which in part bypass appetite satiety regulatory loops and can result in food overconsumption.[16] These physiological mechanisms favoured energy conservation and humans' survival for thousands of years, when food was scarce but, in current obesogenic environments, favour weight gain.[17] Obesity is a trait influenced by the complex interplay between food processing, gut microbiota composition and function, genetic variants, metagenomics and the environment[18,19] and patterns at the individual level may partly explain why some people are more prone than others to develop obesity.

Interventions at the population level

The multifactorial nature of obesity emphasizes the need for macro-policy interventions across multiple sectors to modify the obesogenic environments in order to prevent weight gain and increase the opportunity for people living with obesity to reduce weight.[20] A number of interventions are WHO best buys or recommended interventions (Box 10.2). Tackling the obesogenic environments also requires behavioural change at scale as well as whole-of-government action (e.g. legal, fiscal and regulatory policies to address commercial determinants of NCDs) and requires support from the private sector. These issues are considered in more detail in other chapters.

BOX 10.2 SUMMARY OF WHO BEST BUYS, EFFECTIVE INTERVENTIONS, OTHER RECOMMENDED INTERVENTIONS, AND ENABLING INTERVENTIONS THAT HAVE AN IMPACT ON OBESITY

Best buys

- Implement community-wide public education and awareness campaigns for physical activity.

Effective interventions

- Reduce sugar consumption through effective taxation on sugar-sweetened beverages.

Other recommended interventions

- Promote and support exclusive breastfeeding for the first six months of life.

- Implement subsidies to increase the intake of fruits and vegetables.
- Limit portion and package size.
- Implement nutrition education and counselling in preschools, schools, workplaces, hospitals etc. to increase the intake of fruits, vegetables and whole-grain foods.
- Implement nutrition labelling.
- Implement mass media campaigns on healthy diets, including social marketing to reduce the intake of total fat, saturated fats, free sugars and salt, and promote the intake of fruits, vegetables and whole-grain foods.
- Ensure that macro-level urban design addresses residential density, connected street networks including sidewalks, cycle lanes and access to public transport.
- Implement a whole-of-school programme that includes quality physical education and availability of adequate facilities and programmes.
- Provide convenient and safe access to quality public open space and adequate infrastructures to support walking and cycling.
- Implement multi-component workplace physical activity programmes.
- Promote physical activity through organized sports groups and clubs, programmes and events.

Enabling interventions

- Implement the WHO global strategy on diet, physical activity and health.
- Implement the WHO recommendations on the marketing of foods and non-alcoholic beverages to children.

Interventions at the individual level

The provision of equitable access to integrated healthcare services for the management of obesity should be part of universal health coverage. After a careful medical evaluation, people living with obesity should receive individualized care plans that address the causes and provide support for behavioural change (e.g. nutrition, eating behaviours, physical activity, sedentary behaviours) and adjunctive therapies, which may include psychological, pharmacologic and surgical interventions.[21] Achieving maximum weight loss in the shortest possible time is *not* the key to successful treatment; evidence suggests that a 5–10% weight loss in adults is often sufficient to obtain substantial health benefits from decreasing obesity-related comorbidities. During childhood and adolescence, the aims of treatment are to slow down weight gain while ensuring normal growth, prevent premature complications and improve quality of life. More research is currently needed to shift the focus of obesity management toward focusing on health and psycho-social outcomes rather than weight alone.

Counselling on a healthy diet, including favouring drinking water over consumption of sweetened soft drinks,[22] and regular physical activity should be included in routine primary health care services. While this can lead to significant weight loss (or weight control in youth) among some patients living with obesity, particularly if provided through specialist care and long follow-up, advice and counselling on healthy nutrition and physical activity results often in only modest weight changes.[23] Low-calorie diets can result in short-term weight loss, but a majority of individuals regain the weight that they have lost.[24] Chapters 19 on nutrition and Chapter 25 on physical activity describe healthy patterns and interventions.

Pharmacotherapy is usually recommended for weight loss and weight-loss maintenance for individuals with BMI ≥30 or BMI ≥27 with adiposity-related complications, to support behavioural and psychological interventions. A recent report suggests that compared to lifestyle alone (which reduced body weight by 3.4%), phentermine-topiramate, orlistat, or naltrexone-bupropion reduced body weight by an additional (3–8%) amount.[25] Newer medications acting on specific mechanisms of appetite regulation result in larger and more sustained weight reduction. For example, the GLP-1 agonist semaglutide reduced body weight by 12.7% (and also reduced blood sugar and CVD risk) in individuals with obesity.[26] Nausea and diarrhoea were the most common adverse events with semaglutide; they were typically transient and mild-to-moderate in severity and subsided with time. Other medications, which act on underlying adipocyte-gut-brain mechanisms, are being developed and may have even larger effects.[27]

Bariatric surgery, including gastric banding, gastric bypass and sleeve gastrectomy, is increasingly used in adults and adolescents where resources are available. Surgery results in large weight loss[28] and induces improvement or even remission of obesity-related conditions such as hypertension and type-2 diabetes, and increases life expectancy.[29] Surgery can be cost-effective when set against the high costs of obesity to the individual and society.[30]

Targets and indicators in the WHO Global NCD Action Plan

Target	To halt the rise in diabetes and obesity between 2010 and 2025. (Combining diabetes and obesity into one target emphasizes the strong relationship between the two that has been described in this chapter.)
Indicators	Age-standardized prevalence of overweight and obesity in persons aged 18+ years (BMI ≥25 for overweight and BMI ≥30 for obesity). Prevalence of overweight and obesity in adolescents (defined according to the WHO growth reference for children and adolescents).

Monitoring

Prevalence and trends of overweight and obesity, as well as physical activity and diet, can be assessed through population-based surveys in adults and children/adolescents (see Chapters 5, 19 and 25 on surveillance tools, diet and physical activity). It is also important to monitor health care for individuals with obesity.

Notes

1. Swinburn BA et al. The global syndemic of obesity, undernutrition, and climate change: the Lancet Commission report. *Lancet* 2019;393:791–846.
2. Key facts. Obesity and overweight. WHO, 2021.
3. Cole TJ et al. Establishing a standard definition for child overweight and obesity worldwide: international survey. *BMJ* 2000;320:1240–3.
4. Adab P et al. Is BMI the best measure of obesity? It works for most people most of the time. *BMJ* 2018;360:k1274.
5. Waist circumference and waist-hip ratio report of a WHO expert consultation. WHO, 2008.
6. Batsis JA et al. Diagnostic accuracy of body mass index to identify obesity in older adults: NHANES 1999–2004. *Int J Obes* 2016;40:761–67.
7. NCD Risk Factor Collaboration. Trends in adult body-mass index in 200 countries from 1975 to 2014: a pooled analysis of 1698 population-based measurement studies with 19.2 million participants. *Lancet* 2016;387:1377–96.
8. NCD Risk Factor Collaboration. Worldwide trends in body-mass index, underweight, overweight, and obesity from 1975 to 2016: a pooled analysis of 2416 population-based measurement studies in 128.9 million children, adolescents, and adults. *Lancet* 2017;390:2627–42.
9. Levels and trends in child malnutrition: UNICEF/WHO/The World Bank Group joint child malnutrition estimates: key findings of the 2021 edition. WHO, 2021.
10. Haslam DW, James PT. Obesity. *Lancet* 2005;366:1197–209.
11. Bhaskaran K et al. Association of BMI with overall and cause-specific mortality: a population-based cohort study of 3.6 million adults in the UK. *Lancet Diabetes Endocrinol* 2018;6:944–53.
12. Jayedi A et al. Central fatness and risk of all cause mortality: systematic review and dose response meta-analysis of 72 prospective cohort studies. *BMJ* 2020;370:m3324.
13. Ritchie SA, Connell JCM. The link between abdominal obesity, metabolic syndrome and cardiovascular disease. *Nutr Metab Cardiovasc Dis* 2007;17:319–26.
14. Popkin BM et al. Towards unified and impactful policies to reduce ultra-processed food consumption and promote healthier eating. *Lancet Diab Endocrinol* 2021;9:462–70.
15. Schwartz MW et al. Obesity pathogenesis: an endocrine society scientific statement. *Endocr Rev* 2017;38:267–96.
16. Koenen M et al. The high incidence of overweight/obesity is closely related to overconsumption of inexpensive and palatable high fat and high refined carbohydrate diets. *Circ Res* 2021;128:951–68.
17. Fildes A et al. Probability of an obese person attaining normal body weight: cohort study using electronic health records. *Am J Public Health* 2015;105:e54–9.
18. Loos RJF et al. The genetics of obesity: from discovery to biology. *Nat Rev Genet* 2022;23:120–33.
19. Mozaffarian D. Obesity – an unexplained epidemic. *Am J Clin Nutr* 2022;115:1445–1450.
20. Report of the Commission on Ending Childhood Obesity. *Implementation plan: Executive summary*. WHO, 2017.
21. Schutz D et al. European practical and patient-centred guidelines for adult obesity management in primary care. *Obes Facts* 2019;12:40–66.
22. Lichtenstein AH et al. 2021 dietary guidance to improve cardiovascular death: a scientific statement from the American Heart Association. *Circulation* 2021;144:e472–87.
23. Weight management: lifestyle services for overweight or obese adults. National Institute for Health and Care Excellence, 2014.
24. Hartmann-Boyce J et al. Association between characteristics of behavioural weight loss programmes and weight change after programme end: systematic review and meta-analysis. *BMJ* 2021;374:n1840.

25 Shi Q et al. Pharmacotherapy for adults with overweight and obesity: a systematic review and network meta-analysis of randomised controlled trials. *Lancet* 2022;399:259–69.
26 Wilding J. et al. Once-weekly semaglutide in adults with overweight or obesity. *NEJM* 2021;384:989–1002.
27 Müller TD et al. Anti-obesity drug discovery: advances and challenges. *Nat Rev Drug Discov* 2022;21:201–23.
28 Adams TD et al. Weight and metabolic outcomes 12 years after gastric bypass. *NEJM* 2017;377:1143–55.
29 Syn NL et al. Association of metabolic–bariatric surgery with long-term survival in adults with and without diabetes: a one-stage meta-analysis of matched cohort and prospective controlled studies with 174'772 participants. *Lancet* 2021;397:1830–41.
30 Harrison S et al. Long-term cost-effectiveness of interventions for obesity: a Mendelian randomisation study. *PLoS Med* 2021;18:e1003725.

11 Cancer

Burden, epidemiology and principles for priority interventions

Hesham Gaafar, May Abdel-Wahab, Pascal Bovet, André Ilbawi

This chapter provides a brief overview of the burden, epidemiology, public health impact and main principles for the prevention and treatment of cancer, one of the four diseases in the WHO Global NCD Action Plan. Cancer has a significant socio-economic impact on individuals and their families. A substantial proportion of cancer cases is attributable to the main modifiable NCD risk factors (e.g. tobacco, unhealthy diet, alcohol, physical inactivity). A small number of cancers (e.g. breast, cervical, colorectal and prostate), that together are responsible for 30% of all cancer cases, are described in more detail in other chapters.

Disease burden

Epidemiological data on cancer are widely available.[1,2,3,4] Cancer causes one in six deaths globally. Lung, prostate, colorectal, stomach and liver cancers are the most common types of cancer in men, while breast, colorectal, lung, cervical and thyroid cancers are the most common among women. As the incidence of cancer sharply increases with age, the lifetime risk of developing cancer is large, e.g. 40–50% among men and 35–45% among women where life expectancy at birth exceeds the age of 75–80 years. Table 11.1 provides data on the leading causes of cancer deaths.[5] Overall, the total number of people, or proportions of the population, with cancer has increased between 1990 and 2019 in all country-income group categories. However, the age-adjusted mortality rates for cancer as a whole (which express the risk of developing cancer irrespective of population growth and age distribution) have decreased in all country-income groups, although there has been an increase for a few specific cancers (e.g. colon cancer in all country-income groups except HICs).

Cancer trends

The projected number of people living with, or dying from, cancer depends on changes in several variables: life expectancy and population growth, exposure to risk factors, screening and treatment. As a result, the total number of cancer cases will increase in the coming years in most populations, particularly in low- and middle-income countries. However, the trends in age-adjusted

DOI: 10.4324/9781003306689-13

Table 11.1 Mortality and fractions of mortality attributable to modifiable risk factors for leading cancers

	All cancers		Lung		Colon		Stomach		Breast		Oesophagus		Prostate		Liver		Cervix	
	1990	2019	1990	2019	1990	2019	1990	2019	1990	2019	1990	2019	1990	2019	1990	2019	1990	2019
Number of deaths (10⁶)	5.75	10.1	1.1	2.0	0.52	1.1	0.78	0.96	0.38	0.70	0.32	0.50	0.23	0.49	0.37	0.48	0.19	0.28
Percent of all deaths																		
All countries	12.3	17.8	2.3	3.6	1.1	1.9	1.7	1.7	0.82	1.2	0.68	0.88	0.50	0.86	0.78	0.86	0.40	0.50
High income	25.1	28.9	5.7	6.4	3.2	3.8	2.3	1.7	2.0	1.9	0.65	0.80	1.4	1.8	0.7	1.2	0.38	0.31
Upper middle income	15.9	22.1	2.9	5.3	1.1	2.3	3.0	2.9	0.70	1.1	1.4	1.6	0.4	0.82	1.7	1.3	0.46	0.56
Lower middle income	5.7	10.7	0.74	1.4	0.40	1.0	0.67	0.84	0.51	1.1	0.22	0.38	0.2	0.50	0.20	0.41	0.34	0.47
Low income	4.0	7.5	0.34	0.69	0.21	0.47	0.48	0.71	0.28	0.68	0.28	0.50	0.2	0.50	0.20	0.35	0.44	0.75
Age-standardized mortality rates (per 100,000)																		
High income	168	135	37	30	21	17	16	7.5	14	9.4	4.4	3.9	9.2	7.5	4.7	5.6	2.7	1.6
Upper middle	158	132	29	31	12	14	30	17	6.8	6.6	14	9.2	5.1	5.3	16	7.5	4.4	3.3
Lower middle	98	97	13	13	7.8	9.5	12	7.8	8.4	9.6	4.1	3.5	5.3	5.6	3.6	3.7	5.4	3.9
Low income	120	114	12	12	7.3	8.1	16	12	8.6	10.3	9.2	8.2	9.4	10.2	6.4	5.4	12	10.4
Attributable fractions (% of cancer mortality contributed by modifiable risk factor)																		
Tobacco	26		66		13		17		5		41		6		16		8	
Dietary risk	7		4		34		7		3		13							
Alcohol	5				9				5		22				19			
Low physical activity	1				5				1									
High BMI	5				8				6		17				12			
Drug use															14			
Unsafe sex	2																	98

Particulate matter (pollution)	4	19
Occupational risk	3	14
Other environmental	1	4

Red colour means an increase between 1990 and 2019; green colour, a decrease.

incidence of different cancers depend on trends in the prevalence of risk factors in populations. Examples include:

- The decrease in tobacco use observed in many countries will lead to a reduction in age-adjusted rates of oral, throat and lung cancers.
- The increase in levels of obesity, together with the increasing consumption of ultraprocessed food, will lead to an increase in age-adjusted rates of colon cancer in many populations.
- Increased vaccination coverage for human papillomavirus (HPV) and hepatitis B virus (HBV) will lead to a decrease in age-standardized incidence of cervical and liver cancers, respectively.

The role of screening programmes is also important. Screening, along with early diagnosis and treatment, has resulted in a 20% decrease in premature mortality from cancer between 2000 and 2015 in HICs, and 5% in LICs.

Interventions at the population level

Table 11.1 shows that around one-half of all cancer deaths could be prevented if modifiable risk factors were eliminated in the whole population (with 36% of all cancer deaths attributable to tobacco and 7% to unhealthy diet). For lung cancer, 66% of deaths are attributable to tobacco use and 19% to air pollution. For cervix cancer, 98% of mortality is attributable to unsafe sex (through HPV infection). These relationships underlie the importance of population-based prevention interventions, which can range from taxing unhealthy products such as tobacco or alcohol to HPV and HBV vaccination. At least 5–10% of all cancers have a strong genetic component.[4] Improved understanding of the genetic causes of cancer is providing new opportunities for cancer prevention (e.g. risk prediction, family counselling) and treatment (e.g. different treatments according to genetic markers) and will continue to do so in future (Chapter 29).

Cancer control programmes

Comprehensive cancer control refers to the broad implementation of ethical and proven measures to actively address the burden of cancer. Approaches should range from prevention, early detection (including early diagnosis and screening) to treatment, palliative care and rehabilitation. This also includes, ideally, a cancer registry and surveillance to strengthen the delivery of services and monitor cancer programmes. Comprehensive cancer control programmes aim to reduce the incidence, morbidity and mortality of cancer and to improve the quality of life of cancer patients. These programmes should engage all levels of the national health system and reach the entire population, from the healthy to those at high risk (e.g. those with a family history) and to patients who are yet to show symptoms, have been diagnosed, are cured or are in the final stages of the disease.[6]

With access to the right treatment, many people with cancer can be cured and/or treated effectively. It is therefore important that countries aim to increase the resources available to cancer control programmes. These programmes should prioritize the early detection of cancers that can be cured through early treatment available in a particular setting and provide palliative/survivorship care for less curable cancers.

Early detection

Early detection of cancer (through clinical presentation, or systematic or opportunistic screening) is important, as is rapid treatment following cancer detection, to maximize the prognosis for the patient. This approach assumes even greater importance in the absence of organized systematic screening programmes targeting the general population.

Organized systematic cancer screening programmes aim to detect early pre-cancer or cancer signs among asymptomatic individuals to reduce cancer incidence and/or outcomes (e.g. case-fatality rates and overall mortality). Such programmes typically target the whole population of a certain age (e.g. screening all women aged 30–49 years with a visual inspection, Pap smear or HPV testing; this is a WHO best buy intervention). These programmes require significant resources, and even in countries with well-run programmes, only 5% of all cancers are detected through screening (the greatest impact being for cervical, breast and colorectal cancers).[4] Screening programmes require high participation rates and quality assurance to be effective. The availability of a test is not sufficient for the establishment of a screening programme (see Chapter 43 on screening and health checks). It is also important to recognize that screening programmes, once initiated, are often very difficult to stop. Many countries therefore pilot their programmes ahead of the full roll-out.

Treatment

Under optimal conditions, many cancers can now be effectively cured or treated in a way that allows many years of productive life. Local and systemic treatment (including a mix of one or several from surgery, radio-, chemo-, hormone- and/or immunotherapy components) can all be effective, but resource constraints may preclude their use in many countries. Rapid advances continue to be made, with up to 40% of all clinical trials in 2020 being in oncology.[4] Robust processes and mechanisms need to be in place to make decisions around if, when and how new treatment should be introduced and sustained (Chapter 45 on medical technologies), and to ensure that once introduced treatment is accessible and affordable for everyone.[7]

Palliative and supportive care

Palliative and supportive care provides for the psychological, social and spiritual needs of the patient and their family, as well as pain relief (including access to opiate analgesia), fatigue, sleep deprivation, cognitive impairment, concerns about relationships and fertility, work and finances, and fear of recurrence issues.[8,9] Patient support groups have the potential to play an important role in supporting people with cancer (Chapter 55).

An integrated approach to cancer services

National cancer control programmes, particularly in low-resource settings, should focus on value for money (i.e. cost-effectiveness and affordability, and not only effectiveness) with the appropriate selection and maintenance of affordable innovative technologies (Chapter 44 and Chapter 45 on access to medicines and medical technologies). An essential package of cancer services can cost only US$ 2–9 per capita in low- and middle-income countries, yet only 40% of national programmes in these countries include cancer in their universal health coverage benefit packages.[10] Diagnosis, treatment and care of people with cancer require investing in well-trained multidisciplinary personnel (including protocols to be in place and being used) as well as the necessary equipment and consumables. Many low- and middle-income countries have an insufficient technical capacity and lack adequately trained staff to deliver a well-functioning cancer control programme.[11]

Patient navigators are an important part of a comprehensive cancer control programme providing assistance to patients through screening, diagnosis, treatment and follow-up. This includes assisting patients in: (i) communicating with healthcare providers; (ii) setting up appointments for medical visits; (iii) getting financial, legal and social support; (iv) liaising with insurance companies and employers; and (v) initiating and/or completing treatment.

Cancer registries

Less than half of all countries report on cause-specific deaths and only a small number of people with cancer are included in high-quality population-based cancer registries. Cancer registries systematically collect, store and manage data on persons who have been diagnosed with and/or treated for cancer.[12] When implemented effectively, cancer registries can be cost-saving institutions.[13] Yet, only one in three countries has high-quality incidence data.

Registries can be categorized as population-based cancer registries (PBCRs) or hospital-based cancer registries (HBCRs). PBCRs focus on a particular geographical area, generating data for epidemiological and public health purposes, including monitoring trends, distribution and priority setting. HBCRs collect data within a particular facility (or several or all hospitals of a region), often using data for administrative, research and educational functions. Findings from PBCRs may have broader generalizability to the whole population but with less detailed data, while findings from HBCRs may have lower generalizability to the whole population (as not all cancer patients access hospitals) but can include more detailed information (e.g. detailed information on treatment, follow-up, etc.).

Frameworks need to be developed that encourage diagnostic and treatment services (both public and private) to share relevant data (e.g. biopsy results, staging, outcomes) while ensuring there are adequate levels of data protection. It is crucial that data are held securely so that healthcare workers can confidently encourage patients to provide informed consent to share personal data so that registries can maximize their potential as a resource for monitoring and evaluating health services, and for research.

Data on both PBCRs and HBCRs should be linked with well-functioning civil mortality registration systems in the entire population (e.g. vital statistics) to obtain reliable information on deaths and causes of death, but this is available in less than half of the world population. Civil registration data for the whole population (including age distribution) are also necessary to produce estimates of cancer frequency at the population level. In addition, cancer registries should be linked to, among others, vaccine and cancer screening registries for maximal utility.

Two of the indicators in the WHO NCD Global Monitoring Framework are dependent on functional cancer registries, allowing for reporting at national, regional and global levels (Chapter 35).

Monitoring

SDG target 3.4.1

A one-third relative reduction in mortality from cardiovascular disease (CVD), cancer, diabetes or chronic respiratory disease by 2030 against a 2015 baseline.

Other relevant WHO NCD Global Monitoring Framework targets and indicators

Target	Indicator
As per SDG target 3.4.1.	• Unconditional probability of dying between the ages of 30 and 70 from CVD, cancer, diabetes or chronic respiratory diseases.
An 80% availability of affordable basic technologies and essential medicines, including generics required to treat major NCDs in both public and private facilities.	• Availability and affordability of quality, safe and efficacious essential NCD medicines, including generics, and basic technologies in both public and private facilities.

(Continued)

Target	Indicator
Additional indicators.	• Access to palliative care assessed by morphine-equivalent consumption of strong opioid analgesics (excluding methadone) per death from cancer. • Availability of cost-effective and affordable vaccines against HPV. • Number of third doses of HBV vaccine administered to infants. • Proportion of women aged 30–49 years screened for cervical cancer at least once and for lower or higher age groups according to national programmes or policies.

Examples of disease-specific targets and indicators are included in the other cancer chapters.

Notes

1 Lifetime risk of developing or dying from cancer. *Cancer Org*, 2020.
2 Global cancer observatory. IARC, 2022.
3 Global health observatory. WHO, 2020.
4 WHO report on cancer: setting priorities, investing wisely and providing care for all. WHO, 2020.
5 Global Burden of Disease 2019 Cancer Collaboration. Cancer incidence, mortality, years of life lost, years lived with disability, and disability-adjusted life years for 29 cancer groups from 2010 to 2019: a systematic analysis for the Global Burden of Disease Study 2019. *JAMA Oncol* 2022;8:420–24.
6 Comprehensive cancer control. International Atomic Energy Agency. https://www.iaea.org/topics/comprehensive-cancer-control.
7 Jan S et al. Action to address the household economic burden of non-communicable diseases. *Lancet* 2018;391:2047–58.
8 Quality health services and palliative care: practical approaches and resources to support policy, strategy and practice. WHO, 2021.
9 Cancer care: beyond survival. *Lancet* 2022;399:1441.
10 Health benefit packages survey 2020/2021: main findings. WHO. https://www.who.int/data/stories/health-benefit-packages-a-visual-summary.
11 Trapani D et al. Distribution of the workforce involved in cancer care: a systematic review of the literature. *ESMO Open* 2021;6:100292.
12 Cancer surveillance. The Cancer Atlas, https://canceratlas.cancer.org/the-burden/the-burden-of-cancer/.
13 Cancer registries: the core of cancer control fundamentals of population-based registries. IARC, 2021. https://gicr.iarc.fr/about-the-gicr/the-value-of-cancer-data/Brochure_HD.pdf.

12 Breast cancer

Burden, epidemiology and priority interventions

Miriam Mutebi, Karla Unger-Saldaña, Ophira Ginsburg

In 2020, an estimated 2.3 million people were diagnosed with breast cancer, making it the commonest cancer worldwide (11.7% of all new cases of cancer,[1] with a lifetime risk for women to be diagnosed with breast cancer in up to 13% in some countries).[2] Strong health services and systems are required to ensure that women with breast cancer are diagnosed early and receive effective treatment, including surgery, radiation and systemic therapy.

Disease burden

Breast cancer resulted in 700,000 deaths globally in 2019 (up from 381,000 in 1990) (IHME), with increasing proportions of deaths caused by breast cancer increasing over the last 30 years in all regions, except high-income countries (HICs), partly in line with changes in the age structure of these populations. Age-standardized breast cancer mortality has decreased markedly in HICs, moderately in middle-income countries (MICs), but increased in low-income countries (LICs), in part reflecting screening, diagnosis and cancer care across different parts of the world (Table 12.1).

Breast cancer deaths were attributable, in 2019, to high body mass index (6.5% of cases), alcohol (5.4%), tobacco (5.1%), dietary risk (3.2%) and low physical activity (1.2%) (IHME).

Risk factors

Ninety-nine percent of breast cancers are in women, with incidence increasing with age. In HICs, most breast cancer cases occur in post-menopausal women, although larger proportions of all cancer deaths are found at younger ages in low- and middle-income countries, when women are pre-menopausal or under age 50, largely reflecting younger populations in these countries. There are no known viral or bacterial infections linked to the development of breast cancer.

Reproductive history alters the risk of breast cancer, with an increased risk among those with early age at menarche (<12 years), older age at first pregnancy (>30), late menopause, and among women who have not had children,

DOI: 10.4324/9781003306689-14

Table 12.1 Mortality attributable to breast cancer among females (IHME)

	Global		HICs		Upper MICs		Lower MICs		LICs	
	1990	2019	1990	2019	1990	2019	1990	2019	1990	2019
Proportion of all deaths (%)	1.7	2.7	4.1	3.9	1.5	2.5	1.1	2.4	0.6	1.4
Age-standardized mortality (per 100,000)	18	16	24	17	13	12	16	12	15	18

or who have not breastfed.[3] Exclusive breastfeeding for six months is associated with up to a 20% lower risk of breast cancer in the mother, and for every 12 months of breastfeeding the relative risk of breast cancer is reduced by 4.3%.[4] Oral hormone replacement therapy is also associated with an increased risk, although the degree of risk depends on whether it is combined with oestrogen and progesterone or oestrogen alone and the risk declines after discontinuation.[5] The use of oral contraceptives is also associated with a modest increased risk of breast cancer.[6] Other risk factors include alcohol consumption, increased body mass index and low physical activity, particularly among post-menopausal women.[7] It is important to recognize that even if all the modifiable risk factors above were removed, the risk of developing breast cancer would only be reduced by about one-third.

While a family history of breast cancer increases the risk of developing breast cancer, the majority of breast cancer cases are not linked to a known family history of the disease.[8] Inherited mutations (e.g. of BRCA1, BRCA2, and PALB-2 genes) can increase the risk of breast cancer by up to 60 times.[9] Benign proliferative lesions of the breast such as atypical ductal hyperplasia and lobular carcinoma in situ are not invasive breast cancers but increase the risk of invasive breast cancer.[10]

Breast cancer in men is often associated with a number of rare inherited conditions.[11] Because 99% of breast cancer cases are in women, this chapter uses the term 'women' when describing those affected.

Interventions at the population level

Interventions to reduce exposure to the risk factors common to the four main NCDs are also applicable to breast cancer (i.e. tobacco use, alcohol consumption, unhealthy diet and low physical activity). These interventions are described in other chapters.

Screening and early diagnosis

WHO has defined two distinct but related strategies for the early detection of cancer: screening of asymptomatic women using population-wide programmes and early diagnosis of symptomatic patients.

Screening

Screening programmes with access to high-quality treatment result in a decrease in breast cancer-specific mortality of approximately 20%.[12] Mammography is used to identify pre-cancerous lesions and preclinical breast cancer among asymptomatic individuals.[13] Screening once every two years for women aged 50–69 years, linked with timely diagnosis and treatment, is identified as an effective intervention in the WHO Global NCD Action Plan. WHO recommends that population-based screening programmes for women aged 40–49 years should only be implemented where health systems are adequately resourced,[14] with the women being fully involved in deciding whether to be screened after a discussion on benefits and harm. Countries need to finalize their recommendations for the optimal age range for screening based on international guidance, resources available, the age-adjusted incidence of breast cancer and other factors. As with all screening programmes, there will be a substantial number of false-positive cases requiring unnecessary diagnostic investigations, as well as treatment of breast cancers that would not have caused clinical problems in the future (see Chapter 43 on screening).

Early diagnosis

An early cancer diagnosis is an early identification, diagnostic workup, referral and treatment of patients who present symptomatically.[15] Having organized cancer screening programmes in place for asymptomatic women does not preclude having strong systems that allow for early diagnosis of symptomatic women, since between 60% and 70% of women with breast cancer present symptomatically even in countries that have well-organized mammography programmes in place. The Breast Health Global Initiative recommends that in low- and middle-income countries, where the majority of women start treatment in advanced stages, efforts to strengthen early diagnosis should be prioritized over screening until timely access to quality diagnostic services and treatment are in place.[16] It relies on effective health systems where primary care personnel can adequately suspect cancer among patients presenting with breast symptoms, there is timely access to quality diagnostic tests (breast imaging studies and biopsy), and prompt referral is made to cancer centres for treatment. Early cancer diagnosis strategies include training of first-contact physicians to suspect cancer, fast-track pathways and, in general terms, strengthening of health systems.[17]

Diagnosis of breast cancer

Diagnosis of breast cancer requires examination of tissue taken by biopsy and assessment of local and distant spread (metastases). Breast cancer is not a uniform entity but a spectrum of conditions or subtypes which respond to treatment in different ways. In addition to a histological assessment of the grade of the tumour (where resources allow), immunohistochemistry and molecular techniques will identify the molecular subtype as well as other markers and indicators to guide treatment. These investigations require considerable expertise and quality control.

Staging is important to determine the optimal treatment for each woman and give an indication of her prognosis. Breast cancer staging comprises the following: (i) the size of the invasive tumour; (ii) lymph node involvement (to determine presence, absence and degree of loco-regional spread; and (iii) clinical, laboratory and/or imaging to determine the presence or absence of distant disease (e.g. bone, lung, liver).

Hormone receptors and other markers associated with each cancer define four main subtypes,[18] determined by oestrogen or progesterone receptors (HR+ or HR−), with around two-thirds of breast cancer being HR+, and HER2 protein (HER2+ or HER2−), with around 20% being HER2+. Drugs that lower levels of these hormones or block oestrogen receptors or deplete the amount of oestrogen produced can therefore be used to treat these cancers.

Treatment

Treatment can be local (surgery and/or radiation) and/or systemic (chemo-, hormone- or targeted-therapy). Treatment is guided by the cancer's stage and other tumour features mentioned above, whether the woman is pre- or post-menopausal, her general state of health, and her views on the treatment that she wishes to receive (i.e. 'patient preference').

Treatment most often requires surgery to: (i) remove the cancer (through breast-conserving surgery or mastectomy); (ii) find out whether the cancer has spread to the lymph nodes under the arm; (iii) reconstruct the breast's shape after the cancer is removed; and/or (iv) relieve symptoms of advanced cancer. This can occasionally involve the removal of the ovaries for HR+ tumours in pre-menopausal women. In rare cases, bilateral mastectomy and oophorectomy are considered to prevent rather than treat breast cancer (e.g. for women with BRCA1/BRCA2 mutations).

Radiation is used: (i) after breast-conserving surgery to reduce the likelihood of cancer recurrence; (ii) after a mastectomy, especially if the cancer was large or if the cancer has spread locally to the axillary nodes; and/or (iii) when there are metastases.[19]

Chemotherapy (e.g. doxorubicin) can be used before or after surgery and/ or when the tumour has spread to other organs.

Hormone therapy for HR+ cancers includes medicines that block oestrogen receptors (e.g. tamoxifen, which costs around US$ 100 per year) or lower the body's oestrogen levels (e.g. anastrozole, around US$ 1000 per year).

Targeted agents such as trastuzumab, a monoclonal antibody, are used to treat HER2+ breast cancer, but its high cost (around US$ 20,000–50,000 per year) precludes its use in many settings. Other targeted agents such as those that modulate the immune system (e.g. pembrolizumab) can boost the immune response in triple-negative breast cancers (those that lack oestrogen and progesterone receptors, and are HER2−), but the cost can exceed US$ 50,000–100,000 for a year's treatment.

Pain relief and medication to reduce the side effects of the cancer, and its treatment are paramount. Psychological support is also crucial, and many patients benefit from self-help/support groups. It is important to allow each woman to take her approach to manage her condition. As with all cancers, treatment is a partnership between professionals across a range of disciplines and the patient with shared decision-making.

Rehabilitation is important, including for example, physiotherapy to restore function to the arm, occupational therapy and/or breast reconstruction after mastectomy.

Follow-up

This will depend on the type of cancer, the treatment offered and the response to treatment. However, patients should usually be monitored every 3–6 months for the first 2–3 years, then every six months for five years, and annually thereafter. Follow-up should include clinical examination, mammograms (including of the other breast) and other investigations as required.

Prognosis

The stage of breast cancer determines the prognosis. Overall, the five-year disease-free survival in the best settings can be as high as 99% for women with localized cancer and 86% for one that is regional but drops significantly to 29% where there is a distant spread.[20] Five-year breast cancer-specific survival rates are lower in middle-income countries (e.g. 68% in Thailand, 66% in India and 40% in South Africa),[21] which is largely the result of late diagnosis and limited access to quality care.[22]

Palliative care

The treatments described above all have a role to play to a greater or lesser extent in palliative care. However, pain relief and treatment for other symptoms, as well as psychological support, must be the cornerstone. Palliative care specialists and hospice care are critical resources for end-of-life care. The support of family and friends is of course essential.[23]

Health system response

The diagnosis and management of breast cancer require a robust health system. This includes well-trained staff across a range of disciplines, the availability of the different treatments described above and access to the required medical devices.[24] As women with breast cancer need to access primary, secondary and tertiary care, countries therefore need to develop networks of care, with centres of excellence that can provide high-quality multidisciplinary care,[25] as well as ensure that treatment is included in universal health care packages at no (or minimal) cost to the woman.

The WHO Global Breast Cancer Initiative

The WHO Global Breast Cancer Initiative aims to reduce global breast cancer mortality by 2.5% per year, thereby potentially averting 2.5 million breast cancer deaths globally between 2020 and 2040. The initiative prioritizes strengthening early diagnosis and access to quality treatment, focusing on three elements: (i) health promotion for early presentation of women and early suspicion by the primary health workers, with a goal of achieving a diagnosis of >60% of invasive breast cancers at stage I or II; (ii) timely diagnosis, with a goal of ensuring that evaluation, imaging, tissue sampling and pathology is completed within 60 days; and (iii) comprehensive management, with a goal of >80% of women with breast cancer undergoing multimodality treatment.

Monitoring

Where population-based cancer registries are available, data on frequency, stage, type of cancer and survival rates should be collected to assess the effectiveness of care for those with breast cancer. When registries are not available, breast cancer mortality and data from hospitals (e.g. a number of admissions, pathology reports, survival rates) provide some information that can be useful. Monitoring the completion of diagnostic workup after abnormal screening is essential, and evaluating the effectiveness and impact of screening programmes should be encouraged.

Notes

1 Breast cancer overtakes lung cancer in terms of number of new cancer cases. International Agency for Research on Cancer and WHO, worldwide press release 294, 4 February 2021.
2 Surveillance, Epidemiology, and End Results (SEER) Program. National Cancer Institute, https://seer.cancer.gov/statfacts/html/breast.html.
3 Collaborative Group on Hormonal Factors in Breast Cancer. Menarche, menopause, and breast cancer risk: individual participant meta-analysis, including 118 964 women with breast cancer from 117 epidemiological studies. *Lancet Oncol* 2012;13:1141–51.
4 Collaborative Group on Hormonal Factors in Breast Cancer. Breast cancer and breastfeeding: collaborative reanalysis of individual data from 47 epidemiological studies in 30 countries, including data from 47 epidemiological studies in 30 countries, including 50302 women with breast cancer and 96973 women without the disease. *Lancet* 2002;360:187–95.
5 Collaborative Group on Hormonal Factors in Breast Cancer. Type and timing of menopausal hormone therapy and breast cancer risk: individual participant meta-analysis of the worldwide epidemiological evidence. *Lancet* 2019;394:1159–68.

6 Mørch LS et al. Contemporary hormonal contraception and the risk of breast cancer. *NEJM* 2018;378;1265–6.
7 Arthur S et al. The combined association of modifiable risk factors with breast cancer risk in the women's health initiative. *Cancer Prev Res* 2018;11:317–26.
8 Colditz GA et al. Family history and risk of breast cancer: nurses' health study. *Breast Cancer Res Treat* 2012;133(3):1097–104.
9 Hu C et al. A population-based study of genes previously implicated in breast cancer. *NEJM* 2021;384:440–51.
10 Hartmann LC et al. Benign breast disease and the risk of breast cancer. *NEJM* 2005;353:229–37.
11 Giordano SH. Breast cancer in men. *NEJM* 2018;378:2311–20.
12 Trapani D et al. Global challenges and policy solutions in breast cancer control. *Cancer Treat Rev* 2022;104:102339.
13 Guide to early cancer diagnosis. WHO, 2017.
14 Position paper on mammography screening. WHO, 2014.
15 Guide to cancer early diagnosis. WHO, 2017.
16 Ginsburg O et al. Breast cancer early detection: a phased approach to implementation. *Cancer* 2020;126:2379–93.
17 Harrison CJ et al. Transforming cancer outcomes in England: earlier and faster diagnoses, pathways to success, and empowering alliances. *J Healthc Leadersh* 2019;11:1–11.
18 Cancer stat facts: female breast cancer subtypes. National Cancer Institute. https://seer.cancer.gov/statfacts/html/breast-subtypes.html.
19 Cancer treatment: brachytherapy. IAEA. https://www.iaea.org/topics/cancer-treatment-brachytherapy.
20 Survival rates for breast cancer. American Cancer Society. https://www.cancer.org/cancer/breast-cancer/understanding-a-breast-cancer-diagnosis/breast-cancer-survival-rates.html.
21 Allemani C et al. Global surveillance of trends in cancer survival 2000–14 (CONCORD-3): analysis of individual records for 37 513 025 patients diagnosed with one of 18 cancers from 322 population-based registries in 71 countries. *Lancet* 2018;391:1023–75.
22 Anderson BO et al. The global breast cancer initiative: a strategic collaboration to strengthen health care for non-communicable diseases. *Lancet Oncol* 2021;22:578–81.
23 Planning and implementing palliative care services: a guide for programme managers. WHO, 2016.
24 WHO list of priority medical devices for cancer management. WHO, 2017.
25 Setting up a cancer centre: a WHO-IAEA framework. IAEA & WHO, 2022.

13 Cervical cancer

Burden, epidemiology and priority interventions

Nick Banatvala, Neerja Bhatla, Silvina Arrossi and Nathalie Broutet

Cervical cancer is a common cancer among women globally, with an estimated 604,000 new cases,[1] and the lifetime risk of being diagnosed with cervical cancer is 3% in some high-income countries (HICs).[2] Incidence is strongly related to the acquisition of human papillomaviruses (HPV). Differences in HPV vaccination coverage, screening and treatment underlie the large differences in incidence and mortality observed across countries. Strong health services are required to ensure high HPV vaccination coverage and that women are regularly screened for cervical abnormalities and receive adequate and effective treatment, including pre-cancer treatment, surgery, radiation and systemic treatment as needed.

Disease burden

According to IHME, cervical cancer accounted for 0.48% of all deaths (i.e. 281,000) globally in 2019, up from 0.28% in 1990 (Table 13.1). Table 13.1 shows that mortality attributable to cervical cancer, as a proportion of all deaths, increased in low- and middle-income countries but decreased in HICs. The age-standardized mortality rates (per 100,000 population) were: (i) much lower in HICs than in low- and middle-income countries, and (ii) decreased between 1990 and 2019, although less strongly in these countries than HICs, reflecting improvements in the prevention and management of cervical cancer as well as in socio-economic conditions.[3] The age-standardized incidence of cervical cancer in the world is 13 per 100,000 women, with a tenfold variation between regions (4 per 100,000 women in Western Asia to 40 per 100,000 in Eastern Africa).[1]

Risk factors

Persistent infection with oncogenic human papillomaviruses (HPV), the most common sexually transmitted infection, is the primary cause of cervical cancer. The peak time for acquiring HPV infection for both women and men is in the second decade of life, shortly after becoming sexually active. There are more than 100 types of HPV, of which at least 14 are high-risk genotypes for cervical cancer and 2 of them (genotypes 16 and 18) cause 70% of cervical cancers.

DOI: 10.4324/9781003306689-15

Table 13.1 Mortality attributable to cervical cancer (IHME)

	HICs 1990	HICs 2019	Upper MICs 1990	Upper MICs 2019	Lower MICs 1990	Lower MICs 2019	LICs 1990	LICs 2019
Proportion of all deaths (%)	0.38	0.31	0.46	0.56	0.34	0.47	0.44	0.75
Age-standardized mortality (per 100,000)	2.7	1.6	4.4	3.3	5.4	3.9	12	10.4

While most cervical infections with HPV resolve spontaneously and cause no symptoms, persistent infection can cause cervical cancer. It takes 15 to 20 years for cervical cancer to develop in women with normal immune systems but only 5 to 10 years in women with weakened immune systems, such as those with untreated HIV infection or recipients of immunosuppressive drugs. Other risk factors for HPV persistence and development of cervical cancer include coinfection with other sexually transmitted agents, such as herpes simplex, chlamydia and gonorrhoea, and tobacco smoking. Women living with HIV have a risk several times higher of persistent HPV infection. They are six times as likely to develop cervical cancer and are more likely to develop it at a younger age than women in the general population.[4]

Effective primary prevention (HPV vaccination) and secondary prevention (screening and treating pre-cancerous lesions) can prevent most cervical cancer cases.[5] In addition, cervical cancer is largely curable, particularly if detected early and adequately treated.

Prevention and control

An understanding of the natural history of cervical cancer highlights the importance of prevention and control following a comprehensive, life-course approach.

HPV vaccination and other primary preventive measures

HPV vaccination is a WHO best buy. It is estimated that 90% HPV vaccine coverage among girls under 15 years of age by 2030 would avert more than 45 million cervical cancer deaths over the next hundred years.[6]

For many years, the recommendation has been that two doses should be offered to all girls aged 9–14 years, i.e. before they become sexually active. HPV vaccination is currently included in the national immunization schedules of nearly 60% of countries, with wide variation between high-income countries (over 80%) and low-middle-income countries (around 30%) and even lower in low-income countries. Bivalent, quadrivalent and nonavalent HPV vaccines (against two, four and nine strains) are currently available. The WHO Scientific Advisory Group of Experts (SAGE) on Immunization has, however, recently concluded that single-dose schedules provide comparable efficacy

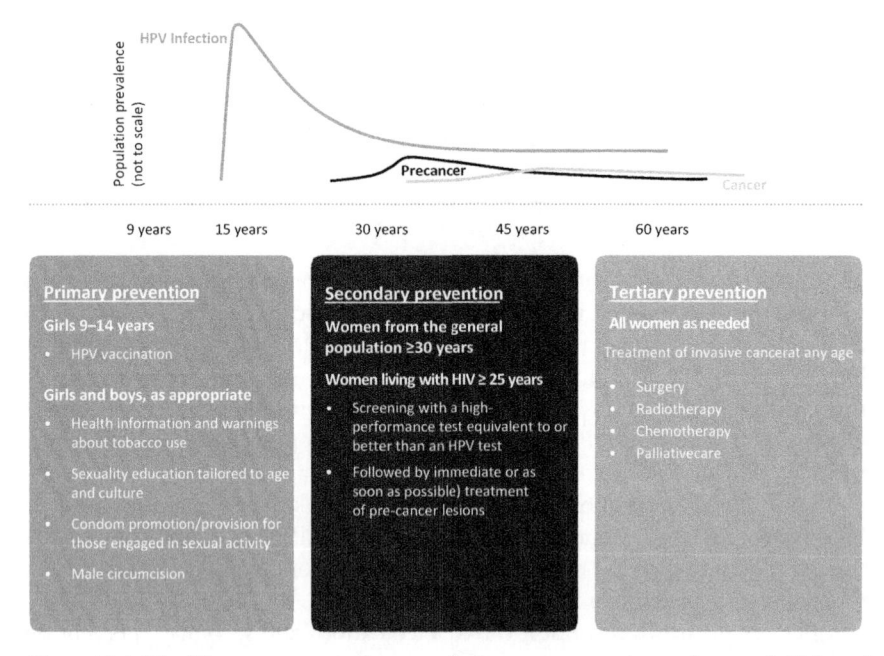

Figure 13.1 The life-course approach to cervical cancer prevention and control. (Adapted from WHO, 2020, Introducing and scaling up testing for HPV as part of a comprehensive programme for prevention and control of cervical cancer: a step-by-step guide).

with recommendations as follows: (i) one- or two-dose schedule for girls aged 9–14; (ii) one- or two-dose schedule for young women aged 15–20; (iii) two doses with a six-month interval for women >21. Those immunocompromised (including those with HIV) should receive three doses if feasible, and if not at least two doses, as there is limited evidence regarding the efficacy of a single dose in this group.[7]

In addition to HPV vaccination, a comprehensive prevention strategy should encompass age-appropriate information on sexual and reproductive health tailored to the age group, safer sexual practices (delaying the age of sexual activity, minimizing the number of sexual partners, using condoms, male circumcision where appropriate) and not using tobacco.[8]

Screening and treatment of pre-cancer lesions

All countries should implement cervical cancer population-based screening. Countries with cervical cancer screening programmes range from nearly 100% in the South East Asia region to around 21% in the African region.[9] However, before embarking on a cervical cancer (or indeed any other) screening programme, treatment must be in place and available for all who need it. It is unethical to screen for cervical cancer and pre-cancer without having treatment and care in place.

Three methods for screening pre-cancer in women aged 30–49 years (and 25–49 for women living with HIV) are also WHO best buys.[10] They are:

- HPV testing with timely treatment of pre-cancerous lesions. Key strengths of HPV testing include its simplicity (including that specimens can be self-collected), reproducibility of results (i.e. not rater-dependent) and the need for repeat tests only every 5 to 10 years (because of high specificity and strong negative predictive value). In many countries HPV testing is followed by triage, then histological confirmation and treatment as needed.
- Cervical cytology by Papanicolaou (Pap) smears every 3–5 years linked with timely treatment of pre-cancerous lesions. When cytology results are suggestive of pre-cancer, the diagnosis of pre-cancer (also known as cervical intraepithelial neoplasia or CIN) is based on subsequent colposcopy and histological results of a biopsy. Treatment is then offered to women with CIN2+ histology results.
- Visual inspection of the cervix with acetic acid (VIA) linked with timely treatment of pre-cancerous lesions. This alternative approach is an option in resource-constrained settings. Although it is affordable, relatively easy to establish and provides point-of-care results (meaning that treatment or referral decisions can be taken in the same visit), its limitations include high inter-operator variability, problematic sensitivity and the need for high-intensity quality assurance efforts. Its sensitivity can be even more variable in older women.

Most countries still use cytology or VIA; however, less than 40% of countries have coverage at the level required to meet the global strategy target of 70% (see below), and in many countries remain at around 5%. Recent WHO guidance is recommending that screening programmes move away from VIA and cytology to HPV DNA testing as this has greater sensitivity and specificity.[11] The high negative predictive value forms the basis of the recent recommendations for only two-lifetime screens at the ages of 35 and 45 years for women living in limited resource situations. Women who test negative at these two-time points are unlikely to develop cervical cancer. A number of low- and middle-income countries are negotiating HPV DNA tests (to around US$ 8), making it potentially more cost-effective than VIA or cytology. The option of self-sampling for the collection of HPV tests enhances the possibility of reaching the target of 70% coverage in more remote communities.[12]

HPV positivity can have a psycho-social impact due to potential stigma, impact on sexual life, fear of cancer and uncertainty about the meaning of results.[13] It is very important to provide women with clear and culturally adapted information and counselling regarding HPV testing and the meaning of results. Mobile technologies could be used to communicate with women, raise awareness on cervical cancer screening, provide counselling and reduce the psycho-social impact of HPV infection.[14]

WHO recommends prioritizing screening in women aged 30–49 years (25–49 for women living with HIV) and women after 50 if they have never been screened, using HPV tests with a screening interval of five to ten years in the general population of women and of three to five years in women living with HIV.[15,16] However, the American Cancer Society recommends that HPV testing should be carried out five-yearly between the ages of 25 and 64 years, and this is also the policy of England's cervical cancer screening programme. As more data emerge in vaccinated populations, the screening interval may increase in these programmes as well. Also, the upper age cut-offs may change in the future.

Treatment options for pre-cancerous lesions CIN include ablative treatment with thermal ablation or cryotherapy or large loop excision of the transformation zone (LEEP/LLETZ) when the patient is not eligible for ablative treatment. The availability of portable battery-powered devices for thermal ablation, and more recently for LLETZ, is changing the landscape for screen-and-treat programmes. Similarly, the development of portable colposcopes can allow screening, triage and treatment programmes to be carried out even at last-mile facilities, where health workers can be trained to take pictures and upload them for evaluation by a specialist. The addition of artificial intelligence is the next frontier which will enable instant decision-making on the need for referral/treatment.

Treatment of invasive cancer

With high-quality care, long-term survival and/or cure can be achieved using surgery and/or radiotherapy in around 90% of women with early-stage cervical cancer. If cervical cancer has spread to surrounding tissues or organs and/or the regional lymph nodes, a combination of radiotherapy and chemotherapy is used although long-term survival is considerably reduced. Where a cure is not possible, palliative care should be provided.

The importance of an effective health system

National cervical cancer programmes should be fully integrated into universal health coverage, with primary care as the main entry point to ensure access to high coverage. In 2019, only 30% of low-income countries reported having the required diagnostic and treatment infrastructure (advanced imaging, pathology, surgery, chemotherapy, radiotherapy) available in the public health system, compared to 90% in high-income countries.[17] It is important to ensure adequate maintenance of equipment and uninterrupted supply chains.

The global strategy for the elimination of cervical cancer as a public health problem

In 2020, the World Health Assembly endorsed a global strategy for the elimination of cervical cancer as a priority public health problem, with elimination (defined as a threshold of four cases of cervical cancer per 100,000 women-years) to be achieved by the end of this century. The global strategy's key elements are: HPV vaccination; screening and treatment of pre-cancerous lesions; and diagnosis and treatment of invasive cervical cancer, including palliative care.[18] The impact of national vaccination programmes, population-based cervical cancer screening and access to quality treatment requires that coverage and quality of services are improved and scaled up in many countries.[19]

The global strategy includes actions and targets for: (i) HPV vaccination; (ii) screening and treating pre-cancerous lesions; (iii) diagnosis and treatment of invasive cervical cancer, as well as palliative care.

Achieving the targets described below in low- and middle-income countries by 2030 would result in:

- A fall in median cervical cancer incidence rate by 42% by 2045, and by 97% by 2120, averting more than 74 million new cases of cervical cancer.
- Median cumulative number of cervical cancer deaths averted will be 300,000 by 2030, over 14 million by 2070, and over 62 million by 2120.
- An estimated US$ 3.2 returned to the economy for every dollar invested through 2050, through increases in women's workforce participation, with this figure rising to US$ 26 when societal benefits are included.

Monitoring progress

Relevant global targets for cervical cancer

By 2030, 90% of girls fully vaccinated with the HPV vaccine by 15 years of age. (Global elimination strategy).[a]	• HPV vaccination coverage disaggregated by age at vaccination and the number of doses.
By 2030, 70% of women screened using a high-performance test by 35 years of age and again by 45 years of age. (Global elimination strategy).[a]	• Screening rate of the target population (women aged 30–49 years or 25–49 for women living with HIV): percentage of women aged 30–49 (25–49 for women living with HIV) who have been screened for the first time in the previous 12-month period.
	• Positivity rate: percentage of screened women aged 30–49 years (25–49 for women living with HIV) with a positive screening test result in the previous 12-month period.
	• Coverage rate: percentage of women aged 30–49 years (25–49 for women living with HIV) who have been screened with a high-performance test at least once between the ages of 30 and 49 years (25–49 for women living with HIV), and the percentage screened at least twice.

By 2030, 90% of women identified with cervical disease are treated.	• Treatment rate: percentage of screening-test-positive women receiving treatment in the previous 12-month period.
By 2030, 90% of women with HPV infection or pre-cancer are treated.	Note: countries that do not treat screen positives may consider using as an indicator the percentage of women with cervical disease receiving treatment 12 months after being screened positive.
By 2030, 90% of women with invasive cancer are managed.	
(Global elimination strategy).	
An 80% availability of the affordable basic technologies and essential medicines, including generics, required to treat major NCDs in both public and private facilities.	• Availability and affordability of quality, safe and efficacious essential noncommunicable disease medicines, including generics, and basic technologies in both public and private facilities.
(Target 9 of the WHO Global NCD Action Plan).	

a   Also reflected in national system response indicators in the WHO Global NCD Action Plan.

The recommendation of a single-dose vaccination schedule described above will enable the vaccine target described above to be reached more rapidly.

In addition to the indicators listed above, national comprehensive cervical cancer programmes should implement population-based cancer registries to measure cervical cancer age-specific incidence and mortality. Population-based cancer registries are important to track the above targets and to monitor and evaluate service provision, including across different socio-economic and ethnic groups.

Notes

1 Cervix uteri fact sheet. IARC/WHO, 2021. https://gco.iarc.fr/today/data/factsheets/cancers/23-Cervix-uteri-fact-sheet.pdf.
2 Surveillance, Epidemiology, and End Results (SEER) Program. National Cancer Institute. https://seer.cancer.gov/statfacts/html/breast.html.
3 Sathishkumar K et al. Trends in breast and cervical cancer in India under National Cancer Registry Programme: an age-period-cohort analysis. *Cancer Epidmiol* 2021;74:101982.
4 Global strategy to accelerate the elimination of cervical cancer as a public health problem. WHO, 2020.
5 Brisson M et al. Impact of HPV vaccination and cervical screening on cervical cancer elimination: a comparative modelling analysis in 78 low-income and lower-middle-income countries. *Lancet* 2020;395:575–90.
6 Canell K et al. Mortality impact of achieving WHO cervical cancer elimination targets: a comparative modelling analysis in 78 low-income and lower-middle-income countries. *Lancet* 2020; 395: 591–603.

7. One-dose human papillomavirus (HPV) vaccine offers solid protection against cervical cancer. WHO, 2022.
8. Human papillomavirus (HPV) and cervical cancer. WHO, 2020.
9. Assessing national capacity for the prevention and control of noncommunicable diseases: report of the 2019 global survey. WHO, 2020.
10. Bouvard et al. The IARC perspective on cervical cancer screening. *NEJM* 385;20:1908–18.
11. WHO guideline for screening and treatment of cervical pre-cancer lesions for cervical cancer prevention, 2nd ed, WHO, 2021.
12. Gupta S. Self-sampling for human papillomavirus testing: increased cervical cancer screening participation and incorporation in international screening programs. *Front Public Health* 2018;6:77.
13. Arrossi S et al. Psycho-social impact of positive human papillomavirus testing in Jujuy, Argentina results from the Psycho-Estampa study. *Prev Med Rep* 2020;18:101070.
14. Sanchez Antelo V et al. A counseling mobile app to reduce the psychosocial impact of human papillomavirus testing: formative research using a user-centered design approach in a low-middle-income setting in Argentina. *JMIR Form Res* 2022;6:e32610.
15. WHO guideline for screening and treatment of cervical pre-cancer lesions for cervical cancer prevention: use of mRNA tests for human papillomavirus (HPV). WHO, 2021.
16. Human papillomavirus (HPV) nucleic acid amplification tests (NAATs) to screen for cervical pre-cancer lesions and prevent cervical cancer: policy brief. WHO, 2022.
17. Assessing national capacity for the prevention and control of NCDs: report of the 2019 global survey. WHO, 2020.
18. Global strategy to accelerate the elimination of cervical cancer as a public health problem. WHO, 2020.
19. Ginsburg O et al. The global burden of women's cancers: a grand challenge in global health. *Lancet* 2017;389:847–60.

14 Colorectal cancer

Burden, epidemiology and priority interventions

Jean-Luc Bulliard, Samar Alhomoud, Dieter Hahnloser

Colorectal cancer consists of cancer of the colon and the rectum and accounts for approximately 10% of new cancers globally.[1] The lifetime risk of developing colorectal cancer is as high as 4.3% in men and 4.0% in women.[2] As colorectal cancer is quite strongly associated with several of the NCD risk factors described in this book, there is significant potential for prevention. In addition, several screening tests are available and early treatment has a high rate of success.

Disease burden

According to IHME, colorectal cancer accounted for 1.9% (approximately 1.1 million) of all deaths worldwide in 2019 (increasing from 1.1% [0.52 million] in 1990), partly owing to growing and aging populations. Table 14.1 shows that the age-adjusted mortality rates of colorectal cancer decreased between 1990 and 2019 in high-income countries (HICs) but have otherwise slightly increased.

Globally, the total number of persons developing colorectal cancer is expected to rise in the decades ahead and colorectal cancer is expected to become the most common cancer by 2070, with 4.7 million new cases per year.[3] The increasing incidence will be largely driven by the increasing and aging populations, particularly in low- and middle-income countries, and by the increasing prevalence of some of the modifiable risk factors described below. Conversely, the incidence of colorectal cancer is expected to level off or even continue to decrease in HICs, given the stable age structure of the population, public health efforts to reduce exposures to modifiable risk factors, screening programmes and access to treatment. This, however, needs to be tempered with recent evidence of increasing rates of colorectal cancer in younger adults, possibly caused by changes in, or interactions between, diet, sedentary lifestyles and the rising prevalence of obesity.[4]

Risk and preventive factors

The aetiology of colorectal cancer is multifactorial. Around 70–75% of colorectal cancer occurs sporadically and is associated with modifiable risk factors.[5] The

DOI: 10.4324/9781003306689-16

Table 14.1 Mortality for colorectal cancer (IHME)

	Global		HICs		Upper MICs		Lower MICs		LICs	
	1990	2019	1990	2019	1990	2019	1990	2019	1990	2019
Proportion of all deaths (%)	1.1	1.9	3.2	3.8	1.1	2.3	0.4	1.0	0.2	0.5
Age-standardized mortality rates (per 100,000)	14	14	21	17	12	14	8	10	7	8

main non-modifiable risk factors include male gender, older age and heritability.[6] As the two most common forms of hereditary colorectal cancer (hereditary non-polyposis colon cancer and familial adenomatous polyposis coli) only account for <5% of all colorectal cancer, there remains much to be understood on the interplay between genetics and the modifiable risk factors described below.[7]

Modifiable risk factors include high consumption of processed food (e.g. processed meat, a diet low in whole grain), alcohol, low physical activity, tobacco use and obesity. Protective factors include a diet high in whole grains, dietary fibre and calcium (e.g. from dairy products or calcium supplements) and regular physical activity.[4] There is reasonable evidence that non-starchy vegetables and fruits, and foods containing vitamins C and D, have a protective effect. According to IHME estimates in 2019, 51% of deaths from colorectal cancer were attributable to behavioural risk factors, including 33% due to unhealthy diet, 13% to tobacco use, 9% to alcohol, 8% to high body mass index (BMI) and 5% to low physical activity (note: the sum of the attributable fractions estimated separately for each risk factor exceeds the attributable fraction for all as the effects of risk factors are not independent of each other). The relationship between colorectal cancer and the composition of microorganisms in the gut (microbiota) is an area of considerable research, which may have preventive and treatment implications in the future.[8] Differences in the prevalence of risk factors and provision of health care between countries and over time mean that age-standardized rates of both incidence and mortality for colorectal cancer can vary by up to ten-fold across countries.[9]

Long-term use of low-dose non-steroidal anti-inflammatory drugs, including aspirin or ibuprofen (which inhibit the enzyme COX-2) is also associated with a reduced incidence and mortality of colorectal cancer and pre-malignant adenomas (relative risk 0.6–0.8), possibly by reducing the risk of colorectal cancers that overexpress COX-2, but not the risk of colorectal cancers with a weak or absent expression of COX-2.[10]

Interventions at the population level

The strong association of colorectal cancer with the modifiable risk factors described above emphasizes the importance of many of the WHO best buys or recommended interventions that make an impact across the full range of NCDs described in several chapters in this book.

Screening

Colorectal cancer is preceded by pre-cancerous lesions (polyps), which can be identified during colonoscopy, biopsied and for smaller lesions removed at the same time. This has important implications when designing screening services/programmes and choosing which tests to use in these programmes. In order to be effective, population-based screening programmes should be implemented in a stepwise manner (including starting with a pilot phase), aim at high coverage of the target population, and be based on quality screening tests and treatment services.[11] Most experience with screening programmes has been in HICs.[12]

Screening tests. Most screening programmes use stool-based testing based on a faecal occult blood test (FOBT) or a faecal immunochemical test (FIT), with programmes increasingly moving from the inexpensive but less accurate FOBT to the more sensitive and reliable FIT. A positive screening test requires follow-up with colonoscopy or flexible sigmoidoscopy. A small number of screening programmes use flexible sigmoidoscopy or colonoscopy as a screening rather than a diagnostic tool. This has the advantage of allowing biopsies of suspected malignant or potentially malignant lesions (e.g. polyps that have evolved or are likely to evolve into cancer) to be removed at the time of screening. Other screening tools include direct visualization tests (e.g. computed tomography colonography), multi-target stool DNA tests, serum-based DNA tests (e.g. methylated septin 9 genes) and urine-based (metabolomic) tests, but they are not currently used for routine population-based screening. Despite the opportunities provided by screening, uptake is often suboptimal.[13] Screening programmes provide the opportunity for improving the health literacy of participants on options for the prevention and control of colon and other cancers.

Age and frequency of screening. The optimal age range target of a screening programme maximizes cost-effectiveness and will therefore vary between countries depending on the incidence of disease, health care capacity and competing priorities. Most screening programmes target individuals aged between 50 and 74 years, but the United States Preventive Services Task Force has recently recommended that the starting age for screening be reduced from 50 to 45 years. Other programmes, such as the one in the UK, start screening at the age of 60 years.[14] FOBT and FITs are usually undertaken annually or every two years. Computed tomography colonography and flexible sigmoidoscopy are conducted less frequently, typically every five years and every ten years for colonoscopy. For people over the age of 75 years, the decision to be screened should be based on resources available as well as the preferences of the individual and their life expectancy, overall health and prior screening history.

A recent review of colorectal cancer screening recommendations across the world identified 15 guidelines (six published in North America, six in Europe, four in Asia and one from the World Gastroenterology Organization). The majority of guidelines recommend screening average-risk individuals between the ages of 50 and 75, using colonoscopy (every 10 years), flexible sigmoidoscopy (every 5 years) or FOBT, mainly FIT (annually or biennially). There are disparities throughout the different guidelines relating to the use of colonoscopy, rank order between tests, screening intervals and optimal age ranges for screening.[15] Population-based colorectal cancer screening, at age >50 years, linked with timely treatment is an intervention recommended by the WHO Global NCD Action Plan.

Resources for population-based screening programmes. Colorectal cancer screening programmes require significant resources for testing large numbers of people and ensuring adequate and timely follow-up of individuals with a positive test, particularly when compared with the greater frequency of other diseases (including NCDs) that could be prevented and treated more cost-effectively and/or more affordably.[16] Screening programmes require sustainable availability of diagnostic procedures (including quality clinical services for undertaking colonoscopy or flexible sigmoidoscopy and histopathology services) and availability of timely treatment (i.e. surgery and/or chemotherapy for cancer cases as well as surgery for the (infrequent) complications of colonoscopy). As a result, well-organized population-based screening programmes, even if cost-effective, may not be affordable and/or not of sufficient priority in a number of countries. Nevertheless, the increasing incidence of colorectal cancer in many low- and middle-income countries means that population screening programmes are likely to become more widespread in the coming years.[17] As with other population-based screening programmes, once established, it is often very difficult to discontinue a programme.

Opportunistic screening for high risk individuals. The priority here is to screen the first-degree relatives of those with a strong family history of colorectal cancer, including, where possible, the determination of a genetic cause. This should be done from the age of 18 years of age at regular intervals, provided resources are available for diagnosis, treatment and follow-up.

Treatment

Preventive treatment. Low-dose non-steroidal anti-inflammatory medications and/or aspirin may be considered in individuals with hereditary colorectal cancer syndromes, as this reduces the overall risk of colorectal cancer.[18]

Early-stage colorectal cancer (so-called 'cancerous polyps') can be removed by colonoscopy and usually requires no further treatment.

Colon cancer. Patients with colon cancer that has not spread to distant sites (most frequently the lungs and the liver) usually have surgery. Where lymph nodes are involved or there is a distant spread, chemotherapy (called adjuvant chemotherapy) is given for around 3–6 months after surgery. The type and duration of chemotherapy depend on the histological cancer type, age and comorbidities of the patient. Where resources permit, microsatellite instability (MSI) in tumour cells should be determined to guide treatment and prognosis.

Rectal cancer. Patients with rectal cancer need often a multi-disciplinary approach including neoadjuvant (before surgery) chemo- and/or radiotherapy to decrease the size of the tumour (making surgery easier, including reducing the chance of having to operate on the anal sphincter, which is a high-risk procedure) and reduce the likelihood of local recurrence. Rectal cancer treatment is however centralized, in many countries, in experienced high-volume centres. Discussion in multidisciplinary tumour boards is crucial to personalize treatment for rectal cancer. If a patient has an excellent response to neoadjuvant treatment and presents a complete clinical response with no visible cancer, an expectative approach without surgery is possible in selected patients.

Follow-up. Patients should be followed up for five years to monitor for recurrence (which can occur in up to 50% of patients) in order to allow for early re-intervention. There is insufficient evidence to give aspirin to patients post-surgery.

Survival. In optimal settings, five-year survival after treatment for colorectal cancer may be as high as 95% for stage I, 85% for stage II, but only 70% for stage III and below 20% for stage IV.[19] MSI is a predictor of a better outcome.[20] Treatment of colorectal cancer stages I and II with surgery +/- chemotherapy and radiotherapy are therefore included as an effective intervention in the WHO Global NCD Action Plan.

Palliative care. Basic palliative care for cancer is a WHO effective intervention, including home-based and hospital care with multi-disciplinary teams and access to opiates and essential supportive medicines.

Monitoring

A comprehensive health information system that can provide ongoing routine quality data is important to develop and evaluate locally-tailored preventive and treatment programmes for colorectal cancer, track set targets and assess service provision, including across socio-economic and other relevant population sub-groups.

When resources allow, population-based cancer registries enable the collection of standardized data (e.g. cancer staging, accurate diagnosis and histology, survival time from diagnosis) that are required to track age-specific incidence and mortality as well as the impact of preventive and screening programmes.

Notes

1 Sung HS et al. Global Cancer Statistics 2020: GLOBOCAN estimates of incidence and mortality worldwide for 36 cancers in 185 countries. *CA Cancer J Clin* 2021;71:209–49.
2 How common is colorectal cancer? American Cancer Society. https://www.cancer.org/cancer/colon-rectal-cancer/about/key-statistics.html.

3. Soerjomataram I, Bray F. Planning for tomorrow: global cancer incidence and the role of prevention 2020–2070. *Nat Rev Clin Oncol* 2021;18:663–72.
4. Loomans-Kropp HA, Umar A. Increasing incidence of colorectal cancer in young adults. *J Cancer Epidemiol* 2019:9841295.
5. GBD 2019 Colorectal Cancer Collaborators. Global, regional and national burden of colorectal cancer and its risk factors, 1990–2019: a systematic analysis for the Global Burden of Disease Study 2019. *Lancet Gastroenterol Hepatol* 2022;7:627–47.
6. International Agency for Research on Cancer. Colorectal cancer screening. Lauby-Secrétan B et al, editors. *IARC Handb Cancer Prev* 2019, 17:1–300. Lyon: IARC Press.
7. Gunter MJ et al. Meeting report from the joint IARC–NCI international cancer seminar series: a focus on colorectal cancer. *Ann Oncol* 2019;30:510–19.
8. Wong SH, Yu J. Gut microbiota in colorectal cancer: mechanisms of action and clinical applications. *Nat Rev Gastroenterol Hepatol* 2019;16:690–704.
9. Arnold M et al. Global patterns and trends in colorectal cancer incidence and mortality. *Gut* 2017;66:683–91.
10. Rothwell PM et al. Long-term effect of aspirin on colorectal cancer incidence and mortality: 20-year follow-up of five randomised trials. *Lancet* 2010;376:1741–50.
11. WHO report on cancer: setting priorities, investing wisely and providing care for all. WHO, 2020.
12. Basu P et al. Status of implementation and organization of cancer screening in the European Union Member States—Summary results from the second European screening report. *Int J Cancer* 2018;142:44–56.
13. Kanth P, Iandomi JP. Screening and prevention of colorectal cancer. *BMJ* 2021;374:n1855.
14. Lin S et al. Screening for colorectal cancer: updated evidence report and systematic review for the US Preventive Services Task Force. *JAMA* 2021;325:1978–97.
15. Bénard F et al. Systematic review of colorectal cancer screening guidelines for average-risk adults: Summarizing the current global recommendations. *World J Gastroenterol* 2018;24:124–38.
16. Lambert RC et al. Mass screening for colorectal cancer is not justified in most developing countries. *Int J Cancer* 2009;125:253–56.
17. Khuhaprema T et al. Organised colorectal cancer screening in Lampang Province, Thailand: preliminary results from a pilot implementation programme. *BMJ Open* 2014;4:e003671.
18. Burn J et al. Cancer prevention with aspirin in hereditary colorectal cancer (Lynch syndrome), 10-year follow-up and registry-based 20-year data in the CAPP2 study: a double-blind, randomised, placebo-controlled trial. *Lancet* 2020;395:1855–63.
19. Araghi M et al. Colon and rectal cancer survival in seven high-income countries 2010–2014: variation by age and stage at diagnosis (the ICBP SURVMARK-2 project). *Gut* 2021;70:114–26.
20. Li K et al. Microsatellite instability: a review of what the oncologist should know. *Cancer Cell Int* 2020;20:16.

15 Prostate cancer

Burden, epidemiology and priority interventions

Dario Trapani, Mariana Siqueira, Manju Sengar, Dorothy C Lombe

Prostate cancer is the commonest cancer among men, with almost 1.5 million new cases globally in 2019.[1] The lifetime risk for men to be diagnosed with prostate cancer can be as high as 13% in some countries.[2] Few preventive factors are identified, which limits primary prevention. Where strong health services are available, survival is high when cancer is diagnosed at early stages. Treatment can range from active surveillance to surgery, radiation and systemic therapy.

Disease burden

Table 15.1 shows that 1.6% of all deaths among men (486,000 deaths) were attributed to prostate cancer worldwide in 2019 with no marked differences across regions. In 2019, the age-standardized mortality rates were highest in low-income countries (LICs), where rates have increased between 1990 and 2019, possibly because of delayed diagnosis and treatment, and in high-income countries (HICs), where rates have decreased, possibly because of better treatment and diagnosis, particularly with the wide use of the prostate-specific antigen (PSA) test used for screening.

The average age at diagnosis is 66 years, with prostate cancer being unusual in men under 40 years. The burden of prostate cancer seems to vary across racial groups. For example, in the USA, African Americans are twice as likely as white individuals to develop or die from prostate cancer. In contrast, Asian American men have the lowest incidence and mortality rates of prostate cancer.[3] Differences in outcomes across ethnical groups are likely to be explained by variations in access to care.[4]

Risk factors

Age is the main risk factor for prostate cancer. IHME estimates that 6% of all prostate deaths are attributable to smoking. Approximately 1.5% to 3.5% of all prostate tumours are associated with mutations of the BRCA1 and BRCA2 genes (and in larger proportions of individuals in some populations with

DOI: 10.4324/9781003306689-17

Table 15.1 Mortality for prostate cancer among men (IHME)

	Global		HICs		Upper MICs		Lower MICs		LICs	
	1990	2019	1990	2019	1990	2019	1990	2019	1990	2019
Percent of all deaths (%)	0.9	1.6	0.9	1.6	0.7	1.5	0.4	0.9	0.4	0.9
Age-standardized rates (per 100,000)	18	15	25	18	13	13	12	12	21	24

elevated frequency of carriers of mutated genes).[5] BRCA2 mutations increase the risk of prostate cancer by up to eight times.[6]

Interventions at the population level

There are no evidence-based interventions at the population level for reducing the incidence of prostate cancer, with the exception of tobacco control.

Systematic screening programmes

There has been much debate over the years around the use of PSA as a screening tool for prostate cancer among asymptomatic men.[7] PSA is a protein produced by normal, as well as malignant, cells of the prostate gland that is detected in the blood of men. There is evidence that systematic screening programmes of asymptomatic men based on PSA result in little or no overall reduction in mortality from prostate cancer.[6] In addition, many studies have shown that PSA screening among asymptomatic men leads to significant over-diagnosis because of the high numbers of 'false positives', and this results in unnecessary diagnostic invasive procedures (e.g. biopsy) and treatment (e.g. surgery) and related acute and longer-term side effects (e.g. incontinence and erectile dysfunction).

When considering the merits of population screening among asymptomatic men, it is important to be aware that up to one-fifth of men with prostate cancer have a normal PSA level,[9] and that autopsy reports from men that have died from other causes show evidence of undiagnosed, clinically non-relevant, indolent, localized prostate cancer in up to one-third of men aged <50 years and more than two-thirds of men ≥70 years. This underlines the fact that the evolution of prostate cancer can be slow, particularly in older men. Equally, it is important to be aware that a delay in diagnosis is a determinant of poorer outcomes among men who present later with advanced cancer. The US Preventive Service Task Force does not recommend population-based, universal screening by PSA, but suggests individualizing the discussion in men aged 50–69 years.[8]

It has been estimated that PSA-based screening among non-symptomatic men would avert <1 death from prostate cancer per 1000 men screened over ten years.[7] Systematic PSA screening is therefore not recommended from a public health perspective. Alternative screening tests for PSA, including biochemical markers have been proposed, but none has been shown to have sufficient sensitivity, specificity or be sufficiently cost-effective.

Screening of high-risk individuals

Where resources are available, individuals that have a strong family history of prostate cancer, or other cancers that are associated with BRCA and similar mutations, such as breast and ovarian cancer, may be referred for genetic counselling to assess whether regular PSA screening is appropriate, given the issues described above.[9] There has been some interest in whether the drug dutasteride, which is used for treating benign prostatic enlargement, reduces the incidence of prostate cancer among men who are at increased risk for the disease, but the current evidence is that it does not.[10]

Interventions at the individual level

Diagnosis

Prostate cancer does not usually cause symptoms until the cancer has grown large enough to cause urinary symptoms (including but not limited to: difficulty starting or frequent urination, weak or slow urinary stream and evidence of blood in the urine). These are to a large extent the same symptoms caused by benign prostatic hypertrophy, a condition that does not evolve into cancer and which is present in a large number of older men.

Diagnosis of prostate cancer and assessment of local spread is made on the basis of physical examination (including digital rectal examination), PSA, ultrasound and/or MRI and confirmed with histological results from one or more biopsies. Prostate cancer can be detected through digital rectal examination in 20% of cases.[9]

Diagnostic imaging (e.g. X-ray, scintigraphy, CT/PET scans) is important in determining the size and spread of the tumour and whether there is evidence of metastases, which most often are in the bones. In resource-constrained settings, risk-based imaging algorithms can help to optimize resources, for example, imaging only those with symptoms that suggest spread.[11]

Histology, using the Gleason score (i.e. a specific histologic pattern) along with tumour size, cancer spread and PSA level combine to determine optimal treatment, likely outcome and approach to follow-up.

Treatment and management

Prostate cancer is a highly curable disease if diagnosed timely. Treatment for prostate cancer includes surgery, radiotherapy and hormone therapy, along with a number of supportive treatments. Almost all the patients diagnosed with localized disease (i.e. stages 1 and 2) are alive at 5–10 years. When diagnosed at an advanced stage (e.g. stage 4), survival rates drop significantly, with one-third or less being alive after five years. Comorbidities, delayed diagnosis and inadequate treatment result in lower survival rates.[12] As prostate cancer is often slow-growing, it can be appropriate in older men or those with other serious illnesses to monitor the disease closely (clinically, radiologically and biochemically) rather than embark on treatment. Differences in outcomes from prostate cancer are likely to be partly explained by variations in access to care.

Active follow-up of cases enables patients with a low Gleason score and with smaller tumours to be enrolled in active surveillance programmes to avoid overtreatment. Active follow-up requires the necessary resources, systems and services to be in place, which is not the case in many settings.[13] Deferring initial treatment may also be considered for patients regardless of the stage of the cancer where multiple comorbidities exist to avoid treatment that is unlikely to improve the overall prognosis. This approach of 'watchful waiting' requires close monitoring, for example using PSA testing quarterly in the first year followed by six-monthly thereafter with the radiological investigation as required.

Surgery (radical prostatectomy through open surgery or laparoscopy) is commonly indicated in men with the localized disease – i.e. when it has not spread outside the prostate itself. There is increasing use of robotic-assisted surgery. Laparoscopic approaches can accelerate the recovery time and reduce blood loss.[9] The robot-assisted approach used in some centres seems to deliver similar outcomes as standard surgery, but at a generally higher cost, but robust evidence on outcomes, as well as post-operative urinary and sexual dysfunctions, is still limited.[14] Radical prostatectomy is major surgery and requires the right facilities and high levels of skill. Complications include those that can result from any major procedure as well those specific to prostate surgery, including removal or damage to local nerves that can result in additional, and often permanent, urinary or sexual dysfunction.

Radiotherapy can be used in the following instances:
- Treatment of localized prostate cancer. Cure rates for these types of cancers can be similar to men treated with radical prostatectomy.
- As part of initial treatment (sometimes along with hormone therapy) for cancers that have spread beyond the prostate gland to local tissue.
- Where the cancer is not removed completely or returns following surgery.
- Where the cancer is advanced, in order to help prevent or relieve symptoms, including as part of palliative care.

Hormone therapy is used to reduce levels of androgens, such as testosterone, which stimulates the growth of prostate cancer cells. While hormone therapy does not cure prostate cancer, it can in some patients prevent disease progression, reduce cancer-related symptoms and improve survival and quality of life. It is used in the following circumstances:

- Where the cancer has spread too far to be cured by surgery or radiation.
- Where there is a recurrent disease after surgery or radiotherapy.

- As an adjuvant therapy to initial treatment alongside radiotherapy (to reduce the risk of recurrence in aggressive and/or widespread disease).
- Before radiation to try to reduce tumour size.

Chemotherapy is sometimes used where prostate cancer has spread and the cancer is not responsive to hormone therapy. While it also does not cure prostate cancer, where facilities are available, chemotherapy may be helpful when given at the same time as hormone therapy.

Immunotherapy and other novel treatments that specifically target prostate cancer cells are used to treat advanced prostate cancer stages that are no longer responding to hormone therapy and/or chemotherapy. While they also do not cure prostate cancer, they can extend survival for a few months and improve disease control. They may, for example, include immunotherapy, radionuclides and DNA-targeting agents for men with BRCA mutations. These medicines are expensive but where resources are available can be used to treat the advanced disease that has becomes resistant to other forms of treatment.

Localized treatments such as cryotherapy and high-intensity focused ultrasound are sometimes used in selected patients instead of surgical treatments.

Palliative care is a critical element across the patient journey and requires access to effective pain control, including opiates, radiotherapy for bone pain and staff skilled in end-of-life support and care.

Interventions and treatment for prostate cancer are included in a range of WHO guidance on cancer management.[15,16] As with the management of all NCDs, an effective health system is critical and access to healthcare must be affordable to patients.

Monitoring

When resources allow, population-based cancer registries enable the collection of standardized data (e.g. cancer staging, accurate diagnosis and histology, survival time from diagnosis) that are required to track age-specific incidence and mortality as well as the impact of preventive and screening programmes.

Notes

1 Fitzmaurice C et al. Global, regional, and national cancer incidence, mortality, years of life lost, years lived with disability, and disability-adjusted life-years for 29 cancer groups, 1990 to 2016: a systematic analysis for the Global Burden of Disease Study. *JAMA Oncol* 2018;4:1553–68.
2 Surveillance, epidemiology, and end results (SEER) program. National Cancer Institute. https://seer.cancer.gov/statfacts/html/breast.html.
3 Hur J, Giovannucci E. Racial differences in prostate cancer: does timing of puberty play a role? *Br J Cancer* 2020;123:349–54.
4 Dess RT et al. Association of Black race with prostate cancer-specific and other-cause mortality. *JAMA Oncol* 2019;5:975–83.
5 Pilarski R. The role of BRCA testing in hereditary pancreatic and prostate cancer families. *Am Soc Clin Oncol Educ Book* 2019;39:79–86.

6. Etzioni R et al. Overdiagnosis due to prostate-specific antigen screening: lessons from U.S. prostate cancer incidence trends. *J Natl Cancer Inst* 2002;94:981–90.
7. Ilic D et al. Prostate cancer screening with prostate-specific antigen (PSA) test: a systematic review and meta-analysis. *BMJ* 2018;362:k3519.
8. Grossman DC et al. Screening for prostate cancer: US preventive services task force recommendation statement. *JAMA* 2018;319:1901–13.
9. EAU Guidelines Office, Arnhem, the Netherlands. http://uroweb.org/guidelines/compilations-of-all-guidelines/.
10. Andriole GL et al; REDUCE Study Group. Effect of dutasteride on the risk of prostate cancer. *NEJM* 2010;362:1192–202.
11. Cotait Maluf F, Gillessen S. Consensus on the screening, staging, treatment, and surveillance of localized, recurrent, and metastatic prostate cancer: the first global prostate cancer consensus conference for developing countries. *JCO Glob Oncol* 2021;7:512–15.
12. Allemani C et al; CONCORD Working Group. Global surveillance of trends in cancer survival 2000–14 (CONCORD-3): analysis of individual records for 37 513 025 patients diagnosed with one of 18 cancers from 322 population-based registries in 71 countries. *Lancet* 2018;391:1023–75.
13. Kang SK et al. Active surveillance strategies for low-grade prostate cancer: comparative benefits and cost-effectiveness. *Radiology* 2021;300:594–604.
14. Ploussard G et al. A 5-year contemporary nationwide evolution of the radical prostatectomy landscape. *Eur Urol Open Sci* 2021;34:1–4.
15. WHO model list of essential medicines, 22nd list, WHO, 2021.
16. WHO list of priority medical devices for cancer management. WHO, 2017.

16 Chronic respiratory diseases

Burden, epidemiology and priority interventions

Nils E. Billo, Nick Banatvala, Pascal Bovet, Asma El Sony

Chronic respiratory diseases (CRDs) are diseases of the airways and other structures of the lung. CRDs include chronic obstructive pulmonary disease (COPD), asthma, bronchiectasis, pneumoconiosis (lung diseases related to occupational exposures, e.g. silicosis and asbestosis), and other rarer lung diseases (e.g. interstitial lung disease and pulmonary sarcoidosis) as well as other chronic respiratory diseases such as pulmonary hypertension and allergic rhinitis.[1,2] More than 500 million people are affected by these conditions globally.

Definitions

COPD is a chronic inflammatory lung disease that causes obstructed airflow to the lungs.[3] Symptoms include breathing difficulty, cough, production of mucus (sputum) and wheezing (stridor). COPD is mainly caused by long-term exposure to particulate matter and irritating chemicals, including tobacco smoke and air pollution (ambient or indoor solid fuel smoke) and dust.[4] People with COPD have an increased risk of developing cardiovascular disease, including pulmonary hypertension, lung cancer and other conditions (including sleep apnoea). Emphysema (characterized by air-filled cavities/spaces in the lung, which results in fewer alveoli [air sacs] needed for oxygen/carbon dioxide exchange) and chronic bronchitis (characterized by an inflammation of the linings of the bronchial tubes that causes sputum production and coughing) are the most common underlying conditions of COPD, and often occur together. COPD is a progressive disease that can lead to fatal respiratory failure. With proper management (removing exposure to tobacco smoke and particulate matter in addition to medical treatment, for example antibiotics to treat pneumonia and oxygen therapy, in severe cases), the symptoms of COPD can be controlled for many years in the majority of people, enabling a reasonable quality of life, and a reduced risk of complications.

Asthma is a chronic inflammatory disease of the lung airways, which affects people of all ages, with a prevalence of around 10% in children (more in high-income countries [HICs], less in low- and middle-income countries).[5] Asthma is characterized by recurring airflow obstruction episodes with bronchospasms, airwall thickening and increased mucus production. Symptoms

DOI: 10.4324/9781003306689-18

include episodes of wheezing, coughing, chest tightness, and shortness of breath, which can occur from a few times a day to a few times per month. The exact causes of asthma are unclear but asthma is often associated with environmental factors (e.g. outdoor/indoor particulate matters, allergens) and a variety of triggers (dust mites, farm animals, viral infections, tobacco smoke, fire cooking, some foods, physical exercise, etc.).[6] There is no known cure for asthma, but episodes can be prevented or, when they occur, fairly easily controlled with medical treatment.

Pneumoconiosis refers to a group of lung diseases caused by the inhalation and retention of, and reaction of the lung tissue to dusts linked to the workplace and environmental exposures. Pneumoconiosis includes asbestosis, silicosis and coal workers' pneumoconiosis. There is generally a long delay – up to ten years or more – between exposure and onset of disease, so most new cases or deaths from pneumoconiosis (including associated lung cancer) reflect the working conditions of the past and often occur later in life, often when individuals have retired.

Disease burden

Table 16.1 shows mortality estimates for CRDs in 1990 and 2019 (IHME).

Globally, CRDs accounted for 7% of all deaths (nearly 4 million) worldwide. COPD contributed to 83% of all CRD deaths in 2019 and asthma to 13% of them. In many countries, the proportion of CRD deaths can be expected to increase over time because of growing and aging populations. Decreases in age-standardized mortality rates for COPD and asthma are in large part due to decreasing exposure to risk factors as a result of public health interventions (e.g. tobacco control, measures to mitigate ambient and indoor air pollution) and improved case management (e.g. asthma). While the global number of deaths due to pneumoconiosis is fairly small, they are entirely preventable.

Table 16.1 Mortality for CRD, including COPD, asthma and pneumoconiosis (IHME)

	Global		HICs		Upper MICs		Lower MICs		LICs	
	1990	2019	1990	2019	1990	2019	1990	2019	1990	2019
Proportion of all deaths (%)										
All CRDs	6.6	7.0	4.6	5.8	10.4	7.5	5.6	8.1	2.4	3.7
COPD	3.7	5.8	3.7	4.9	9.7	6.9	3.8	6.0	1.5	2.6
Asthma	1.0	0.8	0.5	0.2	0.6	0.3	1.6	1.6	0.9	1.0
Pneumoconiosis	<0.1	<0.1	<0.1	<0.1	<0.1	<0.1	<0.1	<0.1	<0.1	<0.1
Age-standardized mortality rates (per 100,000)										
All CRDs	88	51	30	24	132	50	122	89	95	72
COPD	73	42	24	20	123	46	87	68	65	53
Asthma	12	6	4	1	7	2	31	16	27	16
Pneumoconiosis	<1	<1	<1	<1	<1	<1	<1	<1	<1	<1

Risk factors

In 2019, 40% of all COPD deaths were attributable to smoking, 18% to ambient particulate matter, 13% to occupational particulates, 10% to household air pollution, 9% to low temperature, 9% to ozone and 7% to second-hand smoke (IHME). These high attributable fractions related to a few modifiable risk factors emphasize the high potential impact of prevention measures to reduce the occurrence of CRDs, and mainly COPD. For asthma, high BMI contributed to 16% of global asthma deaths, smoking 12% and occupational asthmagens 7% (IHME). In view of their risk factors (including tobacco use, indoor and ambient air pollution), CRDs are often associated with poverty. CRDs, as a result of occupational exposure, is also an important public health issue in certain groups (e.g. coal mines, construction workers, etc.) and although they have decreased over the years they still occur, particularly in marginalized and vulnerable communities.

Interventions at the population level

WHO best buys and other recommended interventions to address tobacco use, are described in Chapters 18 and 33. The following WHO recommendations interventions are specific to CRDs:

- Access to improved stoves and cleaner fuels to reduce indoor air pollution.
- Interventions to prevent occupational lung diseases, e.g. exposure to silica and asbestos.
- Influenza vaccination for patients with COPD is also considered a recommended intervention.

Interventions for reducing air pollution beyond those above are not currently included in the WHO best buys and other recommendations interventions but will be reviewed when the best buys are next updated. A WHO Clean Household Energy Solutions Toolkit (CHEST) was published in 2018[7] and provides tools that countries can use to implement recommendations on household fuel combustion.[8] Further details on air pollution are provided in Chapter 27.

Interventions at the individuals level

The burden of CRDs on the health system is very significant given that up to a third of all patients who attend primary health care present with a cough as a primary symptom and many will have a CRD. Long-term sequelae following COVID-19 infection may add to this burden. Access to appropriate investigations is important in order to diagnose COPD, asthma or another CRD, as well as other causes of cough such as heart disease and cancer, and in order to ensure appropriate treatment. This is important because of the seriousness of these conditions (including the risk of sudden death) and given that treatment is often long term. Despite this, health systems are often poorly resourced when it comes to the effective management of CRD, e.g. standardization of services with adequate diagnostic equipment, medicines, protocols and trained staff, especially in low- and middle-income countries. For example, salbutamol and corticoid inhalers are generally available in primary care public health facilities in only around half of the low-income countries.[9]

The diagnosis of COPD and asthma is usually based on symptoms, lung function tests such as spirometry and peak flow meter (tests used to help diagnose and monitor certain lung conditions by measuring how much air can be exhaled in one forced breath), and response to treatment over time. Basing the diagnosis on clinical symptoms alone may lead to over- or underdiagnosis of these conditions. Spirometry is often not available in low-resource settings (although simple peak flow meters are more likely to be available) and so the diagnosis may be missed or, at least, not documented appropriately. Pneumoconiosis is mainly diagnosed on the basis of the history of exposure, radiological imaging, lung function tests and biopsy.

There is no cure for COPD but early diagnosis and treatment are important to slow the progression of symptoms and reduce the risk of flare-ups.

Treating asthma and symptomatic relief for both asthma and COPD are included in WHO's best buys and other recommended interventions, i.e.:

- Symptom relief for patients with asthma with inhaled salbutamol (which rapidly relaxes muscles of the airways).
- Symptom relief for patients with COPD with inhaled salbutamol.
- Treatment of asthma using low-dose inhaled beclomethasone (a steroid) and a short-acting beta-agonist (e.g. salbutamol).

In addition, patients with asthma or COPD should be advised to:

- Quit smoking (where they smoke).
- Reduce their exposure to particulate matter, including improved stoves and cleaner fuels.
- Be vaccinated against pneumonia, influenza and coronavirus (in addition to vaccination for diseases that can result in pulmonary complications and are part of immunization schedules).

Additional interventions for the management of COPD include pulmonary rehabilitation and treatment of comorbidities such as cardiovascular disease, lung cancer, osteoporosis, muscle weakness and depression. Those with asthma and COPD need support to understand triggers to avoid, how to manage their symptoms and signs, and when and how to get emergency support, as an untreated asthma attack can be rapidly fatal.

It is important that CRDs are managed in a way that is integrated across public health programmes and primary and secondary care. Access to affordable good quality essential medicines for the treatment of asthma and COPD is critical. Progress to achieve this important goal within WHO's universal health coverage policy has been very limited in many low-income countries. Healthcare systems and their healthcare personnel, national professional societies and patient advocacy organizations need to increase their efforts to ensure improved access to medicines and that patients use their medicines and inhalers correctly and as prescribed. Relevant issues around universal health coverage and strengthening health systems are provided in Chapters 38 and 42.

Further guidance on CRDs is available from a number of authoritative publications including:

- The WHO package of essential NCD interventions for primary healthcare, which provides guidance on the diagnosis and treatment of asthma and COPD.[10]
- WHO's practical approach to lung health (PAL), which provides a syndromic approach to the management of patients who attend primary health care services for respiratory symptoms.[11] It largely emphasizes tuberculosis but also addresses other respiratory diseases. It is a multi-step process built on the development and implementation of guidelines for clinical respiratory disease practice with clearly defined coordination between different levels of the health system.
- The Global Initiative For Asthma (GINA), a collaboration launched by WHO and the US National Heart, Lung, and Blood Institute that aims to increase awareness of asthma among health professionals, health authorities and the general public; improve diagnosis, management and prevention; and stimulate research. It publishes annually updated evidence-based strategies for asthma management and prevention, which can be adapted for local use.[12]
- The Global Initiative for Chronic Obstructive Lung Disease (GOLD), which provides guidance for the management of COPD.[13]
- The WHO Model Essential Medicines List, which includes treatment options for asthma and COPD.[14]

Monitoring

Several indicators are useful to assess the capacity to investigate and treat CRDs, including the availability of diagnostic devices (spirometry, peak flow meter) and medicines including salbutamol and corticosteroid inhalers; the proportion of patients with COPD/asthma on treatment, proportion 'under control'; and proportions with exacerbations, lost to follow-up, treated by emergency departments, hospitalized for CRDs and who died.[15] Vital statistics, where available, can provide information on CRD mortality. Surveys are useful for assessing services provision and understanding trends (e.g. SARA,

Table 16.2 Examples of WHO global targets and indicators relevant for CRDs

Domain	Element	Target 2025 (baseline 2010)	Indicator
National systems' response.	Essential NCD medicines and basic technologies to treat major NCDs.	An 80% availability of the affordable basic technologies and essential medicines, including generics required to treat major NCDs in both public and private facilities.	Availability and affordability of quality, safe and efficacious essential NCDs medicines, including generics, and basic technologies in both public and private facilities.
Behavioural risk factors.	Tobacco control.	A 30% relative reduction in prevalence of current tobacco use in persons aged 15+ years.	Prevalence of current tobacco use among adolescents. Age-standardized prevalence of current tobacco use among persons aged 18+ years.

Chapter 5 on surveillance); such surveys should include public as well as private providers.

The WHO Global NCD Action Plan includes targets and indicators that are relevant to all main NCDs, including CRDs (Table 16.2). These and other indicators, for example, air pollution are described in more detail in other chapters.

Notes

1. GBD 2019 Diseases and Injuries Collaborators, Global burden of 369 diseases and injuries in 204 countries and territories, 1990–2019: a systematic analysis for the Global Burden of Disease Study 2019. *Lancet* 2020;396:1204–22.
2. Global surveillance, prevention and control of chronic respiratory diseases: a comprehensive approach. WHO, 2007.
3. Christenson SA et al. Chronic obstructive pulmonary disease. *Lancet* 2022;399:2227–42.
4. Global initiative for chronic obstructive lung disease, 2021.
5. García-Marcos L et al. The burden of asthma, hay fever and eczema in children in 25 countries: GAN phase I study. *Eur Respir J* 2022;60:2102866.
6. Global strategy for asthma management and prevention. Global Initiative for Asthma, 2021.
7. Clean household energy solutions toolkit (CHEST). WHO, 2018.
8. WHO global air quality guidelines: particulate matter (PM2.5 and PM10), ozone, nitrogen dioxide, sulfur dioxide and carbon monoxide. WHO, 2021.
9. Bissell K et al. Access to essential medicines to treat chronic respiratory disease in low-income countries. *Int J Tuberc Lung Dis* 2016;20:717–28.
10. Package of essential noncommunicable (PEN) disease interventions for primary health care. WHO, 2020.

11 Practical approach to lung health – Manual on initiating PAL implementation. WHO, 2008.
12 Reddel HK et al. Global initiative for asthma (GINA) strategy 2021 - Executive summary and rationale for key changes. *Am J Respir Crit Care Med* 2022;1:17–35.
13 Global initiative for chronic obstructive lung disease. https://goldcopd.org/.
14 Halpin DMG et al. Global initiative for the diagnosis, management, and prevention of chronic obstructive lung disease. The 2020 GOLD science committee report on COVID-19 and chronic obstructive pulmonary disease. *Am J Respir Crit Care Med* 2021;203:24–36.
15 Billo NE. Role of the global alliance against respiratory diseases in scaling up management of chronic respiratory diseases-summary meeting report. *J Thorac Dis* 2017;9:2337–38.

Part 3
Social determinants and risk factors for NCDs and priority interventions

17 Social determinants of health and NCDs

Ruth Bell, J Jaime Miranda, Jean Woo, Michael Marmot

Social determinants of health (SDH) are the conditions in which people are born, grow, live, work and age and the distribution of power, money and resources that drive these conditions. Examples of SDH include nutrition, education, housing, the built and natural environment, employment and working conditions, income/wealth, health care and the systems and policies that influence these conditions of daily life. In short, they are the causes of ill health – and for NCDs, this includes the upstream factors underlying the main environmental, behavioural, biological and psychosocial risk factors.

The WHO Commission on Social Determinants of Health[1] provided a framework (Figure 17.1) that has been widely used and adapted to identify opportunities for interventions to improve overall population health and reduce health inequities in many different contexts.[2,3,4,5]

SDH and health inequalities

Inequalities in SDH shape health inequities – the unfair and avoidable differences in health seen within and between countries. Health inequities within countries arise from differential experiences and exposures between groups in society, including by gender, ethnicity, socioeconomic position and geographical area of residence. Socioeconomic disadvantage is associated with a higher risk of premature mortality, NCDs and NCD risk factors, depending on underlying SDH in countries at different stages of development.[6,7] For example, educational level has been found to modify the association of household wealth with obesity, suggesting that education may break the link between increasing wealth and increasing obesity as countries develop.[8] Understanding the socioeconomic distribution of obesity in low- and middle-income countries is vital in developing appropriate context-specific responses to obesity-related NCDs.[9] Similarly, the risk of type-2 diabetes is consistently higher for individuals with the lowest vs highest level of education, occupation and income.[10] It is also well-established that a low socioeconomic position is associated with a substantial reduction in life expectancy.[11]

Tackling SDH is a constant theme that runs through the WHO Global NCD Action Plan. Both Objectives 3 and 4 explicitly refer to underlying social determinants.

DOI: 10.4324/9781003306689-20

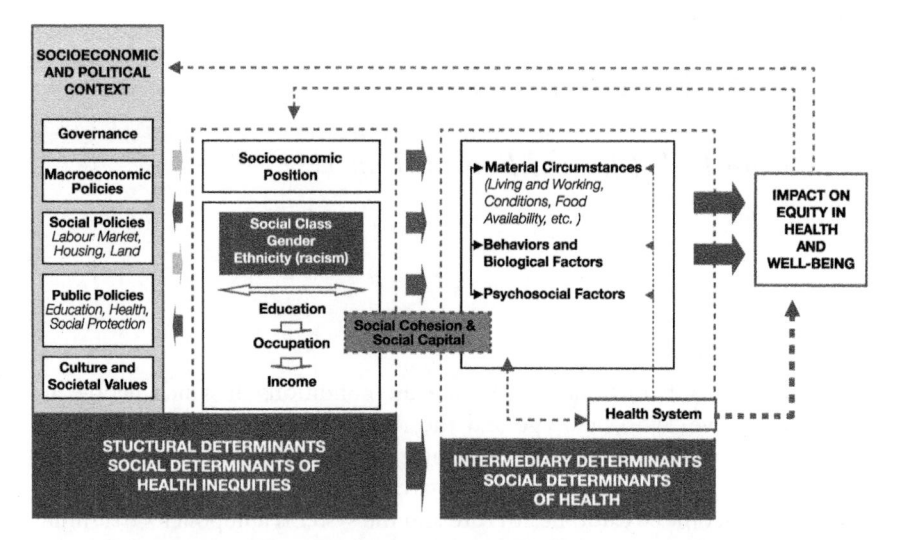

Figure 17.1 Conceptual Framework of the WHO Commission on Social Determinants of Health. (From: Solar O, Irwin A. A conceptual framework for action on the social determinants of health. Social Determinants of Health Discussion Paper 2 (Policy and Practice). WHO, 2010).

The impact of SDH on NCDs

Health inequities in NCD outcomes are linked to differential exposures to social determinants, which also structure the social distribution of health-related risk behaviours (such as unhealthy diet, tobacco use, harmful use of alcohol and insufficient physical activity). Psychosocial stress, such as stress associated with living in poverty, is linked with cardiovascular disease, both directly through biological pathways and indirectly through behavioural pathways. Unequal access to preventive health care is an additional important cause of inequities in NCD outcomes.

NCDs and the life-course

SDH act at all stages of life, from conception through childhood and onwards to older ages. Added to this, early life experiences track through life to affect health at older ages. This means that at any age, health reflects both past and present living conditions. Therefore, a life-course approach is important in understanding short- and longer-term risks for NCDs and for developing policies and interventions for NCD prevention (Chapter 37).

For example, poor maternal nutrition before and during pregnancy affects foetal development in ways that impact health in adulthood, including by increasing metabolic risk for NCDs.[12] Maternal and child nutrition and access to resources for a healthy life impact on the physical, cognitive, emotional and behavioural domains of early child development. Poor nutrition, and inadequate care and stimulation in the early years of life create conditions that limit children's opportunities to reach their full developmental potential.[13] Early life development disadvantages can track through to social and health disadvantages at older ages, including disadvantages in educational outcomes, reasoning ability, employment opportunities, income and access to resources for a healthy life, mental disorders and behavioural risks associated with NCDs. The onset of many NCDs occurs at younger ages in low- and middle-income countries, which is further accompanied by a longer duration of disease and a higher rate of complications including multimorbidity. This is compounded by limited access to preventative and treatment care and reliance on household caregiving including emotional and financial hardships. For these reasons, the early years are seen as a priority area for interventions to improve population health and reduce health inequities,[13,14] including NCDs.

Tackling SDH

The multiple dimensions of poverty (which include lack of money but also deprivation associated with health care, education, living standards, working conditions, housing and environmental conditions, among others) need to be addressed to improve health and prevent NCDs in the entire population. So must the social gradient, since it is not only the poorest in society who suffer preventable illness from NCDs and premature mortality but also those further up the social gradient.

Addressing the complex challenges of improving population health and reducing health inequalities requires responses at national, regional and local levels. National policies should therefore address SDH to tackle health inequities linked to NCDs. The health system, or indeed any system acting alone, cannot address the full breadth of SDH, and a whole system is needed with actions on SDH in multiple sectors across the life-course.

A key response to the social gradient in NCDs and related health behaviours is termed 'proportionate universalism'. This means that policies should be universal (i.e. targeting the whole population) but deployed at a scale and intensity proportionate to needs among different population sub-groups.[13] For example, smoke-free policies for enclosed workplaces and public places benefit everyone exposed in those places, while more targeted initiatives are needed to prevent the initiation of smoking among young people and to help smokers quit.

More broadly, social protection policies provide a safety net for those experiencing poverty, while targeted interventions can include active labour policies in areas of low employment. An umbrella review of macro-level determinants of health and health inequities reported that more generous welfare policies are associated with better health outcomes.[15]

Six areas for action were identified by the 2010 Marmot Review in England to improve health and reduce health inequities in relation to NCDs (Table 17.1).

Table 17.1 The six areas for action in the Marmot Review with examples of action for the prevention and control of NCDs

Areas for action	Areas relevant to NCDs	Examples of action
Give every child the best start in life.	Good nutrition for all children.	• Face-to-face education and peer counselling to support breastfeeding. • Conditional cash transfers. • Healthy food in school meals. • Growing vegetables in school gardens.
Enable all children, young people and adults to maximize their capabilities and have control over their lives.	Reduce stress-related risk behaviours (e.g. smoking, substance misuse and eating junk foods).	• Invest in education and lifelong learning, particularly in more deprived areas and communities. • Invest in reducing access to unsafe substances, including tobacco and alcohol, among adolescents.
Create fair employment and good work for all.	Reduce work stress and physical occupational hazards. Reduce in-work poverty.	• Apply management and occupational health standards in all workplaces. • Introduce healthy living wage legislation. • Economic and active labour market policies to increase opportunities for employment.
Ensure a healthy standard of living for all.	Reduce poverty and inequality.	• Establish a minimum income for healthy living for people of all ages. • Universal and generous welfare policies. • Reducing the impact of inflation on the poor. Subsidies and social welfare policies (including targeted safety nets such as cash transfers, food, and in-kind transfers, and school feeding programmes) can be used to protect the poorest from rising prices.
Create and develop healthy and sustainable places and communities.	Improve availability of healthy foods. Increase opportunities for outdoor physical activity. Reduce outdoor air pollution. Reduce indoor air pollution.	• Town planning to regulate the number of fast-food outlets near schools and in deprived areas. • Food policy taxes for products of limited or no nutritional value. • Improve the quality and amount of green space in urban areas with fewer and lower quality of accessible green space. • Transport and planning policies to encourage modal shift to active transport. • Regulate vehicle emissions. • Municipal waste management e.g. ban burning organic waste in favour of recycling organic waste.

(Continued)

Table 17.1 (Continued)

Areas for action	Areas relevant to NCDs	Examples of action
		• Incentivize replacement of traditional use of wood or charcoal for home cooking with less polluting alternatives (e.g. biogas).
		• Invest in and incentivize energy-efficient heating and ventilation in homes and buildings.
Strengthen the role and impact of ill-health prevention.	Ensure availability, accessibility and acceptability of preventive health care to all.	• Outreach programmes to widen access to preventive health care.

Regional and local authority or municipal areas are well suited to adopting a system-wide approach to addressing SDH, since local partners can convene meetings to bring together all relevant local sectors and actors, including public services, the health sector, voluntary organizations, the business sector and community organizations. In addition, local partners are nearer to the people, in a good position to understand local needs and advise about them, and include locally trusted organizations. In so doing, they are key actors and facilitators in augmenting social cohesion and enhancing social capital.

A crucial component of efforts to tackle NCDs and inequities in NCDs at the local level is community empowerment to enable community participation in making changes in local areas. A randomized control study in village settings in Bangladesh, where a third of adults have type-2 diabetes or intermediate hyperglycaemia, found that community mobilization through a participatory learning and action process significantly reduced the combined prevalence of type-2 diabetes and intermediate hyperglycaemia.[16] The intervention also strengthened health literacy, built self-efficacy among individuals and communities, and reduced gender barriers to physical activity.[17] In Peru, a community-wide salt substitution strategy built with inputs from local voices using a social marketing strategy showed population-wide reductions in blood pressure.[18]

Achieving multiple benefits from interventions is important in strengthening communities and in sustaining the benefits of interventions. Crucially, partners working together can achieve progress towards their own sectoral goals as well as contribute to those of their partners. Understanding each other's language, recognizing shared agendas, looking for multiple wins and agreeing on indicators of progress are important elements in addressing SDH.

132   *Ruth Bell et al.*

The Milan Urban Food Policy Pact demonstrated how cities and urban areas can lead to change in ways that have multiple benefits. This pact is an international commitment by cities around the world to develop sustainable urban food policies; it has specific goals, including sustainable, healthy and safe food for all, and a monitoring framework. As an example, the municipal authority of Curitiba, Brazil, developed programmes that enabled low-income families to access healthy food at affordable prices, while strengthening local agricultural producers, through co-operatives, to access local markets, bringing economic benefits as well as healthier food to the local area.[19]

Monitoring

Monitoring and evaluation are important to guide policy and programmes to reduce inequities in NCDs through action on the SDH. A set of indicators across the social determinants may include indicators relevant to early years development, education, employment, income, housing, transport, environment, the strength of community, access to health care, health behaviours, health and wellbeing. More generally, disaggregation of data by gender, ethnicity, socioeconomic position, disability and geography provides information about the extent and depth of inequities.

Data availability and quality are highly variable in countries around the world. The 2030 Agenda for Sustainable Development, with a focus on promoting health equity, has provided extra impetus in developing national data systems to monitor progress across its 17 goals. In response, WHO has developed a stepwise approach to monitoring health equity and SDH with guidance for monitoring.[20] Meanwhile, lack of data need not be a barrier to taking action to promote health equity. When data are not available at the national level, locally collected information can provide the basis for developing local initiatives and monitoring progress.

Notes

1 WHO commission on social determinants of health, final report: closing the gap in a generation: health equity through action on the social determinants of health. WHO, 2008.
2 Just societies: health equity and dignified lives. Report of the Commission of the Pan American Health Organization on Equity and Health Inequalities in the Americas. PAHO, Washington, 2019.
3 Build back fairer: achieving health equity in the Eastern Mediterranean Region. WHO EMRO Commission on Social Determinants of Health in the Eastern Mediterranean Region, 2021.
4 Health inequalities in Taiwan. Health Institute of Health Equity, Ministry of Health, Taiwan, 2016.
5 Build back fairer: reducing socioeconomic inequalities in health in Hong Kong. Chinese University of Hong Kong and UCL Institute of Health Equity, 2020.

6. Sommer I et al. Socioeconomic inequalities in non-communicable diseases and their risk factors: an overview of systematic reviews. *BMC Public Health* 2015;15:914.
7. Miranda JJ et al. Understanding the rise of cardiometabolic diseases in low- and middle-income countries. *Nat Med 2019*;25:1667–79.
8. Aitsi-Selmi A et al. Education modifies the association of wealth with obesity in women in middle-income but not low-income countries: an interaction study using seven national datasets, 2005–2010. *PlosOne* 2014;9:e90403.
9. Jiwani SS et al. The shift of obesity burden by socioeconomic status between 1998 and 2017 in Latin America and the Caribbean: a cross-sectional series study. *Lancet Glob Health* 2019;7:e1644–54.
10. Agardh E et al. Type 2 diabetes incidence and socio-economic position: a systematic review and meta-analysis. *Int J Epidemiol* 2011;40:804–18.
11. Stringhini S et al. Socioeconomic status and the 25 × 25 risk factors as determinants of premature mortality: a multicohort study and meta-analysis of 1·7 million men and women. *Lancet* 2017;389:1229–37.
12. Wilkins E et al. Maternal nutrition and its intergenerational links to non-communicable disease metabolic risk factors: a systematic review and narrative synthesis. *J Health Popul Nutr* 2021;40:20.
13. Strategic review of health inequalities in England post-2010. *Fair society, healthy lives: (the Marmot review)*. London, 2010; Institute of Health Equity.
14. Hurley KM et al. Early child development and nutrition: a review of the benefits and challenges of implementing integrated interventions. *Adv Nutr* 2016;7:357–63.
15. Naik Y et al. Going upstream – an umbrella review of the macroeconomic determinants of health and health inequalities. *BMC Public Health* 2019;19:1678.
16. Fottrell E et al. Community groups or mobile phone messaging to prevent and control type 2 diabetes and intermediate hyperglycaemia in Bangladesh (DMagic): a cluster-randomised controlled trial. *Lancet Diab Endocrinol* 2019;7:200–12.
17. Morrison J et al. Participatory learning and action to address type 2 diabetes in rural Bangladesh: a qualitative process evaluation. *BMC Endocr Disord* 2019;19:118.
18. Bernabe-Ortiz A et al. Effect of salt substitution on community-wide blood pressure and hypertension incidence. *Nat Med* 2020:26:374–78.
19. Forster T et al (editors). *Milan urban food policy pact. Selected good practices from cities.* Fondazione Giangiacomo Feltrinelli, Milan, 2015.
20. Hosseinpoor AR et al. Measuring health inequalities in the context of sustainable development goals. *Bull WHO* 2018;96:654–59.

18 Tobacco use

Burden, epidemiology and priority interventions

Pascal Bovet, Nick Banatvala, Jude Gedeon, Armando Peruga

Tobacco use is the leading, fully preventable cause of mortality globally. A number of interventions are highly effective in reducing tobacco use but in most countries are not fully implemented.

Disease burden

Table 18.1 shows that tobacco use accounted for 15.4% of all deaths globally (8.7 million) in 2019, up from 14.5% (6.8 million) in 1990 (IHME). Secondhand smoke accounted for 1.3 million tobacco-related deaths in 2019. The increase in proportionate mortality decreased between 1990 and 2019 in high-income countries (HICs) but increased in lower-middle-income countries, partly owing to tighter control measures in the former than the latter. The age-standardized mortality rates attributable to tobacco use have decreased markedly in all income country regions, which reflects the decreasing prevalence of smoking in all populations between 1990 and 2019 (largely due to tobacco control policy).

At the global level, tobacco-related deaths in 2019 were attributable, mainly, to cardiovascular diseases (CVD) (36.7%), cancer (29.9%), chronic respiratory diseases (20.6%) and respiratory infections (7.0%) (IHME).

Prevalence of tobacco use

The age-standardized prevalence of tobacco smoking ranged between 7% and 65% in men and between 1% and 40% in women across countries, corresponding to 1.14 billion current smokers smoking 7.41 trillion cigarette-equivalents in 2019.[1] Globally, 15% and 8% of boys and girls aged 15 years had smoked at least one cigarette during the past 30 days, with large differences between countries.[2] The overall prevalence of tobacco smoking has decreased substantially between 1990 and 2019 (by 28% in men and 38% in women). However, the total number of smokers globally has increased slightly over the last 30 years (from 0.99 billion in 1990 to 1.14 billion in 2019), largely because of population growth. The greatest declines in smoking prevalence have occurred in men and women of Latin America and the Caribbean. In

DOI: 10.4324/9781003306689-21

Table 18.1 Mortality attributable to tobacco use (IHME)

	Global 1990	Global 2019	HICs 1990	HICs 2019	Upper MICs 1990	Upper MICs 2019	Lower MICs 1990	Lower MICs 2019	LICs 1990	LICs 2019
Number of deaths (million)	6.8	8.7	2.0	1.8	2.9	4.9	1.7	2.6	0.18	0.26
Proportion of all deaths (%)	14.5	15.4	23.0	18.9	19.4	20.4	9.5	12.5	3.7	5.2
Age-standardized rates (per 100,000)	178	109	152	78	209	123	176	122	121	87

contrast, the smallest declines have happened among women in Central Asia and men and women in North Africa and the Eastern Mediterranean. Yet, the prevalence of tobacco use has increased, between 1990 and 2019, in a minority of countries in all regions, particularly in Eastern Europe, Central Asia and Middle East countries, and generally more often among women than men. Likewise, the prevalence of tobacco use among adolescents has decreased in a majority of countries between 2010 and 2018 but increased in a few countries in different regions.[2]

Socioeconomic impact

Tobacco use not only brings suffering, disease and death, but it also impoverishes families and national economies. The global economic cost of smoking (from health expenditures and productivity losses) was estimated to be as high as US$ 1.4 trillion in 2012, i.e. around 2% of the world's annual gross domestic product.[3] In addition, tobacco use results in substantial expenses for the treatment of smoking-related diseases and loss of revenue, making smoking an important cause of impoverishment for many smokers.

Interventions to reduce tobacco use in the population

The WHO Framework Convention on Tobacco Control (WHO FCTC) and the Protocol to Eliminate Illicit Trade in Tobacco Products (Chapter 33) aim to protect present and future generations from tobacco by establishing an evidence-based minimal legal set of demand and supply reduction provisions that Parties (countries) sign up to deliver. It is essential that countries have well-functioning national mechanisms for coordination of the WHO FCTC implementation.

To support countries in implementing the demand reduction measures of the WHO FCTC, WHO has developed the MPOWER package (**M**onitoring tobacco consumption, **P**rotecting people from tobacco smoke, **O**ffering help to quit tobacco use, **W**arning about the dangers of tobacco, **E**nforcing bans on tobacco advertising, promotion and sponsorship, **R**aising taxes on tobacco).

Interventions at the population level

(★ indicates a best buy, + indicates effective or recommended interventions as defined in the WHO Global NCD Action Plan for both population and individual level interventions).

Measures that reduce the demand for tobacco products

- *Raising tobacco taxes*★ to increase real tobacco prices is the most powerful single measure to curb the demand for tobacco products. Any increase or decrease in the price of cigarettes is rapidly associated with a commensurate change in the prevalence of cigarette use. WHO advises that the proportion of total tax should exceed 70% of the retail sale price of a tobacco product. Unfortunately, tobacco tax remains relatively low in a majority of countries across the world. In 2020, only 13% of the global population lived in countries protected by tax accounting for 75% or more of the sale price of the most popular brand of cigarettes. When implementing tobacco taxation, key principles include: (i) making taxation as simple as possible, e.g. by applying a specific excise tax to tobacco products, in addition to the other usual sale and trade taxes; (ii) ensuring that excise tax increases regularly to reduce the affordability of tobacco products, and is at least adjusted for inflation; (iii) applying tax in a way that minimizes incentives for tobacco users to switch to cheaper brands, e.g. the same excise tax to all cigarettes. Detailed guidance on developing, implementing and enforcing tobacco taxation is available.[4]
- Develop comprehensive legislation to ban or restrict tobacco advertising, promotion and sponsorship (TAPS)★ in all media, including plain packaging, and a ban of insidious sponsorship under the pretence of corporate social responsibility.
- Protect by law from secondhand smoke exposure in all indoor workplaces, public places and public transport★. This should be extended to as many public and private settings as possible, particularly those attended by minors (e.g. sports premises, cultural and social venues, cars).
- Implement plain/standardized packaging and/or large graphic health warnings on all tobacco packages.★ The WHO FCTC states that the area for pictorial warnings should cover ≥50% of the main sides of tobacco product packets.
- Implement regularly effective mass media campaigns to educate the public about the harms of smoking/tobacco use and secondhand smoke.★

Measures to reduce the supply of tobacco products

- Implement measures to minimize illicit trade in tobacco products+ (e.g. tracing and tracking of cigarette packets based on packet unique identifiers).
- Ban cross-border advertising, including using modern means of communication.+

- Ban the sale of tobacco products by and to minors.
- Ban added flavours (which can make tobacco use more attractive, particularly to young people).
- Limit retail sale and display of tobacco products by:
  - Ensuring that tobacco products for sale cannot be accessed directly by customers but only through vendors (who can check a client's age).
  - Banning the sale of individual cigarettes. Single-stick sales facilitate smoking among non-affluent youth and those beginning smoking.
  - Banning tobacco vending machines (as they are both advertising points and usually accessible to minors).
- Promote economically viable alternative livelihoods for tobacco workers and growers as part of moving away from tobacco farming. Tobacco growing is often associated with child labour, health risks for farmers and deforestation, thereby contributing to climate change and jeopardizing food security.

The demand and supply measures mentioned above are addressed in more detail in Chapter 33 on the WHO FCTC.

Interventions at the individual level

- Provide cost-covered, effective and population-wide support (including brief advice, national toll-free quitline services) for tobacco cessation to all those who want to quit.[+]

Interventions for smoking cessation at the individual level are essential for rapidly decreasing the tobacco-related disease burden, given that public health measures can take years to curb the tobacco prevalence in populations. Simple advice to quit smoking that is given by health professionals results in smoking cessation in a small proportion of smokers, yet this measure is highly cost-effective given the low cost of this measure; this advice should be part of usual health care for all smoking patients.[5] Nicotine replacement therapy (e.g. nicotine gums or patches) and other pharmacological interventions (e.g. bupropion or varenicline) reduces symptoms of nicotine withdrawal among smokers who want to quit smoking, and can double a smoker's odds of quitting successfully, particularly when used in adjunction to counselling.[6] However, behavioural and pharmacological interventions result in one-year cessation in <20% of treated cigarette smokers at best. This emphasizes the importance of well-organized tobacco cessation programmes with trained personnel who can provide quality care for smokers who wish to quit. The frequent failure of smoking cessation attempts emphasizes the need for repeated cessation attempts.

Electronic cigarettes

Electronic nicotine and non-nicotine delivery systems (EN&NNDS), also known as electronic cigarettes, supply an aerosol for inhalation by the user that contains some toxicants. Therefore, they are not harmless. Under typical conditions of use, however, the total amount of potentially toxic substances emitted from unadulterated EN&NNDS is generally lower than in cigarette smoke, except for some metals. Although long-term effects on morbidity and mortality have not yet been studied sufficiently, EN&NNDS are not safe for young people, pregnant women and adults who have never smoked. While EN&NNDS increase health risks, non-pregnant adult smokers can reduce their overall risk if they switch entirely from combustible cigarettes to the use of unadulterated and appropriately regulated EN&NNDS alone, particularly if this is a step toward total abstinence from both tobacco and EN&NNDS. Moderate evidence shows that some smokers may successfully quit tobacco by using some types of ENDS, while others experience no difference or are even prevented from quitting. While some types of ENDS may help some smokers to quit combustible cigarettes under certain circumstances,[7] the evidence is insufficient to issue a blanket recommendation to use any type of ENDS as a cessation aid for all smokers.[8]

The way industry undermines efforts to tobacco control

Chapter 56 on the private sector describes issues around industries that are not aligned with public health goals and policies and laws that influence behaviours and can reduce the NCD burden. The WHO FCTC defines the tobacco industry as tobacco manufacturers, wholesale distributors and importers of tobacco products. The tobacco industry uses a range of tactics to undermine tobacco control measures, using its economic power, lobbying and marketing machinery, and manipulation of the media to discredit scientific research and influence governments in order to propagate the sale and distribution of its products.[9] As part of this, the tobacco industry continues to fund a range of tobacco industry front groups and inject large philanthropic contributions into social programmes worldwide to create a positive public image under the guise of corporate social responsibility.[10] Most recently, WHO has described a set of SCARE tactics to influence the political economy of tobacco, including: **s**muggling and illicit trade, **c**ourt and legal challenges, **a**nti-poor rhetoric, **r**evenue reduction, and **e**mployment impact. A number of organizations have dedicated websites providing up-to-date information on the activities and tactics of the tobacco industry.[11,12,13]

Monitoring

Monitoring tobacco use and patterns (e.g. which tobacco products or e-cigarettes are used, how frequently, cessation attempts) and associated variables (e.g. individual, family and social co-variates) relies on population-based surveys of children and adults. Surveys can also be conducted by telephone or through other electronic media. Surveys should be conducted regularly (e.g. every 5–10 years) to monitor trends over time. Simple and standardized survey methodology has been developed to provide information on tobacco use, e.g. WHO STEPS (adults), the Global School-based Student Health Survey (age 13–15 years), and the School-based Global Youth Tobacco Survey (age 13–15 years). These survey instruments are described in more detail in Chapter 5 on surveillance tools. Useful information, and trends over time, can also be derived from sales/taxation data (acknowledging that sales data do not account for smuggled or counterfeit cigarettes).

Relevant global targets and indicators for tobacco control

A 30% relative reduction in the prevalence of current tobacco use in persons aged 15+ years (NCD GBD target).	Prevalence of current tobacco use among adolescents.
	Age-standardized prevalence of current tobacco use among persons aged 18+ years.
Strengthen the implementation of the WHO FCTC in all countries (SDG Target 3.a).	Age-standardized prevalence of current tobacco use among persons aged 15+ years (SDG target 3.a.1).

Way ahead

While many countries have implemented several tobacco control measures and the prevalence of tobacco use (at least cigarette smoking) is decreasing in many countries, but not in all, it is estimated that 100 million deaths would have been avoided between 2009 and 2017 if increased tax, ban on TAPS and ban on smoking in enclosed premises had been implemented strictly worldwide since 2009.[14] A 1-unit increase in the MPOWER composite score reduces the prevalence of smoking by 0.2 percentage points and cigarette consumption by 23 cigarettes per capita per year.[15] Among the 41 countries that had adopted at least one highest-level MPOWER policy between 2007 and 2010, the number of smokers dropped by 14.8 million, with 7.4 million smoking-attributable deaths averted during that period.[16] There remains a huge need to accelerate the full implementation of the tobacco control measures worldwide.

Notes

1 GBD 2019 Tobacco Collaborators. Spatial, temporal, and demographic patterns in prevalence of smoking tobacco use and attributable disease burden in 204 countries and territories, 1990–2019: a systematic analysis from the Global Burden of Disease Study 2019. *Lancet* 2021;397:2337–60.
2 Ma C et al. Prevalence and trends in tobacco use among adolescents aged 13–15 years in 143 countries, 1999–2018: findings from the Global Youth Tobacco Surveys. *Lancet Child Adolesc Health* 2021;5:245–55.
3 Goodchild et al. Global economic cost of smoking-attributable diseases. *Tob Control* 2018;27:58–64.
4 WHO technical manual on tobacco tax policy and administration. WHO, 2021.

5 Stead LF et al. Physician advice for smoking cessation. *Cochrane Database Syst Rev* 2013;5:CD000165.
6 Silagy C et al. Nicotine replacement therapy for smoking cessation. *Cochrane Database Syst Rev* 2004;3:CD000146.
7 Balfour DJK et al. Balancing consideration of the risks and benefits of E-cigarettes. *Am J Public Health* 2021;111:1661–72.
8 WHO report on the global tobacco epidemic 2021: addressing new and emerging products. WHO, 2021.
9 Big tobacco: exposing its deadly tactics. Campaign for Tobacco-Free Kids, 2010.
10 Tobacco Industry Front Group: the International Tobacco Growers' Association. Campaign for Tobacco-Free Kids, 2011.
11 Tobacco Industry Interference. The Global Centre for Good Governance in Tobacco Control and WHO FCTC Secretariat (web site).
12 Tobacco Tactics. University of Bath, United Kingdom (web site).
13 Truth Tobacco Industry Documents. University of California San Francisco (web site).
14 Flor LS et al. The effects of tobacco control policies on global smoking prevalence. *Nat Med* 2021;27:239–43.
15 Ngo A et al. The effect of MPOWER scores on cigarette smoking prevalence and consumption. *Prev Med* 2017;105S:S10–14.
16 Levy DT et al. Smoking-related deaths averted due to three years of policy progress. *Bull WHO* 2013;91:509–18.

19 Unhealthy diets

Burden, epidemiology and priority interventions

Francesco Branca, Pascal Bovet, Namukolo Covic, Elisabetta Recine

An unhealthy diet is a leading modifiable cause of noncommunicable diseases (NCDs), particularly cardiovascular disease (CVD). A number of population-based interventions in multiple sectors can encourage the adoption of healthy diets by individuals.

Disease burden

According to IHME (Table 19.1), 14.1% (7.9 million) of all deaths in 2019 were attributable to dietary risks (the specific dietary risks considered by IHME in these estimates are listed in the next paragraph), with 86% of these diet-related deaths being attributable to cardiovascular disease (CVD), 8% to cancer and 6% to diabetes. The proportions of deaths attributable to dietary risks increased between 1990 and 2019 in all countries except high-income countries (HICs), which partly reflects aging populations. However, the *age-standardized* rates of mortality attributable to dietary risks decreased in all regions (with the largest decreases in HICs and upper-middle-income countries [MICs]), partly reflecting improvements in some components of the diet over time[1] and improving prevention and control of outcomes due to dietary risks (e.g. CVD), particularly in HICs. Of note, these estimates do not account for malnutrition, underweight, mineral deficiencies and high body mass (BMI) (see Chapter 10 on obesity).

The overall dietary risk described in Table 19.1 combines several specific dietary risks. IHME has estimated that the proportions of all deaths in 2019 that could have been prevented for different dietary risks were (proportions of all CVD deaths that would be prevented are mentioned in parentheses): high sodium 3.3% (9.2%); low whole grains 3.3% (8.6%); low legumes 2.0% (6.0%); low fruit 1.9% (4.5%); high red meat 1.6% (4.0%); high trans fat 1.1% (3.5%); low fibre 1.1% (2.9%); low nuts and seeds 1.0% (3.0%); low vegetables 0.94% (2.8%); low polyunsaturated fats (PUFA) 0.61% (1.9%); low seafood omega 3 fatty acids 0.60% (1.8%); high processed meat 0.54% (1.1%); high sweetened beverages 0.43% (1.1%); low milk 0.29%; and low calcium 0.24%. Notwithstanding the primary goal to improve the overall quality of diet for improved health, these estimates show the potential impacts that could result from interventions on these specific dietary risks.

DOI: 10.4324/9781003306689-22

Table 19.1 Mortality attributable to dietary risks (IHME)

	Global 1990	Global 2019	HICs 1990	HICs 2019	Upper MICs 1990	Upper MICs 2019	Lower MICs 1990	Lower MICs 2019	LICs 1990	LICs 2019
Proportion of all deaths (%)	11.6	14.1	18.8	13.4	14.9	17.5	7.7	13.0	3.6	6.2
Age-standardized mortality (per 100,000)	154	101	126	58	175	111	162	132	136	114

Key elements of a healthy diet

Briefly, a healthy diet includes the following: [2,3]

- Breastfeeding infants and young children.
- Balancing energy intake and expenditure to achieve and maintain a healthy body weight.
- Consumption of: (i) at least five portions a day of fruits and vegetables, whole grains (rather than refined grains) and legumes; (ii) proteins from plants (legumes), fish/seafood, meat and poultry, and limit red and processed meat; and (iii) liquid plant oils (e.g. olive, sunflower, soybean) rather than tropical oils (coconut, palm, and palm kernel), animal fats (e.g. butter and lard) and partially hydrogenated oils, and consuming low-fat dairy products instead of high-fat ones, given the high saturated fat content in the latter vs the former.
- Minimizing intake of: (i) beverages and foods containing free sugars (sodas and fruit juices) to keep daily intake of free sugars <10% of total energy intake, or possibly <5% for maximum health benefits and foods with high levels of added salt to keep daily intake <5 g (approx. 2 g sodium) per day.
- Avoiding highly processed foods (as these tend to be high in energy, sugar, fats and salt), and avoiding or limiting alcohol intake.

Broader determinants

It has been estimated that a healthy diet, which would be based predominantly on fresh and unrefined products is not affordable for around 3 billion people, a challenge across all regions of the world.[4]

There are complex and important relationships between globalization, trade, a country's geographic location, access to global and domestic markets (including volatility in prices), and production, distribution and supply chains that can have a major impact on people's ability to access food for a healthy diet.[5,6] For example, obtaining affordable fresh, frozen, or other adequately packaged fruit and vegetables on a regular basis throughout the year is obviously more difficult in some places than others. In addition, changes in the food environment have led to an increase in the consumption of industrially processed foods in many countries.

In addition, a number of determinants affect the population's and an individual's choice of food. These include: (i) biological determinants such as hunger, appetite and taste; (ii) economic determinants such as cost and income; (iii) physical determinants such as access, availability, education, knowledge, skills and time; (iv) social determinants such as class, culture and social context; (v) psychological determinants such as mood, stress and guilt; and (vi) attitudes, beliefs and knowledge about food.[7]

National Food-Based Dietary Guidelines

National Food-Based Dietary Guidelines (FBDGs) provide context-specific guidance on healthy diets and lifestyles, informed by sound scientific evidence and responding to a country's public health and nutrition priorities, food production and consumption patterns, sociocultural influences and accessibility, among other factors. FAO has collected and analyzed FBDGs from over 100 countries worldwide, adapted to their nutrition situation, food availability, culinary cultures and eating habits.[8]

FGDGs can also be used to highlight sustainability considerations that policymakers, food producers and consumers can make to promote alignment between a healthy diet and what a sustainable diet should be, i.e. one that promotes all dimensions of individuals' health and wellbeing; has low environmental pressure and impact; is accessible, affordable, safe and equitable; and is culturally acceptable.[9]

Interventions at the population level

Improving diets requires action across all components of food systems. Food systems include all the elements (environment, people, inputs, processes, infrastructures, institutions, etc.) and activities that relate to the production, processing, distribution, preparation and consumption of food, and the outputs of these activities, such as socio-economic and environmental outcomes.

Changing diets requires action across: (i) supply chains (including production systems, storage and distribution, processing and packaging, retail and markets); (ii) the food environment (food availability and access, promotion, advertising and information, food quality and safety); and (iii) consumer behaviours (preferences on foods to acquire, prepare, cook, store and eat).[10,11]

While a number of processed foods (e.g. breakfast cereals, industrially produced bread, etc.) may be fortified/supplemented with a number of potentially healthy nutrients (vitamins, minerals) and can be convenient to consumers (e.g. shorter preparation time), many have high contents of fats, sugars and salt, which can trigger weight gain, hypertension, cancer, CVD and other conditions.

A number of key food system interventions for a healthy diet are described below as well as in other chapters (e.g. Chapter 10 on obesity, Chapter 20 on cholesterol, fats and trans fats, Chapter 21 on salt, Chapter 22 on sugary drinks, and Chapter 26 on alcohol), which also include details on WHO technical packages such as SHAKE (salt reduction), SAFER (alcohol) and REPLACE (trans fats).

Reformulation of processed foods

This is an effective and efficient way to reduce the intake of energy, saturated fats, trans fat, sugars and salt in processed foods. The reformulation of processed foods by industry enables people to avoid making particular efforts to change their usual eating habits. Approaches to the reformulation of selected foods can be mandatory or voluntary. Chapter 23 on food reformulation provides further detail.

Nutrition labelling

Nutrition labelling enables consumers to better select the products they buy. In addition to factual information (e.g. content of macro or micronutrients, e.g. calories, sugar, saturated fats, salt, etc.), interpretive labels (e.g. front-of-pack warning labels with a star rating or colour-coded systems) can be used to facilitate informed choices by consumers. Chapter 24 on nutrition labelling provides further detail.

Fiscal policies

Fiscal and pricing policies, including taxes and subsidies, are valuable tools for promoting healthy diets. There is increasing evidence that raising taxes for the retail price of sugar-sweetened beverages by 10–20% can reduce their consumption (Chapter 22 on sugar-sweetened beverages). There is similar evidence that subsidies for producing fresh fruits and vegetables that reduce prices by 10–30% are effective in increasing their consumption.[12] While taxes on unhealthy foods have been challenged for having a regressive effect, they are most likely to decrease health inequalities.[13] Chapter 41 on fiscal measures provides more detail.

Marketing

The pervasive marketing of processed foods and drinks high in energy, free sugars or salt influences food preferences, purchases and consumption patterns, particularly in children. Marketing techniques have evolved from using traditional media, such as television, radio and billboards, to digital media including social media, sponsorship, product placement, sales promotion, cross-promotions using celebrities, brand mascots or characters popular with children, websites, packaging, nutrition labelling, point-of-purchase displays, e-mails and text messages. Voluntary and legal instruments have been used to restrict marketing food and beverages to children, with various scopes (e.g. age of children, target foods and beverages, target marketing approaches).

Following the endorsement of the 2010 WHO set of recommendations on the marketing of foods and non-alcoholic beverages to children,[14] several voluntary pledges were made and a few mandatory regulations were established. Nevertheless, marketing to children remains highly pervasive, including in areas where children gather. Policy and regulator action should therefore be developed and implemented as there is evidence that they are effective in limiting the marketing of unhealthy food to children.[15]

Public food procurement

Regulation is important to encourage the public sector to provide foods and beverages in public settings (e.g. hospitals, schools, workplaces, nursing homes, and correctional facilities) that contribute to a healthy diet.[16] Supply chains need to be developed or adapted to ensure the regular provision of fresh foods and food operators need to be adequately trained. These settings have an important role in promoting nutrition literacy.

Communication campaigns

Simple messages need to be developed, carefully aimed at behaviours that require the greatest attention. FBDGs can be used to help develop communication messages for the population, for example through food guides, often using pictorial forms such as food pyramids and food plates as well as providing entry points for different food systems actors to contribute to attaining healthier diets. Development of FBDGs should be promoted in all countries (currently only nine African countries have FBDGs). Online practical tools, such as the USDA programme My Plate, can also be helpful.

Communication campaigns are, however, expensive to implement and have to compete with the much larger investment in food marketing by the food industry (Chapter 50 on communication). While their impact is generally modest,[17] they are important as complementary interventions to the strategies described above.

Interventions at the individual level

Dietary counselling at the healthcare level is an important component of the management protocol for several chronic diseases, mainly CVD, hypertension, obesity and diabetes (this is discussed in other chapters in the compendium).[18,19]

For a number of population and individual interventions, cost-effectiveness analyses have been conducted, and they form part of the WHO best buys and recommended interventions (Box 19.1).

Box 19.1 shows a menu of cost-effective interventions recommended by the WHO to change diets at the population and individual levels.[20]

BOX 19.1 WHO BEST BUYS, EFFECTIVE INTERVENTIONS, AND OTHER INTERVENTIONS TO CHANGE DIETS AT THE POPULATION AND INDIVIDUAL LEVELS

Best buys

- Reduce salt intake through reformulation of food products to contain less salt, and set target levels for maximum amounts of salt in foods and meals.
- Reduce salt intake through the establishment of a supportive environment in public institutions such as hospitals, schools, workplaces and nursing homes to enable lower sodium options to be provided.
- Reduce salt intake through behaviour change communication campaigns and mass media.
- Reduce salt intake through the implementation of front-of-pack nutrition labelling.

Effective interventions

- Eliminate industrial trans fats through the development of legislation to ban their use in the food chain.
- Reduce sugar consumption through effective taxation on sugar-sweetened beverages.

Other recommended interventions

- Promote and support exclusive breastfeeding for the first six months of life, including promotion of breastfeeding.
- Implement subsidies to increase the intake of fruits and vegetables (compatibly with available resources).
- Replace trans fats and saturated fats with unsaturated fats through food reformulation, nutrition labelling, fiscal policies or agricultural policies.
- Limit portion and package size to reduce energy intake and the risk of being overweight/obese.
- Implement nutrition education and counselling in different settings (e.g. in preschools, schools, workplaces and hospitals) to increase the intake of fruits and vegetables.

- Implement nutrition labelling to encourage consumers to reduce total energy intake, sugars, sodium and fats.
- Implement mass media campaigns on healthy diets, including social marketing to reduce the intake of total fat, saturated fats, sugars and salt, and promote the intake of fruits and vegetables, as well as drinking water instead of sugar-sweetened beverages.

In addition to being an important cause of NCDs, unhealthy, inequitable and unsustainable food systems are at the root of many of the world's most pressing threats to human, animal and planetary health, including negative impacts on the environment with degradation of arable lands, water and oceans, reduced biodiversity, climate change and air quality.[21] Political commitment and action across government and society are critical to meet the challenges and have the potential to result in significant co-benefits for health and broader sustainable development (Chapters 53 and 54 on whole-of-government and whole-of-society).

Monitoring

Monitoring nutrition and the impact of policies is critical. Population surveys (e.g. WHO-STEPS, Chapter 5) are useful to assess dietary patterns in the population through food questionnaires and/or using biological markers (e.g. salt in urine, blood carotene levels). The WHO/FAO GIFT platform is used to disseminate information on individual dietary intake.[22] Monitoring the policies of countries is done, for example, through the WHO Country Capacity Survey, the WHO Global nutrition policy reviews and the WHO Global database on the Implementation of Nutrition Actions.

Regularly assessment of the content of common processed foods should also be done (e.g. sugar, salt, saturated fats, and trans fats), noting that there are often differences between the same product brands between countries and over time.[23]

Notes

1. Imamura F et al. Dietary quality among men and women in 187 countries in 1990 and 2010: a systematic assessment. *Lancet Glob Health* 2015;3:e132–42.
2. https://www.who.int/news-room/questions-and-answers/item/healthy-diet-keys-to-eating-well.
3. Lichtenstein AH et al. Dietary guidance to improve cardiovascular health: a scientific statement from the American Heart Association. *Circulation* 2021;144:e472–87.
4. The state of food security and nutrition in the world 2021 – Transforming food systems for food security, improved nutrition and affordable healthy diets for all. FAO, IFAD, UNICEF, WFP and WHO, 2021.
5. *Managing food price volatility: policy options to support healthy diets and nutrition in the context of uncertainty*. London: Global Panel on Agriculture and Food Systems for Nutrition, Policy brief, 2016.

6. Greb F, Rapsomanikis G. Food price volatility in landlocked developing countries. Ferdi Policy Brief B139, 2015.
7. Pheasant H et al. Health and social behaviour. Chapter 2e Public Health Textbook. UK Faculty of Public Health.
8. What are food-based dietary guidelines? FAO. https://www.fao.org/nutrition/education/food-based-dietary-guidelines.
9. Sustainable healthy diets – guiding principles. FAO & WHO, 2019.
10. This includes several reports by the high level panel of experts on food security and nutrition. UN Committee on World Food Security.
11. Food systems for health: information brief. WHO, 2021.
12. Fiscal policies for diet and prevention of noncommunicable diseases: technical meeting report, 5–6 May 2015, Geneva, Switzerland. WHO, 2016.
13. Implementing fiscal and pricing policies to promote healthy diets: a review of contextual factors. WHO, 2021.
14. Set of recommendations on the marketing of foods and non-alcoholic beverages to children. WHO, 2010.
15. Boyland E et al. Systematic review of the effect of policies to restrict the marketing of foods and non-alcoholic beverages to which children are exposed. *Obes Rev* 2022;23:e13447.
16. Action framework for developing and implementing public food procurement and service policies for a healthy diet. WHO, 2021.
17. Snyder LB. Health communication campaigns and their impact on behavior. *J Nutr Educ Behav* 2007;39(2 Suppl):S32–40.
18. Evert AB et al. Nutrition therapy for adults with diabetes or prediabetes: a consensus report. *Diabetes Care* 2019;42:731–54.
19. Canuto R et al. Nutritional intervention strategies for the management of overweight and obesity in primary health care: a systematic review with meta-analysis. *Obes Rev* 2021;22:e13143.
20. Effective interventions with cost effectiveness analysis ≤ I$ 100 per DALY averted in low- and middle-income countries.
21. Food systems for health. WHO. www.who.int/initiatives/food-systems-for-health.
22. Global individual food consumption data tool. FAO, WHO. https://www.fao.org/gift-individual-food-consumption/en/.
23. Arcand JA et al. Sodium levels in packaged foods sold in 14 Latin American and Caribbean countries: a food label analysis. *Nutrients* 2019;11:369.

20 Cholesterol, saturated fats and trans fats

Burden, epidemiology and priority interventions

Roger Darioli, Pascal Bovet, Nick Banatvala, Kay-Tee Khaw

Unhealthy levels of blood lipids, which are largely associated with an unhealthy diet (particularly saturated fats and trans fat), are a strong cause of atherosclerosis and high blood cholesterol level is a main modifiable metabolic risk factor of cardiovascular disease (CVD), particularly ischaemic heart disease (IHD). Interventions promoting a healthy diet in the whole population can improve population levels of blood lipids, while several blood cholesterol-lowering medications are highly effective among individuals with a high CVD risk.

Dietary fats provide energy as well as essential fatty acids and fat-soluble vitamins. From a health perspective, two major types of fats in food are of particular relevance: *saturated fats* and *unsaturated fats* (monounsaturated or polyunsaturated). High overall fat intake may be associated with excessive total energy intake as there are nine calories in every gram of fat, regardless of the type of fat (i.e. over twice the amount of calories per gram of carbohydrate or protein).

> **BOX 20.1 DIETARY FATS AND CHOLESTEROL AND THEIR RELATIONSHIPS TO CARDIOVASCULAR RISK**
>
> *Saturated fats:* high concentrations are found in animal products such as meat and dairy products and some vegetable oils (e.g. palm oil which accounts for a third of all oil consumed globally, and coconut oil). Saturated fats are generally detrimental to health in large amounts (e.g. >10% of total dietary intake), mainly because they increase the levels of blood cholesterol. However, the relationships between levels, types and sources of saturated fats on health, and their interaction with broader dietary habits, are a complex area of science and public health[1] and are not described further in this chapter.
>
> *Unsaturated fats:* foods with a high content include most vegetable oils, as well as nuts, seeds and oily fish. Unsaturated fats (monounsaturated or

DOI: 10.4324/9781003306689-23

polyunsaturated) are not generally detrimental to cardiovascular health (except trans fats).[2]

Trans fats (also called trans fatty acids): a particular type of unsaturated fats. Natural trans fat is present in low levels (<5%) in the meat and dairy products of ruminant animals. However, most dietary trans fat intake comes from the industrial processing of unsaturated fat to give food a longer shelf life and make the fat more resistant to heating (e.g. allowing oil to be used repeatedly for frying). Industrially-produced trans fat occurs in substantial proportions (e.g. 5–30%) in fried and baked foods (e.g. doughnuts, cakes, pie crusts, biscuits, frozen pizza, cookies, crackers) and margarines. Trans fat is a major cause of atherosclerosis, with a 23% higher risk of IHD for each 2% increase in calories from trans fat.

Cholesterol: a lipid essential to building healthy cells and a precursor of several hormones and steroids. Dietary intake of saturated fats increases the *de novo* production of cholesterol by the body (particularly in the liver) and increases blood cholesterol levels. Dietary intake of cholesterol (e.g. from eggs) has a relatively small role in blood cholesterol levels and CVD risk.[3] High blood cholesterol is the main cause of atherosclerosis and CVD.[4]

Triglycerides: Most of the fats we eat are in the form of triglycerides (TG). They are carried in the blood and used to provide and store energy. TG is also formed in the body from excess calories, alcohol and sugar. High blood TG levels are often a sign of other conditions that increase the risk of IHD,[5] including obesity and metabolic syndrome — a cluster of conditions that includes too much fat around the waist, high blood pressure, high blood TG, low blood HDL-cholesterol, and high blood glucose.

Blood lipids and their relationships to cardiovascular risk

Cholesterol is not water-soluble and is therefore transported in the blood 'attached' to large water-soluble lipoproteins. Around ~80% of all cholesterol in the blood is 'attached' to low-density lipoproteins (LDL): this is the 'LDL-cholesterol' (LDL-C). High blood LDL-C is strongly associated with atherosclerosis and a *higher* risk of CVD, and it is therefore called 'bad cholesterol'. Trials of interventions with statins showed that a reduction of 1 mmol/L (38.7 mg/dL) in LDL-C – in line with an average effect of a low-dose statin treatment- reduces the risk of IHD by 33%.[6] The blood level of 'total cholesterol' (TC) is a good proxy of LDL-C since ~60-80% of all cholesterol in the blood is attached to LDL.

A substantial proportion of cholesterol in the blood (e.g. ~10–30%) circulates in high-density lipoproteins (HDL), which act to remove cholesterol from arterial walls. A high blood level of HDL-C is associated with a *lower* CVD risk and is therefore called 'good cholesterol'. However, trials of medications that increase blood levels of HDL-C have shown no significant reduction in CVD.[7]

Factors associated with unhealthy blood lipid levels (dyslipidaemia)

In addition to an unhealthy diet, abnormal levels of blood lipids (particularly increased levels of TG and decreased levels of HDL-C) are associated with obesity, tobacco use, physical inactivity, diabetes, hypothyroidism and chronic kidney disease. Familial hypercholesterolemia is a genetic condition that affects ~0.3% of the population and which is strongly associated with a premature heart attack.[8]

Disease burden (LDL-C and trans fat)

Approximately 4.4 million (7.8%) of all deaths worldwide were estimated to be attributable to elevated *LDL-C* in 2019, an increase from 3.0 million (6.4%) in 1990 (Table 20.1). These proportions decreased between 1990 and 2019 in high-income countries (HICs) and upper-middle-income countries (MICs) but increased in lower MICs and low-income countries (LICs), partly because

Table 20.1 Mortality attributable to high blood LDL-cholesterol and diet high in trans fat (IHME)

	Global		HICs		Upper MICs		Lower MICs		LICs	
	1990	2019	1990	2019	1990	2019	1990	2019	1990	2019
Metabolic risk: high LDL-C										
Proportion of all deaths (%)	6.4	7.8	14.0	8.0	6.9	9.6	3.9	7.2	1.3	2.7
Age-standardized mortality (per 100,000)	89	56	95	34	86	63	85	73	50	49
Diet high in trans fat										
Proportion of all deaths (%)	1.0	1.1	2.2	1.3	0.9	1.1	0.75	1.27	0.2	0.3
Age-standardized mortality (per 100,000)	13.5	8.2	14.5	5.6	10.8	7.3	15.2	12.6	7.4	6.2

of aging populations. However, the age-adjusted mortality rates (per 100,000 population) attributable to high LDL-C *decreased* in all regions between 1990 and 2019, and the decrease was much larger in HICs (a threefold decrease) than in low- and middle-income countries (only a ~20-30% decrease). This partly reflects a larger decrease in dietary intake of saturated fat (e.g. shift from whole to skimmed milk, or from meat to poultry) and better prevention and control of health outcomes (e.g. IHD) in HICs than in LICs. Correspondingly, the prevalence of high LDL-C (or that of high total cholesterol), often in the range of 10-30% among adults in HICs, has decreased in many, but not all, countries.[9] Approximately 85% of deaths related to increased LDL-C were caused by IHD and 15% by stroke (IHME).

High dietary trans fat accounted for approximately 645,000 deaths (1.1%) worldwide in 2019 (IHME). The age-adjusted mortality rates attributable to trans fats decreased in all regions between 1990 and 2019 and were lowest in 2019 in HICs, where policies to ban or limit industrially-produced trans fat have been increasingly widely implemented[10] and prevention and control of CVD developed. Virtually all of these deaths are due to IHD (IHME).

Interventions at the population level

Interventions around diet, physical activity, obesity, tobacco and alcohol are described in other chapters. WHO effective and recommended interventions that reduce unhealthy diet and can reduce LDL-C and TG blood levels include the following:

- Eliminate industrial trans fat through the development of legislation to ban their use in the food chain.
- Reduce sugar consumption through effective taxation on sugar-sweetened beverages.
- Implement policies such as subsidies to increase the intake of fruits and vegetables.
- Replace trans fat and saturated fat with unsaturated fats through reformulation, labelling, fiscal policies or agricultural policies.
- Limit portion and package size to reduce energy intake and the risk of being overweight or obese.
- Implement nutrition labelling to reduce total energy intake, sugars, sodium and fats, including displaying proportions of total fat and saturated fat, preferably with interpretive information (e.g. traffic light or equivalent systems).
- Implement nutrition education and counselling in different settings (e.g. schools, workplaces, hospitals) to increase the intake of fruits and vegetables as part of a healthy diet.
- Implement mass media campaigns on healthy diets, including social marketing to reduce the intake of total fat, saturated fats, sugars and salt, and promote the intake and fruits and vegetables.

The WHO REPLACE package provides a strategic approach to support countries in reducing trans fat in manufactured food, with the goal of global elimination by 2023.[11] The package includes six actions of action to:

- **RE**view dietary sources of industrially-produced trans fat and the landscape for required policy change;
- **P**romote the replacement of industrially-produced trans fat with healthier fats and oils;
- **L**egislate or enact regulatory actions to eliminate industrially-produced trans fat;
- **A**ssess and monitor trans fat content in the food supply and the changes in trans fat consumption in the population;
- **C**reate awareness of the negative health impact of trans fat among policymakers, producers, suppliers and the public; and
- **E**nforce compliance with policies and regulations.

Interventions at the individual level

Screening. Recommendations vary on who should be screened for high blood cholesterol and how often. The US Preventive Services Task Force for example recommends screening for all people aged 40 to 75 years.[12] Most guidelines recommend that screening is offered to individuals at high risk of CVD (e.g. those with diabetes or with a family history of CVD or high blood cholesterol, including familial hypercholesterolaemia).

Assessing blood lipids. LDL-C is the main marker of interest for CVD risk and can be measured either directly or calculated with the Friedewald formula as = TC minus HDL-C minus TG/2.2 (in mmol/l). Ideally, a complete 'lipid panel' (TC, LDL-C, HDL-C and TG) should be assessed to guide personalized management of patients with dyslipidaemias. Measurement of TC alone is a useful proxy measure of LDL-C where a complete lipid profile cannot be done. Most CVD risk score calculators require information on at least one blood cholesterol marker, e.g. total cholesterol, LDL-cholesterol or LDL-C/HDL-C ratio). Table 20.2 displays blood lipid level categories commonly considered by leading cardiology societies.

Counselling

All individuals who have abnormal blood lipid levels should be advised to adopt a healthy diet, engage in regular physical activity, abstain from using tobacco and maintain a normal weight. Further details are provided in chapters on these risk factors.

Assessing CVD risk

It is important to determine an individual's total (absolute) CVD risk (using CVD risk score calculators) in order to identify individuals who will benefit

Table 20.2 CVD risk categories associated with abnormal blood lipid levels in mmol/l (mg/dl in parentheses)

CVD risk category	TC	LDL-C	HDL-C	TG
Desirable/optimal	<5.2 (<200)	<2.6 (100)	High >1.6 (60)	<1.7 (150)
Near or above optimal		2.6–3.3 (100–129)		
Borderline high	5.2–6.2 (200–239)	3.3–4.1 (130–159)		1.7–5.7 (150–499)
High	≥6.2 (240)	4.1–4.9 (60–190)		5.7–11.4 (500–999)
Very high	≥7.5 (290)	>4.9 (190)	Low <1.0 (40)	≥11.4 (1000)

Grundy SM et al. 2019 Guideline on the management of blood cholesterol: a report of the American College of Cardiology/American Heart Association Task Force on Clinical Practice Guidelines. *Circulation* 2019;139:e1082–143.
Visseren FLJ et al. 2021 ESC guidelines on cardiovascular disease prevention in clinical practice. *Eur Heart J* 2021;42:3227–37.

most from cholesterol-lowering treatment (i.e. those for whom the absolute CVD risk would decrease by a large amount). National guidelines need to take into account resource availability when making recommendations for pharmacologic therapy.

Pharmacological treatment

Treatment to reduce LDL-C (or TC) should be offered to individuals of all ages who have a high CVD risk, including individuals with very high LDL-C levels or who have had a CVD event, and most individuals with diabetes. Chapter 7 on CVD provides more details. Cholesterol-lowering medications are highly effective in reducing blood TC, LDL-C levels and cardiovascular mortality.[13] Statins (HMG-CoA reductase inhibitors) can safely reduce LDL-C by up to 50–60% and are the first-line medication to treat elevated TC/LDL-C blood levels. Generic statins can be fairly inexpensive (e.g. <0.1 US$ per day). Other lipid-lowering drugs include fibrates and bile acid sequestrants (e.g. cholestyramine, questran), but they are less effective than statins and have more side effects than statins. Lipid-lowering medications are generally safe, but myalgia can occur in 1–5 % of those taking statins.[14] When blood levels of TC/LDL-C cannot be sufficiently lowered with a statin alone at maximum dosage, it is possible, where resources allow, to use, in addition to a statin, another cholesterol-lowering drug, such as cholesterol absorption inhibitors (e.g. ezetimibe) or weekly/monthly injectable monoclonal antibody inhibitors of the proprotein convertase subtilisin/kexin 9 (PCSK9 inhibitors, e.g. evolocumab, alirocumab), which are highly effective but expensive.

New cholesterol-lowering medications continue to be developed, including therapies that can be taken less frequently (e.g. monthly) and could increase compliance.[15]

Although this chapter does not address the management of high blood TG, hypertriglyceridaemia is often sensitive to diet (e.g. a diet restricted in sugar and alcohol) and responds fairly well to some medications (including statins and fibrates). Guidelines on the treatment of blood lipids provide more detail on this.

The aim of blood lipid treatment should be to reduce LDL-C by >30% in patients at intermediate CVD risk and by >50% in patients at high or very high CVD risk, depending on available resources. In secondary prevention, an increasing number of guidelines, e.g. the American Heart Association and the European Society of Cardiology, recommend a very low LDL-C target (e.g. 1.8 mmol/l [<70 mg/dl]), which often requires the use of several cholesterol-lowering medications (again, depending on available resources).

Adherence and response to treatment should be evaluated at 1–3 month intervals after starting cholesterol-lowering therapy. Once acceptable levels of LDL-C (or TC) are achieved, monitoring can be reduced to 6–12 monthly intervals. Many studies show large treatment gaps in all countries, with many patients not getting the treatment they require because it is not available, not included in local guidelines, not affordable or not prioritized, and because too often long-term adherence to treatment is suboptimal (e.g. as low as <40%).[16,17] There is an increasing interest in combining lipid-lowering and blood-pressure-lowering medications (and aspirin in secondary prevention) in the form of a one polypill regimen daily, which can simplify treatment, improve adherence and reduce CVD risk at least as well as usual care.[18]

Monitoring

Indicators from the WHO Global Monitoring Framework directly related to blood lipids include:

Biological risk factors.	Age-standardized prevalence of raised TC among persons aged 18+ years (TC ≥5.0 mmol/l or 190 mg/dl); and mean TC concentration.
National health response.	Proportion of eligible persons (age 40+ with a ten-year CVD risk ≥30%, including those with existing CVD) receiving drug therapy and counselling (including glycaemic control) to prevent heart attacks and strokes.
National health response.	Availability and affordability of quality, safe and efficacious essential NCD medicines, including generics, and basic technologies in both public and private facilities.
Additional indicators.	Adoption of national policies that limit saturated fatty acids and virtually eliminate trans fats in the food supply.

Surveys on the quality of health care are useful to enhance the adherence of health professionals to guideline recommendations and benchmarking of care providers.[19]

Notes

1. Forouhi NG et al. Dietary fat and cardiometabolic health: evidence, controversies, and consensus for guidance. *BMJ* 2018;361:k2139.
2. Saturated fats and health. Scientific Advisory Committee on Nutrition, Public Health England, 2019.
3. Tobias DK. What eggsactly are we asking here? Unscrambling the epidemiology of eggs, cholesterol, and mortality. *Circulation* 2022;145:1521–23.
4. Libby P et al. Atherosclerosis. *Nat Rev Dis Primers* 2019;5:56.
5. Burgess S et al. Mendelian randomization to assess causal effects of blood lipids on coronary heart disease: lessons from the past and applications to the future. *Curr Opin Endocrinol Diabetes Obes* 2016;23:124–30.
6. Silverman MG et al. Association between lowering LDL-C and cardiovascular risk reduction among different therapeutic interventions: a systematic review and meta-analysis. *JAMA* 2016;316:1289–97.
7. Woudberg NJ et al. Pharmacological Intervention to modulate HDL: what do we target? *Front Pharmacol* 2018;8:989.
8. Akioyamen LE et al. Estimating the prevalence of heterozygous familial hypercholesterolaemia: a systematic review and meta-analysis. *BMJ Open* 2017;7:e016461.
9. NCD Risk Factor Collaborators (NCD-RisC). Repositioning of the global epicentre of non-optimal cholesterol. *Nature* 2020;582:73–7.
10. Nagpal T et al. Trans fatty acids in food: a review on dietary intake, health impact, regulations and alternatives. *J Food Sci* 2021;86:5159–74.
11. REPLACE trans fat: an action package to eliminate industrially produced trans-fatty acids. WHO, 2019.
12. Mangione CM et al. Statin use for the primary prevention of cardiovascular disease in adults: US Preventive Services Task Force Recommendation Statement. *JAMA* 2022;328:746–53.
13. Silverman MG et al. Association between lowering LDL-C and cardiovascular risk reduction among different therapeutic interventions: a systematic review and meta-analysis. *JAMA* 2016;316:1289–97.
14. Alonso R et al. Diagnosis and management of statin intolerance. *J Atheroscler Thromb* 2019;26:207–15.
15. Wilkins JT et al. Novel lipid-lowering therapies to reduce cardiovascular risk. *JAMA* 2021;326:266–67.
16. Chowdhury R et al. Adherence to cardiovascular therapy: a meta-analysis of prevalence and clinical consequences. *Eur Heart J* 2013;34:2940–48.
17. Marcus ME et al. Unmet need for hypercholesterolemia care in 35 low- and middle-income countries: a cross-sectional study of nationally representative surveys. *PLoS Med* 2021;18:e1003841.
18. Yusuf S et al. Polypill with or without aspirin in persons without cardiovascular disease. *NEJM* 2021;384:216–28.
19. Aktaa S et al. European society of cardiology methodology for the development of quality indicators for the quantification of cardiovascular care and outcomes. *Eur Heart J Qual Care Clin Outcomes* 2020;26:qcaa069.

21 Dietary salt and NCDs

Burden, epidemiology and priority interventions

Pascal Bovet, Michel Burnier, Nick Banatvala, Leo Nederveen

Increased sodium intake is associated in a graded manner with several detrimental health outcomes, particularly high blood pressure (BP), heart disease and stroke. A number of public health interventions can effectively reduce dietary salt intake in populations and significantly reduce the NCD burden.

Disease burden

Globally, IHME estimated that 3.3% of all deaths (approximately 1.9 million) were attributable to high sodium in 2019, up from 2.8% in 1990 (Table 21.1). These proportions increased in low- and middle-income countries but decreased in high-income countries (HICs). The age-standardized mortality rates were highest in upper-middle-income countries (MICs) and lowest in high-income countries (HICs), and were decreasing in all income groups between 1990 and 2019. These differences reflect variant patterns in terms of dietary salt intake, as well as prevention and control of salt-related diseases across countries and over time.

Of all deaths in 2019 attributable to high dietary sodium intake (IHME), 41% could be attributed to stroke, 37% to ischemic heart disease, 9% to hypertensive heart disease, 5% to kidney disease and diabetes and 4% to neoplasms. Of note, estimates of the salt-related burden may vary substantially depending on the assumptions made when modelling the relationships between sodium intake, BP, and disease morbidity and mortality.

Definition of elevated salt intake

WHO defines high sodium consumption as >2 grams of sodium/day, equivalent to >5 g of salt (NaCl) per day for a 2000 kcal diet. In many populations, salt intake averages 9–12 g per day, in several high and middle-high-income countries up to 15 g,[1] with <10–20% of individuals meeting the WHO guidance that establishes an upper limit of <5 g per day.

Assessment of dietary salt intake

Determining individuals' salt intake is challenging. The reference method is based on 24-hour urine collections performed once. Recent recommendations

DOI: 10.4324/9781003306689-24

Table 21.1 Mortality attributable to a diet high in sodium (salt)

	Global		HICs		Upper MICs		Lower MICs		LICs	
	1990	2019	1990	2019	1990	2019	1990	2019	1990	2019
Percent of all deaths (%)	2.8	3.3	3.0	2.1	5.2	5.7	1.4	2.2	0.9	1.4
Age-standardized rates (per 100,000)	36	24	19	9	55	35	28	22	36	27

suggest that 24-hour collections should preferably be repeated at least three times to obtain a valid assessment of sodium intake in a given individual. However, urine collections are cumbersome, resource-intensive and not practical outside the research setting. Dietary recalls and food frequency questionnaires are notably inaccurate and prone to bias. Morning urine spots are easy to perform but they rely on calculations that take into account several other variables. Urine spots are useful to assess mean sodium intake at the population level but lack accuracy at the individual level, particularly at low salt intake values. Salt intake is generally greater in overweight persons and parallels their larger calorie intake for energy balance (when they are not engaged in a hypocaloric diet to lose weight).

Relationship between salt intake, blood pressure and cardiovascular disease

Several recent reviews describe the current knowledge.[2,3] Abundant observational and experimental data unambiguously show a direct linear relation between sodium intake and BP, with a steeper association in the upper range of sodium intake.[4,5] Likewise, observational and experimental evidence shows that a reduction in salt intake is associated with reduced BP and lower CVD incidence and overall mortality.[6] However, some studies have found no reduction or even an increase of CVD and/or total mortality at very low salt intake, showing J- or U-shaped relationships and an increase of renin and aldosterone at low salt intake levels.[7] Some of these studies were funded by the industry and/or had methodological limitations that could alter the associations between sodium intake and disease.[8,9] This may be partly related to biased estimation of salt intake in the low sodium intake range in studies based on spot urines and to reverse causation (i.e. sick people tend to have lower food/salt intake), but activation of the renin-angiotensin system and increased plasma lipids concentrations at very low salt intake levels have also been suggested. The effect of sodium intake on BP levels and CVD incidence accrues over time (cumulative effect) and estimates of the salt-related burden can therefore be underestimated when based on studies with short follow-ups.[10] This underlies that salt reduction strategies should start at an early age, including among children. High salt intake is also associated with BP-independent complications such as proteinuria, renal stones and gastric cancer. In addition, a high sodium intake decreases the efficacy of antihypertensive drugs such as diuretics and blockers of the renin-angiotensin system.

Sources of dietary salt

The main dietary source of sodium is salt, in the form of sodium chloride, but in many parts of the world also in high-sodium sauces and condiments. In many HICs, and increasingly in low- and middle-income countries, a significant proportion of sodium in the diet comes from processed foods, such as cheese, processed meats, bread, soups, salty snacks, salami, stock cubes,[11] which underlies the crucial role of promoting healthy diets based on natural and sustainably produced foods as well as reformulating processed foods rich in salt toward lower salt content. Salt added during cooking or at the table can account for a large proportion of a person's total salt intake, particularly in low-income settings where processed or pre-packaged foods are less available.[12]

Interventions to reduce dietary salt intake in the population

A number of priority actions are available to reduce salt intake in the population.[13,14] The WHO Global NCD Action Plan identifies four best buys aimed at reducing salt intake at the population level. They are:

- Reformulating food products to contain less salt and setting target levels for the amount of salt in foods and meals.
- Reducing salt intake through the implementation of front-of-pack nutrition labelling.
- Reducing salt intake through behaviour change communication and mass media campaigns.
- Establishing a supportive environment in public institutions such as hospitals, schools, workplaces and nursing homes, to enable lower sodium options to be provided.

Reformulating food products to contain less salt and setting target levels for the maximum amount of salt in foods and meals

While the best way to reduce salt consumption is to lower consumption of processed food, which is often high in fats, sugars and salt, reformulation by industry of selected common processed foods that have a particularly high salt content enables people to have a lower salt intake without requiring them to make particular efforts to change their eating habits. Reformulation is more effective when implemented through regulations that set a maximum salt content in selected foods. However, salt reduction in ultraprocessed foods may have less than expected impact if consumption of ultraprocessed foods increases, which emphasizes the need for ambitious salt reduction targets.

Mandatory approaches provide the legal tools and financial and human resources necessary to guarantee appropriate implementation and monitoring mechanisms.[15] Mandatory reformulation can achieve larger salt reductions than voluntary agreements and larger health benefits. The implementation of a regulatory framework implies a level playing field for the food industry (large vs small and medium-sized enterprises) and legislative measures allow for the introduction of financial penalties for non-compliance. Legislation is more difficult to abandon if a new government comes into power.[16]

While the food industry should be encouraged to reduce salt in foods as much as possible, it should ensure that, where appropriate, salt in packets and salt added to foods is supplemented with iodine (an important public health measure to prevent iodine deficiency disorders). Salt is added to processed foods and meals for a variety of reasons but primarily because it is a cheap way of adding flavour to otherwise bland foods. When high-salt foods are consistently consumed, the salt taste receptors are suppressed, creating the habit of eating highly salted foods and leading to greater consumer demand. Inversely, if the salt content in commonly consumed high-salt foods is reduced gradually over months or years (e.g. in bread), consumers tend to not notice the change, e.g. if the reduction is <20% in one step. With time, individuals become increasingly able to rediscover and enjoy a variety of flavours from the same foods.

In 2021, WHO released a set of global benchmarks for sodium levels in >60 different foods,[17] and the Pan American Health Organization released regional targets in 2015, which were updated and 2021. These benchmarks can guide countries in progressively reducing the sodium content in different categories of processed foods (e.g. packaged bread, savoury snacks, meat products, cheese). These benchmarks may substantially accelerate progress toward the WHO goal of a 30% reduction in global salt/sodium intake by 2025 (compared to 2010).

In the UK, where voluntary targets for industry to reformulate their products were developed, adults' salt intake decreased by approximately 15% between 2003 and 2011, suggesting that target-setting across multiple food categories can achieve some meaningful reductions in sodium consumption in the population. However, no further change was observed in the UK between 2011 and 2018, with salt intake in adults remaining >40% higher than the upper limit of <5 g/day. Also, data from some large food manufacturers indicate that the salt content of their products has not decreased, and in some cases, even increased. This indicates the huge challenge of implementing and maintaining favourable changes and achieving the set goals, as well as the need for appropriate legislation.

Reducing salt intake through the implementation of front-of-pack nutrition labelling

Nutritional labelling, including salt content, enables consumers to better select the products they buy. Front-of-pack labels should be government-endorsed and allow consumers to correctly, quickly and easily identify products that contain excessive amounts of critical nutrients, preferably through mandatory front-of-package interpretative warning labels (e.g. as requested by law in Chile and being implemented in an increasing number of countries), since they have proven to effectively reduce a population's calorie intake and purchase of unhealthy foods.[18] Other common front-of-pack labelling systems include traffic light systems or NutriScore.[19,20] Using a smartphone to scan a food's barcode (when barcodes provide such information) is a user-friendly way for informing consumers about detailed food and beverage nutritional value (as well, for some systems, its environment impact, including carbon footprint).

*Reducing salt intake through behaviour change
communication and mass media campaigns*

Health education campaigns must inform the public about how to choose healthy food and raise their awareness about limiting their salt intake. This includes providing information on salt levels in processed foods and how to interpret it, information about the effect of salt on health and encouraging individuals to reduce salt when cooking and at the table. Comprehensive and interpretative information that can be obtained from barcodes on foods has a large potential for educating consumers about choosing healthy foods. Choosing low-salt foods is especially important among individuals with hypertension and/or at increased risk of CVD. Partial substitution of NaCl with KCl may be useful, but KCl tends to have an unpleasant taste if its concentration is high (use of spices and herbs may be useful). A simple and short practical health message for all individuals can be to 'eat plenty of fruit, vegetables, grains and unsalted nuts, drink water (instead of sugary beverages), and less processed foods and pre-packaged meals'. Such public health messaging has multiple benefits as fruit and vegetables contain low amounts of salt, while containing plenty of potassium (which attenuates the detrimental impact of salt on BP) and other nutrients that are also beneficial for NCD prevention and control. In addition a high fruit and vegetables diet will reduce the intake of saturated fats, salt and calories.

*Establishing a supportive environment in public institutions
such as hospitals, schools, workplaces and nursing homes,
to enable lower sodium options to be provided*

There is good potential for reducing salt in the food supply in settings such as schools, workplaces and hospitals, as the management often has control over the foods served. Community settings are a platform for local implementation of both national salt reduction policies and specific salt reduction interventions. The establishment of healthy foods and drinks guidelines (national or for some specific institutions), including salt criteria, is useful. Several countries have developed standards for food providers and defined the maximum levels of salt in foods sold in schools and hospitals.[21]

The WHO SHAKE technical package

The WHO SHAKE technical package for salt reduction provides guidance on the development, implementation and monitoring of salt reduction strategies, and for working with industry to reduce levels of salt in food products. SHAKE[22] consists of five elements:

- **S**urveillance: measure and monitor salt use.
- **H**arness industry: promote the reformulation of foods and meals to contain less salt. The food industry should be encouraged to reduce salt in foods as

much as possible while at the same time ensuring that, where appropriate, salt added to foods is iodized.
- **A**dopt and implement standards for accurate labelling and marketing of food.
- **K**nowledge: educate and communicate to empower individuals to eat less salt.
- **E**nvironment: support settings to promote healthy eating.

The SHAKE package also includes a number of useful country case studies.

Relevant global targets and indicators for salt reduction

A 25% relative reduction in the prevalence of raised BP or contain the prevalence of raised BP, according to national circumstances.	Age-standardized prevalence of raised BP among persons aged 18+ years (systolic/diastolic BP ≥140/90 mmHg) and mean systolic/diastolic BP.

Monitoring

This includes surveillance of salt intake in the population, for example through 24-hour urine collections or morning urine spots in random sub-samples of population-based surveys (e.g. STEPS). It is also important to regularly assess the salt content in selected common processed foods to inform and monitor salt-reduction interventions. It is important to monitor the salt content of foods in each country or region as foods from the same brand often have different levels of salt in different countries.[23] The FLIP Food Information Program has been used successfully in Canada, Latin America and the Caribbean to monitor sodium content through food labels.

WHO has developed a *Sodium Country Score Card* to track the progress of countries in implementing legislative and other measures to reduce dietary sodium intake, including: national policy towards sodium reduction; voluntary approaches to reduce sodium in the food supply; mandatory declaration of sodium on pre-packaged foods; and implementation of one or several of the sodium-related WHO best buys for tackling NCDs.[24]

Notes

1 Salt reduction. WHO, 2020. www.who.int/news-room/fact-sheets/detail/salt-reduction.
2 Cook NR et al. Sodium and health—concordance and controversy. *BMJ* 2020;369:m2440.
3 Graudal NA et al. Effects of low sodium diet versus high sodium diet on blood pressure, renin, aldosterone, catecholamines, cholesterol, and triglyceride. *Cochrane Database Syst Rev* 2020;12:CD004022.
4 Filippini T et al. Blood pressure effects of sodium reduction: dose-response meta-analysis of experimental studies. *Circulation* 2021;143:1542–67.

5 Ma Y et al. 24-hour urinary sodium and potassium excretion and cardiovascular risk. *NEJM* 2022;386:252–63.
6 He GJ et al. Salt reduction to prevent hypertension and cardiovascular disease: JACC state-of-the-art review. *JACC* 2020;75:632–47.
7 O'Donnell M et al. Joint association of urinary sodium and potassium excretion with cardiovascular events and mortality: prospective cohort study. *BMJ* 2019;364:l772.
8 Tsirimiagkou C et al. Dietary sodium and cardiovascular morbidity/mortality: a brief commentary on the "J-shape hypothesis". *J Hypertension* 2021;39:2335–43.
9 Cappuccio FP, Sever PS. The importance of a valid assessment of salt intake in individuals and populations. A scientific statement of the British and Irish Hypertension Society. *J Hum Hypertension* 2019;33:345–48.
10 Neal B, Wu J. Sodium, blood pressure, and the likely massive avoidable burden of cardiovascular disease. *Circulation* 2021;143:1568–70.
11 Bhat S et al. A systematic review of the sources of dietary salt around the world. *Adv Nutr* 2020;11:677–86.
12 Campbell NRC et al. Sodium consumption: an individual's choice? *Int J Hypertens* 2012;2012:860954.
13 Ide N et al. Priority actions to advance population sodium reduction. *Nutrients* 2020;12:2543.
14 Santos JV et al. A systematic review of salt reduction Initiatives around the world: a midterm evaluation of progress towards the 2025 global non-communicable diseases salt reduction target. *Adv Nutr* 2021;12:1768–80.
15 Hyseni L et al. Systematic review of dietary salt reduction policies: evidence for an effectiveness hierarchy? *PLoS ONE* 2017;12:e0177535.
16 Updated PAHO regional sodium reduction targets. PAHO, 2021.
17 New WHO benchmarks help countries reduce salt intake and save lives. WHO, 2021.
18 Taillie LS et al. Changes in food purchases after the Chilean policies on food labelling, marketing, and sales in schools: a before and after study. *Lancet Planet Health* 2021;5:e526–33.
19 Front-of-package labeling as a policy tool for the prevention of noncommunicable diseases in the Americas. PAHO, 2020.
20 Superior efficacy of front-of-package warning labels in Jamaica. PAHO, 2021.
21 Action framework for developing and implementing public food procurement and service policies for a healthy diet. WHO, 2021.
22 SHAKE the salt habit: the SHAKE technical package for salt reduction. WHO, 2016.
23 Arcand JA et al. Sodium levels in packaged foods sold in 14 Latin American and Caribbean countries: a food label analysis. *Nutrients* 2019;11:369s.
24 Sodium Country Score Card. *Global database on the implementation of nutrition action (GINA)*. WHO, 2022.

22 Dietary sugars and NCDs

Burden, epidemiology, and priority interventions

Pascal Bovet, Nick Banatvala, Eric Ravussin, Leo Nederveen

Definition of sugar[1]

Sugar is the generic name for sweet-tasting water-soluble carbohydrates. Sugars (or saccharides) can appear in the form of single carbohydrate building block units (i.e. monosaccharide, such as glucose $C_6H_{12}O_6$) or molecules made of two units (i.e. disaccharide such as sucrose). Glucose (its D-isomer being also called dextrose), fructose (fruit sugar), and galactose (dairy sugar) are main monosaccharides (simple sugars), while common disaccharides include sucrose ('table sugar', glucose + fructose), lactose (glucose + galactose), and maltose (glucose + glucose). Sugars have different sweetness. Compared to sucrose (reference = 1), the sweetness of lactose is ~0.16, maltose ~0.4, galactose ~0.65, glucose ~0.8 and fructose ~1.5. In comparison, non-saccharide substances can be much sweeter: aspartame (dipeptide methyl esther) 180–250, stevia (a naturally occurring vegetal glycoside) 40–300, or sodium saccharin (sulfonyl) 300–700.

Several groups of foods contain substantial concentrations of sugar:

- Intrinsic sugars incorporated within the structure of intact fruit and vegetables (mainly glucose, fructose).
- Milk (lactose and galactose).
- Free sugars (mainly glucose and fructose), defined by WHO[2] as 'added to foods and beverages and those naturally present in honey, syrups, fruit juices and fruit juice concentrates'.

The WHO Manual on Food Drink and Taxation to Promote Healthy Diet[3] defines sugary drinks as:

> all types of beverages containing free sugars and these include carbonated or non-carbonated soft drinks, fruit/vegetable juices and drinks, liquid and powder concentrates, flavoured water, energy and sports drinks, ready-to-drink tea, ready-to-drink coffee, and flavoured milk drinks. The term is sometimes used interchangeably with sugar-sweetened beverages (SSBs), which are defined identically.[4]

DOI: 10.4324/9781003306689-25

Production and per capita consumption

Sugar is found in the tissue of most plants. Honey and fruit are abundant natural sources of monosaccharides (glucose and fructose). Sugar cane and sugar beet are the main sources of disaccharides from which the refined sugar sucrose is extracted industrially. The sugar extracted from corn (corn syrup) is glucose, and is often transformed industrially into fructose.

The average person currently consumes ~24 kg of sugar each year, ranging from <20 kg in Africa (albeit increasing) to >50 kg in North America.[5] A large proportion of sugar in the diet comes from sugary drinks and foods such as confectionery, desserts, cakes, jams, and breakfast cereals. Among adolescents in several European countries, sugar represents approximately a quarter of the total energy intake. Free sugars contribute 80% of this total sugar intake, with soft drinks and fruit juices contributing similar substantial proportions of the total sugar intake.[6]

Physiology of sugar[1]

Disaccharides, similarly to other edible carbohydrates (i.e. polysaccharides found in starches), are hydrolyzed into monosaccharides by the intestine (glucose, fructose or galactose) to: 1) provide energy through cellular aerobic respiration and concomitant production of ATP used by the cells for energy; 2) be converted into glycogen in the liver and skeletal muscle as short-term energy stores; 3) be converted into structural polysaccharides (e.g. pectin for cell walls) or; 4) be transformed in body fat by *de novo* lipogenesis as long-term energy stores.

However, sugar has distinctive characteristics compared to starches when it comes to digestion.

- First, digestion is more rapid for sugars than starch and sugar intake rapidly increases blood glucose levels, which stimulates insulin production by the pancreas to facilitate glucose storage as glycogen and its conversion into body fat.
- Second, the rapid absorption of sugars by the intestine partially bypasses the endocrine regulatory loops (e.g. ghrelin) for appetite and satiety, thus delaying the sensation of having eaten enough, especially when consumed in liquid form, possibly leading to calorie overconsumption.
- Third, sugars trigger neurophysiological dopamine-related 'reward' mechanisms, which further stimulate energy intake.[7]
- Fourth, the quicker increase and fall of insulin, after eating sugar vs starches, leads to reactive low glucose levels, thus driving appetite.
- For example, drinking 500 ml of soft drink/fruit juice and eating 100 g of bread (2 large slices) each provide around 250 calories. Yet, satiety will be much lower following a sugary drink as it is absorbed nearly instantly. Bread (or indeed fruit) will in comparison be absorbed considerably more

slowly. The result is that there is a much greater desire for further food and drink following a sugary drink compared with an intake of a less refined food.

Health effects of high sugar intake and related NCD burden

High sugar intake, including soft drinks and fruit juices, is a significant driver of obesity, diabetes, cardiovascular disease, and tooth decay in children and adults.[8,9,10] High intakes of glucose and fructose are also common causes of hypertriglyceridemia and non-alcoholic fatty liver disease.

Disease burden

Table 22.1 (data from IHME) shows that the proportions of all deaths attributable to a diet high in SSBs increased from low levels in 1990 to higher levels in 2019 in low- and middle-income countries with inverse trends in HICs. This partly reflects the relatively low but rapidly increasing consumption of SSBs in low- and middle-income countries driven by the large and increasing supply of cheap sugar in the world market.[11] The age-standardized mortality rates attributable to a diet high in SSBs decreased in all regions, partly reflecting improving prevention and control of the health consequences of SSBs. Around three-quarters of the SSB-related deaths were attributable to cardiovascular disease (CVD) and one-quarter to diabetes. Of note, estimates in Table 22.1 do not include sugar sources other than SSBs, such as beverages with naturally occurring sugar (e.g. fruit juices) and the many foods that include added sugars.

Recommended dietary intake of sugar

WHO recommends that adults and children reduce their intake of free sugars to <10% of their total energy intake throughout the life-course and ideally to <5%. Public health interventions should therefore aim at limiting dietary intake of free sugars, particularly sugary drinks that have little nutritional value beyond energy supply. For example, a 3 dl glass/bottle of a sugary drink can typically contain as much as ~30–40 g of sugar (i.e. ~120–160 calories), and regular consumption of sugary drinks can contribute up to 20–30% of the total daily calorie intake, particularly among children. Sugar concentration is even

Table 22.1 Mortality attributable to high dietary intake of sugar-sweetened beverages (IHME)

	Global		HICs		Upper MICs		Lower MICs		LICs	
	1990	2019	1990	2019	1990	2019	1990	2019	1990	2019
Proportion of all deaths (%)	0.32	0.43	0.60	0.50	0.38	0.51	0.20	0.37	0.12	0.19
Age-standardized rates (per 100,000)	4.3	3.1	4.1	2.2	4.7	3.3	4.7	3.9	4.7	3.7

larger in fruit juices (natural or reconstituted), e.g. around 9–25 g/100 ml vs soft drinks (9–12 g/100 ml), which implies that consumption of fruit juices (but not that of fresh fruits) should also be limited.

Non-calorie sweeteners, also called non-sugar sweeteners

The food industry is increasingly replacing part or all sugar in sweetened drinks with natural non- or low-calorie sweeteners (e.g. stevia, which provides a very low-calorie intake) and/or artificial sweeteners (e.g. aspartame, which provides virtually no calories), particularly in countries that impose a tax on sugary drinks. Consumption of beverages including non-caloric sweeteners may be associated with a lesser weight gain than ordinary sugar beverages and with no current evidence of adverse health effects,[12,13] but further trials are needed to better assess this question. However, it seems that regular consumption of beverages with a sweet taste (including those with non-caloric sweeteners) can sustain a continued appetence for sugary foods (biscuits, etc.) which can contribute to excess calorie intake and overweight.[14]

Public health interventions to reduce the consumption of sugar

Policies and interventions to promote a healthy diet to reduce NCDs are discussed in Chapter 19. The following measures are specifically aimed at reducing dietary consumption of sugar and, particularly, added sugars. An asterisk appears for interventions recommended by WHO (Appendix 3 of the WHO Global NCD Action Plan).

Promote a healthy diet low in sugar*

- Health education programmes,* including social marketing*, and dietary guidelines, at the national and subnational levels (including workplaces, schools and public places) should promote a healthy diet, including one that is low in sugar, and advocate for drinking water instead of sugary drinks. Making water fountains broadly available in public places and institutions is a useful practical companion intervention.
- Public procurement policies, for example setting nutrition standards for foods and beverages allowed to be provided or sold in and around schools.
- Nutritional labelling*, including sugar content, enables consumers to better select the products they buy.[15] Front-of-pack labels (FOPL) should be government-endorsed and enable consumers to correctly, quickly and easily identify products that contain excessive amounts of critical nutrients, preferably through mandatory front-of-package interpretative warning labels (e.g. as requested by law in Chile and being implemented in an increasing number of countries), since they have been proven to effectively reduce population's calorie intake and critical nutrients purchase.[16] Other common FOPL systems include traffic light systems or NutriScore.[17,18] Using a smartphone to scan a food's barcode (when barcodes provide such information)

is a user-friendly way for determining detailed food and beverage nutritional value (as well as environmental carbon impact for some of these barcode systems).

Reduce the marketing of sugary drinks and foods*

- This includes a ban or restriction on advertising/marketing of unhealthy foods and beverages, including sugary drinks, particularly when targeting children. This can be done through legislation banning advertisements for unhealthy foods and beverages on the internet, social media, television (e.g. during viewing hours by youth), banning the sale of sugary drinks in selected settings (e.g. schools) and restricting the placement of selected unhealthy products in supermarkets.

Reformulation of sugar products toward lower sugar intake*

- Reducing the production and consumption of ultra-processed foods and reformulating the food content of common sugar-rich foods and beverages are cornerstone strategies to reduce sugar intake at the population level. This may imply setting sugar content targets for selected foods and working with industry to achieve these through voluntary means[19] or, preferably, through regulation (e.g. Sugar Act in South Africa). Of note, several food manufacturers are decreasing the sugar level in selected ultraprocessed products sold in some countries, partly under the pressure of public health policy (e.g. sugar tax) and consumers' demand, with substantial differences in sugar content of the same foods across different countries.[20]

Excise tax on sugar-sweetened beverages*

WHO and other authoritative public health bodies recommend applying an excise tax on sugary beverages (also called SSBs, as mentioned above).[21,22] This measure was shown to be cost-effective for reducing the consumption of sugary drinks and the disease burden attributable to obesity, tooth decay and NCDs.[23,24]

- The tax should be sufficiently large to increase the cost of sugary drinks by ≥20% (and if possible, even more[25]) to effectively curb the sale of these drinks (price elasticity of −1: a 10% increase in price leads to a 10% decrease in consumption).[26] Almost 50 countries have implemented a tax on sugary drinks but only a few have implemented a tax that increased beverage costs by ≥20% or even ≥10%.
- A tax on sugary drinks sends a strong message to the population that regular consumption of sugary drinks should be avoided.
- A tax incentivizes the food industry to reduce the sugar content of their products.

- A few countries also impose a tax on fruit juices, given that sugar concentration is at least as high in fruit juices as in soft drinks. In addition, a tax on soft drinks alone may increase the sales of fruit juices. When implementing a tax on fruit juices, it is important to inform the public that it is healthier to consume fresh fruits (which also include fibre and other healthy nutrients) than fruit juices.
- Concerning tax structure, an excise tax per volume enables the price of inexpensive sugary beverages to increase by a large margin. Tax should be regularly adjusted to inflation and nominal economic growth to retain its impact. Tax may apply only to sugary drinks that exceed a certain sugar concentration, e.g. ≥5 g sugar/100 ml, as implemented in some countries.
- Galactose (for which concentration is ~4.5 g/100 ml in milk) is not associated with adverse health effects and unflavoured dairy products should be exempted from tax on sugary drinks.
- Food labelling on macronutrient content (including carbohydrates and free/added sugar) must be mandatory so that fiscal and customs authorities can tax sugary beverages accordingly (while additional interpretative labelling, e.g. a traffic light system, may be more useful to inform consumers, as mentioned above).
- Part of tax revenue may be earmarked to fund health-promoting activities, e.g. water fountains in schools or similar health initiatives. This also enhances tax acceptance by the public.
- It may be useful to promote other fiscal incentives aimed at reducing the price of commercially bottled water to facilitate a consumption shift away from sugary drinks.

Monitoring

Nutritional surveys in adults and children (e.g. STEPS, GSHS – Chapters 4 and 5 on surveillance) can inform on the consumption of sugary drinks and selected foods rich in free sugar. An accurate assessment of the intake of foods and macronutrients (including sugar) requires asking many questions to assess the volume and frequency of consumption of many foods (based on either food frequency questionnaires and/or dietary 24-hour recalls).

Marketing studies on the sales of foods and beverages rich in sugars as well as food composition surveys (based on labelling of commercial foods or through independent food content analysis) are useful to assess food sales and composition differences over time within the same country or between countries.

Notes

1 Nelson DL, Cox MM (editors). *Lehninger principles of biochemistry*, 8th ed. New York, USA: Macmillan Learning, 2021.
2 Guideline: sugars intake for adults and children. WHO, 2015.
3 Implementation manual on food and drink taxation to promote healthy diets. WHO, 2018.

4 Technical briefing: dietary interventions for the Appendix 3 of the Global Action Plan for NCDs. WHO, 2017.
5 OECD-FAO Agricultural Outlook 2020–2029. FAO, 2019.
6 Mesana MI et al. Dietary sources of sugars in adolescents' diet: the HELENA study. *Eur J Nutr* 2018;57:629–41.
7 Berthoud HR et al. Learning of food preferences: mechanisms and implications for obesity and metabolic diseases. *Int J Obes* 2021;45:2156–68.
8 Afshin A et al. Health effects of dietary risks in 195 countries, 1990–2017: a systematic analysis for the Global Burden of Disease Study 2017. *Lancet* 2019;393:1958–72.
9 Te Morenga L et al. Dietary sugars and body weight: systematic review and meta-analyses of randomised controlled trials and cohort studies. *BMJ* 2013;345:e7492.
10 Moynihan PJ et al. Effect on caries of restricting sugars intake: systematic review to inform WHO guidelines. *J Dent Res* 2014;93:8–18.
11 Curbing global sugar consumption. *Effective food policy actions to help promote healthy diets & tackle obesity.* World Cancer Research Fund International, 2015.
12 Toews I et al. Association between intake of non-sugar sweeteners and health outcomes: systematic review and meta-analyses of randomized and non-randomised controlled trials and observational studies. *BMJ* 2019;364:k4718.
13 McGlynn N et al. Association of low- and no-calorie sweetened beverages as a replacement for sugar-sweetened beverages with body weight and cardiometabolic risk: a systematic review and meta-analysis. *JAMA Network Open* 2022;5:e222092.
14 Sylvetsky AC et al. Consumption of low-calorie sweetened beverages is associated with higher total energy and sugar intake among children, NHANES 2011–2016. *Pediatr Obes* 2019;14:e12535.
15 Song J et al. Impact of color-coded and warning nutrition labelling schemes: a systematic review and network meta-analysis. *PLoS Med* 2021;18:e1003765.
16 Taillie LS et al. Changes in food purchases after the Chilean policies on food labelling, marketing, and sales in schools: a before and after study. *Lancet Planet Health* 2021;5:e526–33.
17 Front-of-package labeling as a policy tool for the prevention of noncommunicable diseases in the Americas. PAHO, Washington, 2020.
18 Superior efficacy of front-of-package warning labels in Jamaica. PAHO, Washington, 2021.
19 Sugar reduction and wider reformulation programme: report on progress towards the first 5% reduction and next steps. Public Health England, London, 2018.
20 Lewis N et al. Differences in the sugar content of fast-food products across three countries. *Public Health Nutr* 2020;23:2857–63.
21 Proritizing areas for action in the field of population-based prevention of childhood obesity. WHO, 2012.
22 Fiscal Policies for Diet and Noncommunicable Diseases. WHO, 2015.
23 Itira A et al. Taxing sugar-sweetened beverages as a policy to reduce overweight and obesity in countries of different income classifications: a systematic review. *Public Health Nutr* 2021;24:5550–60.
24 Popkin B et al. Sugar-sweetened beverage taxes: lessons to date and the future of taxation. *PLOS Med* 2021;18:e1003412.
25 Alsukait R et al. Sugary drink excise tax policy process and implementation: case study from Saudi Arabia. *Food Policy* 2020;90:101789.
26 Teng AM et al. Impact of sugar-sweetened beverage taxes on purchases and dietary intake: systematic review and meta-analysis. *Obes Rev* 2019;20:1187–204.

23 Food reformulation for NCD prevention and control

Chizuru Nishida, Rain Yamamoto, Eduardo AF Nilson, Alison Tedstone

Product improvement through reformulation is an important tool to improve the food environment to promote healthy diets and reduce the risks of NCDs. This chapter outlines the characteristics of successful reformulation programmes, along with three examples: industrially produced trans fat elimination from the food supply, reduction of salt/sodium in manufactured food and reduction in the content of sugars in food and beverages.

Reformulation is the process of changing the ingredients or recipe to affect the nutrient composition of a food or beverage product with the objective of making it healthier, usually while trying to minimize the impact on taste and flavour, as well as affordability. If unhealthy food products that are frequently consumed are reformulated toward healthier products (e.g. reduced levels of salt in bread), this can result in improvement in people's diets without individuals having to make a conscious effort to seek out healthier options or being health literate.

An increasing number of countries are introducing legislation to eliminate industrially produced trans fat,[1] and there is growing momentum for implementing reformulation policies and programmes to reduce dietary intake of salt/sodium,[2] sugars, saturated fat and energy both at the individual and population levels. A recent systematic review showed positive impacts of food reformulation on food choices, nutrient intake and health status for reformulation policies on salt/sodium and trans fat and that reformulated products were generally well accepted and purchased by consumers.[3] For example, sodium intakes were lower by 0.57 g/day and trans fat was reduced by 38–85% after reformulation.

Successful reformulation programmes are characterized by:

- Using scientific evidence on the relationship between diet, nutrition and health outcomes.
- Having strong political will from governments, with strong support and advocacy from civil society, professional organizations and academics.
- Focusing on reformulating the main food and beverage sources of the target nutrients or energy in the diet. Dietary surveys and food purchase data can provide information on such food and beverage sources.

DOI: 10.4324/9781003306689-26

- Setting stretching but achievable time-bound targets for specific nutrients (e.g. sodium, sugars, saturated fat) or reductions in energy levels. Insights into what is achievable can be obtained by considering the range of nutrient levels across similar foods (this requires food composition information) or by comparing levels in similar products on the market in countries with established reformulation programmes (e.g. sugar levels in cookies). A balance must be struck between:
  - The socio-economic and public health impact of improving diet.
  - Acceptability of changes in taste or palatability to consumers. For example, experience suggests that a 5–10% reduction in levels of salt or sugar is not detected. Where larger changes are required, incremental steps or other changes, such as recipe improvement through the use of herbs or spices, may be required.
  - Technical constraints associated with the functionality of the nutrient within the food, e.g. the use of salt as a preservative in processed meat. While the food industry will provide advice on functional constraints, their views should always be tested through the involvement of consumer groups and insights from countries that have implemented reformulation programmes as well as, in the case of sodium reduction, regional and international benchmarks such as those established by WHO.[4]

Different countries have used different approaches for setting targets, for example using maximum or average levels of target nutrients per 100 g or 100 ml product. Product categories may be widely or narrowly defined (e.g. all cookies or a particular type of cookies, or all or specific sugar-sweetened beverages [SSBs]). Some countries have set a maximum level per serving which can be particularly useful for restaurants, take-away and food deliveries.

Experiences in implementing reformulation policies in different countries also indicate the following:

- Voluntary reformulation programmes are unlikely to be successful without planned actions to implement legislation, taxation, or other measures if targets are not achieved.
- Where reformulation programmes are not mandatory, engagement should be sought from all food companies including retailers, manufacturers, restaurants, take-away and food delivery chains. Small businesses are unlikely to have the resources for reformulation so may require additional or specific measures. In addition, supportive marketing to promote reformulated products may help encourage reformulation efforts by the food industry.
- Gradual reformulation is often more effective than an abrupt approach especially for sodium and sugar in order to ensure the product remains acceptable to consumers over the course of reformulation.[5] Likewise, targets need refreshing and moving downwards every few years.

- Clear guidance should be available on what could and should be used as alternatives to replace the target nutrient, if needed (e.g. unsaturated fats for trans fat). It is important to provide technical support to those with limited resources and experience such as small and medium-sized enterprises.
- Monitoring and reporting should be undertaken on the progress made by businesses. This is best done independently and transparently. More detail on this is provided at the end of this chapter.

Watch points for reformulation policies include:

- Potential detrimental effects on the nutrient profile of a product can result from reformulation, e.g. where trans fat is replaced with excessive amounts of saturated fat. This can be guarded against through guidance to the food industry and by monitoring. Similarly, it is important that reformulation does not increase the energy density of a product, for example by replacing sugars with fats with a resulting net positive caloric content.
- Government should set clear rules of engagement with food manufacturers to ensure that decisions are made in the interest of public health. Engagement with the food industry should be transparent. Canada, for example, has set a mechanism to ensure transparency of all communications with stakeholders in relation to healthy eating initiatives, including trans fat elimination and salt/sodium reduction; this includes a registry of all meetings and correspondence with officials and a commitment that no correspondence is treated as confidential. Mechanisms to hold food companies accountable for their commitments are also key. For example, an agreement between the Norwegian health authorities and the food industry are evaluated by an independent research body, with results publicly available.
- Other interventions should be undertaken alongside reformulation to contribute to the improvement of the food environment. These include fiscal policies (i.e. taxation, subsidy), policies to restrict marketing, and nutrition labelling policies (including front-of-pack labelling). A good example of implementing a package of comprehensive policy measures can be observed in Chile where a combined programme of marketing restrictions, warning logos on the front-of-pack, and public food procurement, such as in schools are used.

Food fortification alongside reformulation

Fortification is an important tool in reducing micronutrient deficiencies. For example, WHO recommends the iodization of salt to help eliminate iodine deficiency disorders.[6,7] At the same time WHO recommends reducing the intake of sodium (salt) to reduce blood pressure and risk of cardiovascular diseases (CVD), stroke and ischemic heart disease (IHD).[8] These seemingly contradicting policies are in fact compatible, provided that there is a full implementation of universal salt iodization and effective implementation of sodium reduction policies including reformulation and the ability to monitor and adjust iodine concentrations in table/cooking salt in response to any decrease in population sodium intake.

However, food manufacturers may use foods fortified with micronutrients for promotional purposes, which can contribute to excess intake of macronutrients, energy, and salt/sodium, when fortified foods contain high levels of sugars, fats and sodium. Food fortification alone cannot, therefore, be a substitute for diet- and nutrition-related policy actions to address NCDs, and fortified foods should also be included in reformulation policies.

Examples of reformulation policies

Eliminating industrially produced trans fat from the food supply

Industrially produced trans fat is partially hydrogenated unsaturated fats that largely result from the industrial transformation of unsaturated oils to harden them and increase their shelf life. Industrially produced trans fat is strongly associated with an increased risk of CHD (Chapter 20 on cholesterol, fat and trans fat). Elimination of industrially produced trans fat is feasible and achievable and over the last 20 years, governments have successfully used both mandatory and voluntary measures to encourage industry to eliminate industry-produced trans fat, in order to reduce an individual's intake of trans fat to <1% of total energy intake with trans fat being replaced by unsaturated fatty acids.[9] WHO recommends that countries introduce a mandatory national limit of 2 g of industrially produced trans fat per 100 g of total fat in all foods; and a mandatory national ban on the production or use of partially hydrogenated oils as an ingredient in all foods. These best-practice policies can remove virtually all industrially produced trans fat from the food supply.[10,11,12]

In 2021, best-practice trans-fat policies have been implemented in 40 countries (covering 1.4 billion people) and best-practice trans-fat policies in six additional countries (covering an additional 1.7 billion people) will come into effect over the next two years.[13]

REPLACE is a WHO step-by-step guide for the elimination of industrially-produced trans-fatty acids from the global food supply. It provides six areas of action:

- **Re**view dietary sources of industrially produced trans-fat and the landscape for required policy change.
- **P**romote the replacement of industrially produced fat with healthier fats and oils.
- **L**egislate or enact regulatory actions to eliminate industrially produced trans-fat.

- **A**ssess and monitor trans-fat content in the food supply and changes in trans-fat consumption in the population.
- **C**reate awareness of the negative health impact of fats among policy-makers, producers, suppliers and the public.
- **E**nforce compliance with policies and regulations.

WHO has also developed a technical framework and a set of online implementation resources[14] as well as a global laboratory protocol for measuring trans fat in foods.[15] WHO also provides technical support to countries to accelerate best-practice policy development, implementation and enforcement as well as laboratory capacity-building and training.

Reformulation to reduce the amount of salt/sodium in processed food

Excessive intake of salt/sodium increases blood pressure and CVD risk and was accountable for 1.9 million deaths globally in 2019 (IHME). WHO recommends a reduction to <2 g/day sodium consumption (<5 g/day salt) in adults. A 30% reduction in mean population intake of salt/sodium by 2025 (vs 2010) is a global target to be achieved by 2030.

In many high-income countries, and increasingly in low- and middle-income countries, a significant proportion of dietary salt/sodium comes from manufactured foods such as bread, processed meats, cheese, cookies, breakfast cereals, snacks and ready-to-eat products. A cost-effective way to reduce population salt/sodium intake can therefore be through lowering the sodium content of food products that are consumed frequently.[16] Many countries have introduced national reformulation strategies and targets to reduce sodium in manufactured foods.[17] Depending on the foods consumed and the political situation in the country, there is a variation in measures adopted, the food products targeted, and the targets adopted. However, a priority component of a successful reformulation plan is for countries to set time-bound limits for salt/sodium levels in foods and meals for the food industry to implement. In 2021, WHO issued the global sodium benchmarks for various food categories to drive progress in reducing sodium content in foods.

At least 17 countries have reported reductions in population salt intake since 2014, through a variety of policy interventions to reduce salt/sodium intake in their populations including through reformulation, with 12 countries reporting a substantial (>2 g/day) or moderate (1–2 g/day) reduction.[18]

Reformulation to reduce levels of sugars in food and beverages

WHO recommends limiting the intake of free sugars to <10% of total energy intake, and suggests a further reduction in the intake of free sugars to <5% of total energy intake for added health benefits (Chapter 22). A growing number of national authorities have set targets for sugar levels in different food and beverage categories. In the UK, reports show evidence of success in reducing sugar content in some food groups including breakfast cereals, yogurts and ice creams.[19] Randomised controlled studies in children suggest that reductions in the sugar content of SSBs are associated with lower total energy intake and reduced body weight.[20] Chapter 22 provides more detail.

One should be mindful that reducing sugar content in products (e.g. SSBs) will only lead to overall reductions in sugar in the diet if sales and consumption of reformulated products do not change. If sales of reformulated products increase then sugar intake may increase. For example, if cookies are reformulated to contain less sugars, but more cookies are sold, or if individuals consume more other (liquid or solid) products high in sugar, then the total amount of dietary sugars may not decrease or even increase. This can be guarded against by other supportive policies, such as policies to restrict marketing and/or taxation of less healthy products.

Taxation has been used to support the reduction of sugar content in food. For example, following the introduction of a soft drink industry levy in the UK, the proportion of potentially taxable drinks with sugar levels above the lower levy threshold (5 g sugar/100 mL) fell by 43.7%, suggesting that the levy had incentivized manufacturers to reformulate their products.[21] Importantly, all socio-economic groups are likely to accrue the health benefits linked to lower levels of sugars in the diet.

Monitoring

Monitoring the progress of reformulation programmes is important to demonstrate impact and its contribution to broader efforts to prevent and control NCDs, as well as to encourage continued and enhanced action. Data on fats, sugars, and salt/sodium levels in foods are needed in order to monitor progress. They can be obtained from sales, surveys on population intakes, surveys of shop and restaurant declared levels (on labels or menus), and extraction of nutrition data from retail websites. Nutrient information on products is particularly important.

Monitoring is more likely to be meaningful if it is independently done. Involving civil society (e.g. the academia and NGOs) in monitoring is a way of encouraging transparency and maintaining pressure on the food industry. Different countries have taken different approaches. For example, in the UK, Public Health England has reported progress on sugar reduction according to food category, food sector, business, and product level, and found reductions of 13.3% and 12.9% in sugar levels in breakfast cereals and yogurt[23] but no change for confectionery. Brazil has also reported progress in sodium reduction at the food category and product level (8–34% reduction in the average sodium content of over half of food categories).[22]

Impact evaluation (e.g. the impact of reformulation on diet and health outcomes) is important, and needs considering. The impact of sodium reduction through food reformulation has been studied directly and through modelling methodologies in countries including the UK, USA, Australia and Brazil, for example, to assess changes in sodium intake, blood pressure and hypertension and CVD.[23,24,25,26]

Disseminating reports that describe the results of such monitoring and evaluation is also important. The WHO progress report on trans fat elimination describes the global, regional and national situations and progress made over the past year with regard to trans fat reformulation in countries and discusses challenges and opportunities for future action. The report is published annually in a countdown to the 2023 goal of global elimination of industrially produced trans fat. WHO is also planning to issue biannual progress reports on sodium reduction starting in 2022.[13]

Notes

1 TFA Country Score Card. Global database on the implementation of nutrition actions (GINA). WHO, 2022.
2 Sodium Country Score Card. Global database on the implementation of nutrition actions (GINA). WHO, 2022.
3 Gressier M et al. What is the impact of food reformulation on individuals' behaviour, nutrient intakes and health status? A systematic review of empirical evidence. *Obes Rev* 2021;22:e13139.
4 WHO global sodium benchmarks for different food categories. WHO, 2021.
5 Bobowski N et al. A longitudinal comparison of two salt reduction strategies: acceptability of a low sodium food depends on the consumer. *Food Qual Prefer* 2015;40:270–78.
6 Essential nutrition actions: mainstreaming nutrition through the life-course. WHO, 2019.
7 Guideline: fortification of food-grade salt with iodine for the prevention and control of iodine deficiency disorders. WHO, 2014.
8 Guideline: sodium intake for adults and children. WHO, 2012.
9 Guidelines on saturated fatty acid and trans-fatty acid intake in adults and children. WHO (under finalization).
10 Downs SM et al. The effectiveness of policies for reducing dietary trans fat: a systematic review of the evidence. *Bull WHO* 2013;91:262–69.
11 Hyseni L et al. Systematic review of dietary trans-fat reduction interventions. *Bull WHO* 2017;95:821–30.
12 Downs SM et al. The impact of policies to reduce trans fat consumption: a systematic review of the evidence. *Curr Dev Nutr* 2017;1(12):cdn.117.000778.
13 Countdown to 2023: WHO report on global trans-fat elimination. WHO, 2021.
14 REPLACE trans fat-free by 2023: an action package to eliminate industrially-produced trans-fat from the global food supply [website]. WHO, Geneva.
15 Global protocol for measuring fatty acid profiles of foods, with emphasis on monitoring trans-fatty acids originating from partially hydrogenated oils. WHO, 2020.
16 Van Vliet BN, Campbell NRC. Canadian hypertension education program. Efforts to reduce sodium intake in Canada: why, what, and when? *Can J Cardiol* 2011;27:437–45.
17 Rosewarne E et al. A global review of national strategies to reduce sodium levels in packaged foods. *Adv Nutr* 2022;13:1820–33.
18 Santos JA et al. A systematic review of salt reduction initiatives around the world: a midterm evaluation of progress towards the 2025 global non-communicable diseases salt reduction target. *Adv Nutr* 2021;12:1768–80.
19 Scarborough P et al. Impact of the announcement and implementation of the UK soft drinks industry levy on sugar content, price, product size and number of available soft

drinks in the UK, 2015–19: a controlled interrupted time series analysis. *PLoS Med* 2020;17:e1003025.
20 Scientific Advisory Committee on Nutrition. Carbohydrates and health report. London TSO, 2015. https://assets.publishing.service.gov.uk.
21 Sugar reduction: report on progress between 2015 and 2019. Public Health England, 2020.
22 Nilson EAF et al. Sodium reduction in processed foods in Brazil: analysis of food categories and voluntary targets from 2011 to 2017. *Nutrients* 2017;9:742.
23 He FJ et al. Salt reduction in the United Kingdom: a successful experiment in public health. *J Hum Hypertens* 2014;28:345–52.
24 Pearson-Stuttard J et al. Estimating the health and economic effects of the proposed US Food and Drug Administration voluntary sodium reformulation: microsimulation cost-effectiveness analysis. *PLoS Med* 2018;15:e1002551.
25 Coyle D et al. Estimating the potential impact of Australia's reformulation programme on households' sodium purchases. *BMJ Nutr Prev Health* 2021;4:49–58.
26 Nilson EAF et al. Estimating the health and economic effects of the voluntary sodium reduction targets in Brazil: microsimulation analysis. *BMC Med* 2021;19:1–10.

24 Nutrition labelling for NCD prevention and control

Katrin Engelhardt, Chizuru Nishida, Jenny Reid, Bridget Kelly

Unhealthy diets are a leading cause of ill health and mortality, and in 2019 caused 7.9 million deaths globally.[1] The food environment plays a critical role in shaping people's diets, including what kind of food and beverages are produced and processed, how they are labelled, marketed and sold, their price and how and where they are consumed. The current food retail environment offers an unprecedented selection of both packaged and unpackaged foods. Nutrition labelling provides information to consumers on the nutritional properties of food[2] and is an important tool to guide healthy food choices and support the adoption of healthier diets, which help to improve and protect the health of people.[3,4]

The Codex Alimentarius Commission (Codex) is responsible for implementing the Joint FAO/WHO Food Standards Programme and for providing international food-related standards, guidelines and codes of practice, including guidelines on nutrition labelling. Codex standards and guidelines serve as a basis for national legislation to protect the health of consumers and to ensure fair practices in the food trade, and they are used as a reference point for international trade agreements of the World Trade Organization.

This chapter focusses on the following components of nutrition labelling: ingredient lists, nutrient declarations, and supplementary nutrition information (which includes front-of-pack labelling [FOPL]). This chapter also describes nutrition and health claims, which are used to promote the sale, purchase and intake of food.

Ingredient list

The list of ingredients is a mandatory requirement for the label of all pre-packaged foods (except for single-ingredient foods), as described in a general Codex standard. All pre-packaged foods must carry a list of ingredients, in descending order of weight.[5] For example, if sugar is listed first, it contributed the largest amount to the food at the time it was manufactured. Importantly, there are different ways to define sugars. The general naming requirements and other details for ingredient lists are defined by Codex.

Nutrient declarations

Nutrient declarations inform consumers about the energy and nutrient content of the food. Codex requires that the nutrient declaration must appear directly on the package (usually on the back or side).[2] The regulatory requirement for these declarations is determined at country or regional level. The Codex Guidelines on Nutrition Labelling state that where a nutrient declaration is applied the following declarations should be mandatory: energy value, protein, available carbohydrate (excluding dietary fibre), total sugars, fat (including saturated fat), and sodium (or salt). Codex guidelines also state that the amount of any other nutrient considered to be relevant for maintaining a good nutritional status, as required by national legislation or dietary guidelines, should be declared. Some foods may be exempt from displaying a nutrient declaration, for example on the basis of nutritional or dietary insignificance or small packaging (e.g. chewing gum). Although trans fat is not a mandatory nutrient to be included in the list of nutrient declarations, in countries where the intake level of trans fat is a public health concern, trans fat declaration should be considered.

Prior to 2013, saturated fat, sodium and total sugars were not included as mandatory nutrients to be declared. However, as part of the efforts of Codex in implementing the Global Strategy on Diet, Physical Activity and Health[6] and to address the increasing public health problems of obesity and diet-related NCDs, in 2013 Codex endorsed the inclusion of saturated fat, sodium and total sugars as mandatory nutrients to be declared in nutrient declarations. Codex also developed the nutrient reference values relevant to the prevention of NCDs (NRVs-NCD) based on WHO guidelines.

Importantly, if a food carries a nutrition or health claim (further discussed below), e.g. claiming that a food is low or high in a particular nutrient, the amount of the nutrient referred to must be declared.

Supplementary nutrition information

Supplementary nutrition information is intended to increase the consumer's understanding of the nutritional value of their food. It should not be used in place of the nutrient declaration, except for target populations who have a high illiteracy rate and/or comparatively little knowledge of nutrition. FOPL is an example of supplementary nutrition information and can be voluntary or mandatory, in line with national legislation.

There are two main types of FOPL systems: *interpretive* and *non-interpretive*, and there is wide geographic variation in the use of FOPL.

- Interpretive systems provide at-a-glance guidance on the relative healthfulness of the product. They may provide a summary indicator of the overall relative healthfulness or unhealthfulness of food (e.g. symbols, figures, or cautionary text). Examples include the Nutri-Score system (e.g. France)[7] and the Health Star Rating System (e.g. Australia and New Zealand),[8] as well as the multiple traffic light labelling systems (e.g. the

United Kingdom),[9] which provide an interpretation of the number of different nutrients in the food, and the warning system (e.g. Chile)[10] which provides an indicator of high levels of nutrients that increase the risk of diet-related NCDs. In contrast, endorsement logos, such as the Green Keyhole (e.g. Sweden), provide an indicator of the relative healthfulness of a food, with no indication of unhealthfulness.
- Non-interpretive systems, such as Guideline Daily Amount (GDA), convey nutritional content as numbers rather than graphics, symbols or colours, allowing consumers to create their own judgements about food healthfulness.

What FOPL system to use depends on the country's context. Some countries will create their own system, whereas other countries may adopt an existing one. No matter what system is used, the FOPL system should enable appropriate comparisons between foods and facilitate the consumers' understanding of the nutritional value of the food and their choice of food, consistent with the national dietary guidance or health and nutrition policy of the county or region of implementation. Codex has published Guidelines on Front of Pack Nutrition Labelling to assist countries in their development of FOPL systems.[2] The WHO Guiding Principles and Framework Manual for FOPL[11] is a tool to help countries in developing and implementing FOPL, highlighting the importance of multi-sectoral engagement and applying a collaborative approach to developing the FOPL system. These also provide guidance on conducting a contextual analysis, defining the aims, scope and principles of the FOPL system, selecting the appropriate FOPL system (including format and content) design, implementation as well as monitoring and evaluation.

The supplementary nutrition information on labels should be accompanied by consumer education programmes to help increase consumer awareness, understanding and effective use of the information.

Nutrition and health claims

Nutrition and health claims are any representation which states, suggests or implies that a food has particular characteristics relating to its origin, nutritional properties, nature, production, processing, composition or any other quality.[12] Claims can be used to promote the sale, purchase and intake of food. Examples of nutrition claims include products low- or free in fat, sugars or sodium. All nutrition and health claims should be supported by a sound body of scientific evidence. *Health* claims should have qualifying and/or disqualifying conditions for eligibility, and claims should not be made for foods that contain nutrients in amounts that increase the risk of disease or an adverse health-related condition. Codex has defined what 'free', 'low', or 'very low' means for energy, fat, saturated fat, cholesterol, sugars and sodium.[13] Some examples are shown in Table 24.1.

Policies should be implemented at a national or regional level, based on Codex, to regulate the use of nutrition and health claims to avoid their misuse

Table 24.1 Examples of conditions for nutrient content claims[17]

Component	Claim	Condition
Fat	Low	3 g per 100 g (solids) or 1.5 g per 100 ml (liquids)
	Free	0.5 g per 100 g (solids) or 0.5 g per 100 ml (liquids)
Sugars	Free	0.5 g per 100 g (solids) or 0.5 g per 100 ml (liquids)
Sodium	Low	0.12 g per 100 g
	Very low	0.04 g per 100 g
	Free	0.005 g per 100 g

and ensure such claims provide truthful and non-misleading information that is substantiated by scientific evidence.

Other nutrition labelling that may help determine the healthiness of a food

Barcodes on food packages

Most food packages include barcodes, which provide a unique product code and are an important tool to manage the supply chain and food traceability, and when necessary, help with the recall of contaminated batches of a specific product. The use of barcodes on foods has evolved and where available, may allow consumers to use mobile phones to scan them to obtain more details on food products. This could include supplementary nutrition labelling, the product's origin and place of manufacture, as well as the carbon footprint (for its production and transport) in some cases.

Developing nutrition labelling policies

Developing, implementing and monitoring nutrition labelling policies should be government-led and transparent. Nutrition labelling policies should have clear objectives and measurable outcomes. While details of the nutrition labelling policy will depend on the country's context, many have adapted the labelling provisions of Codex texts, including the nutrient declaration provisions.

Nutrition labelling policies will also need to take into account relevant national and regional regulations and agreements and consider the nutrition and health needs of the population. Policies will require collaboration across government departments/authorities including food and drug, food standards, consumer affairs, health, trade and the economy.

Nutrition labels described in this chapter are not intended to be implemented independently from one another, but rather in a coherent and integrated manner (Figure 24.1).

The implementation of nutrition labelling policies in many countries indicates their feasibility and priority. A recently conducted review of factors that may impact the development and implementation of nutrition labelling policies identified elements that support or hinder the development, implementation,

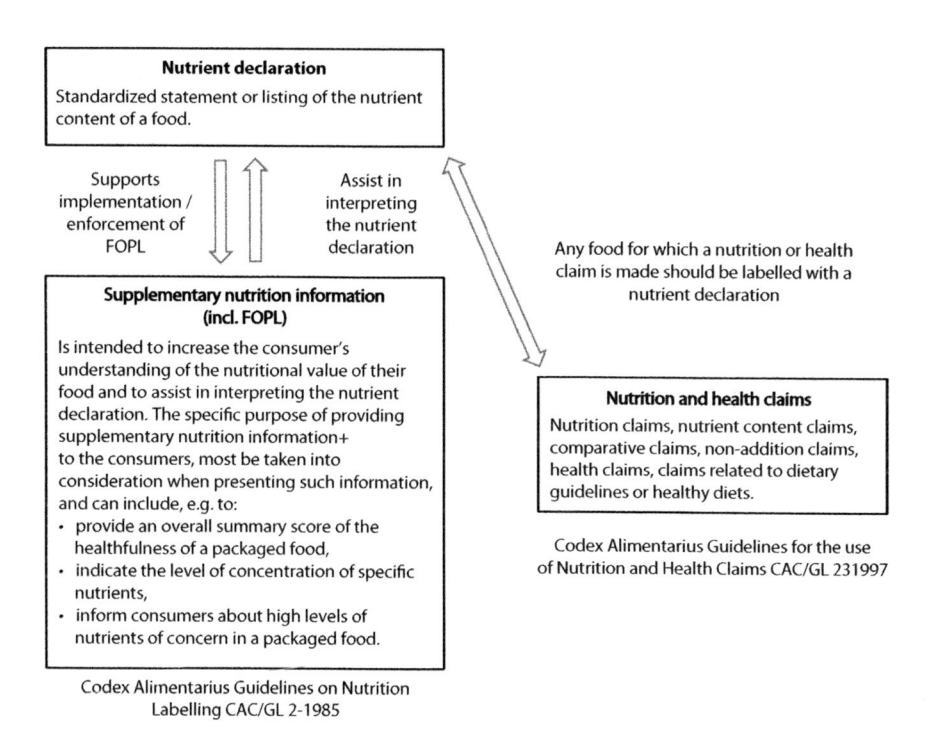

```
┌─────────────────────────────────────────┐
│         Nutrient declaration            │
│ Standardized statement or listing of    │
│ the nutrient content of a food.         │
└─────────────────────────────────────────┘
     ↓↑                    ↖
 Supports          Assist in      ↖
 implementation/   interpreting     ↖
 enforcement of    the nutrient      ↖  Any food for which a nutrition or health
 FOPL  ↓↑          declaration        ↖ claim is made should be labelled with a
                                        nutrient declaration
┌─────────────────────────────────────────┐
│   Supplementary nutrition information   │
│             (incl. FOPL)                │
│ Is intended to increase the consumer's  │
│ understanding of the nutritional value  │        ┌────────────────────────────────┐
│ of their food and to assist in          │        │  Nutrition and health claims   │
│ interpreting the nutrient declaration.  │        │ Nutrition claims, nutrient     │
│ The specific purpose of providing       │        │ content claims, comparative    │
│ supplementary nutrition information+    │        │ claims, non-addition claims,   │
│ to the consumers, most be taken into    │        │ health claims, claims related  │
│ consideration when presenting such      │        │ to dietary guidelines or       │
│ information, and can include, e.g. to:  │        │ healthy diets.                 │
│ • provide an overall summary score of   │        └────────────────────────────────┘
│   the healthfulness of a packaged food, │
│ • indicate the level of concentration   │         Codex Alimentarius Guidelines for the use
│   of specific nutrients,                │         of Nutrition and Health Claims CAC/GL 231997
│ • inform consumers about high levels of │
│   nutrients of concern in a packaged    │
│   food.                                 │
└─────────────────────────────────────────┘
Codex Alimentarius Guidelines on Nutrition
Labelling CAC/GL 2-1985
```

Figure 24.1 Integrating nutrient declarations, supplementary nutrition information and health and nutrition claims.

monitoring, evaluation and enforcement of such policies.[14] Supportive elements include strong political leadership, robust and independent evidence, intersectoral collaboration, transparent processes and pilot-testing of FOPL.[15,16] Barriers include conflict of interests, industry interference and challenges in agreeing on the optimal system in the country concerned.[17] A number of surveys indicate public support for clear and easy-to-interpret labels.[17] The food industry in general prefers voluntary numerical systems over more interpretive systems. Chapter 56 on the private sector describes broader challenges around the alignment of the food and beverage industry with government policies to promote public health.

Effectiveness of nutrition labelling

The impact of nutrition labelling depends on the multiple drivers of nutrition behaviour and food-related decisions, including taste, price, convenience, brand, cultural and/or family preferences. These factors, in addition to the attributes of the label itself, including its content, format and context, influence the extent to which the information on the label will be sought and used by the consumers.

Available evidence on the impact of nutrition labelling mostly comes from studies that assessed the impact of certain labelling design and content elements that may inform the development or revision of labelling policies[18,19,20,21] or the performance of different FOPL systems[22,23] rather than from evaluations of nutrition labelling policies as such. However, policy evaluations are starting to emerge – in particular on a diverse range of nationally implemented FOPL systems, examples include Australia[24] and Chile.[25]

Nutrition labelling has been shown to be an important policy implementation tool for improving consumers' understanding of the nutritional content and quality of the food supply, and for guiding healthier food decisions. It is important that policymakers recognize that nutrition labelling is one (albeit important) part of a comprehensive approach for promoting healthy diets.

The authors gratefully acknowledge the valuable inputs and critical review provided by Philippa Hawthorne and Rebecca Doonan, Ministry of Primary Industry, Government of New Zealand.

Notes

1 GBD 2019 Risk Factors Collaborators. Global burden of 87 risk factors in 204 countries and territories, 1990–2019: a systematic analysis for the Global Burden of Disease Study 2019. *Lancet* 2020;396:1223–49.
2 Codex Guidelines on Nutrition Labelling. CAC/GL 2-1985 (last revised in 2021).
3 Comprehensive implementation plan on maternal, infant and young child nutrition. WHO, 2012.
4 Report of the commission on ending childhood obesity. WHO, 2016.
5 Codex Alimentarius. General Standard for the Labelling of Prepackaged Foods. FAO & WHO. CXS 1-1985 (revised in 2018).
6 Global strategy on diet, physical activity and health. WHO, 2004.
7 Ducrot P et al. Objective understanding of front-of-package nutrition labels among nutritionally at-risk individuals. *Nutrients* 2015;7:7106–25.
8 Department of Health, Australia. Health Star Rating System. http://www.healthstarrating.gov.au/internet/healthstarrating/publishing.nsf/Content/Home.
9 Guide to creating a front of pack (FoP) nutrition label for pre-packed products sold through retail outlets. Department of Health, 2016.
10 Colchero MA et al. The impacts on food purchases and tax revenues of a tax based on Chile's nutrient profiling model. *PLoS One* 2021;16:e026069.
11 Guiding principles and framework manual for front-of-pack labelling for promoting healthy diets. WHO, 2019.
12 Guidelines for Use of Nutrition and Health Claims. Nutrition and Health Claims, CAC/GL 23-1997 (revised in 2004, amended last in 2013).
13 Guidelines for Use of Nutrition and Health Claims, CAC/GL 23-1997.
14 Implementing nutrition labelling policies: a review of contextual factors. WHO, 2021.
15 Corvalan C et al. Structural responses to the obesity and non-communicable diseases epidemic: the Chilean law of food labelling and advertising. *Obes Rev* 2013;14:79–87.
16 Edalti S et al. Development and implementation of nutrition labelling in Iran: a retrospective policy analysis. *Int J Health Plann Manage* 2020;35:e28–44.
17 Signal L et al. Front-of-pack nutrition labelling in New Zealand: an exploration of stakeholder views about research and implementation. *Health Promot J Aus* 2012;23:48–51.
18 Antúnez L et al. How do design features influence consumer attention when looking for nutritional information on food labels? Results from an eye-tracking study on pan bread labels. *Int J Food Sci Nutr* 2013;64:515–27.

19 Arrúa A et al. Warnings as a directive front-of-pack nutrition labelling scheme: comparison with the guideline daily amount and traffic-light systems. *Public Health Nutr* 2017;20:2308–17.
20 Feunekes GIJ et al. Front-of-pack nutrition labelling: testing effectiveness of different nutrition labelling formats front-of-pack in four European countries. *Appetite* 2008;50:57–70.
21 Tórtora G et al. Influence of nutritional warnings and other label features on consumers' choice: results from an eye-tracking study. *Food Res Int* 2019;119:605–11.
22 Croker H et al. Front of pack nutritional labelling schemes: a systematic review and meta-analysis of recent evidence relating to objectively measured consumption and purchasing. *J Hum Nutr Diet* 2020;33:518–37.
23 Ares G et al. Comparative performance of three interpretative front-of-pack nutrition labelling schemes: insights for policy making. *Food Qual Prefer* 2018:215–25.
24 Health Star Rating system (2020). Formal review of the system after five years of implementation (June 2014 to June 2019). http://www.healthstarrating.gov.au/internet/healthstarrating/publishing.nsf/Content/formal-review-of-the-system-after-five-years.
25 Taillie L et al. Changes in food purchases after the Chilean policies on food labelling, marketing, and sales in schools: a before and after study. *Lancet Planet Health* 2021;5:e526–33.

25 Physical inactivity and NCDs

Burden, epidemiology, and priority interventions

Estelle Victoria Lambert, Fiona Bull

Regular physical activity improves physical and mental health.[1,2] For NCDs, physical activity is associated with lower risks of cardiovascular disease (CVD), a number of cancers (including breast and colon), diabetes, as well as maintaining a healthy weight.[3] In addition to health-related benefits, physical activity provides a range of additional social and economic benefits and therefore contributes to a large number of Sustainable Development Goals.[4]

BOX 25.1   DEFINITIONS OF PHYSICAL ACTIVITY AND RELATED TERMS[1]

Physical activity Any bodily movement produced by skeletal muscles that results in energy expenditure. It can be part of work, domestic chores, transportation or during leisure time, including exercise or sports activities.

Physical inactivity Used to refer to participation in low levels of physical activity and specifically at levels that do not meet WHO guidelines. The term physical inactivity is used instead of insufficient physical activity.

Exercise Planned and structured physical activity performed during leisure time with the primary purpose of improving or maintaining physical fitness, physical performance, or health.

Physical fitness A measure of the body's ability to function efficiently and effectively in work and leisure activities, and includes, for example, muscular strength and cardiorespiratory fitness.

Sedentary behaviour Any waking behaviour with very low energy expenditure while sitting, reclining, or lying, for example most desk-based office work, driving a car, and watching television.

DOI: 10.4324/9781003306689-28

Physical activity can be of **light intensity**, such as slow walking (no substantial increase in heart rate or breathing rate), **moderate intensity**, such as fast walking (one has increased heart rate, but can still talk) or **vigorous intensity**, such as running (i.e. one can no longer hold a conversation).

Metabolic equivalent of task (MET), or simply metabolic equivalent – a physiological measure expressing the intensity of physical activities. One MET is the energy equivalent expended by an individual while seated at rest. Light-, moderate- and vigorous-intensity refers to physical activity performed at 1.5–3, 3–6 and more than 6 METS, respectively.

Recommended levels of physical activity

Table 25.1 provides WHO-recommended levels of physical activity for children and adolescents, adults and older adults, as well as for pregnant and postpartum women, and those people living with chronic conditions and disability.

Guidelines on recommended levels of movement, sedentary and sleep for children under the age of five are also available.[5]

Data at global and country levels

Globally, one in four adults and four in five adolescents do not meet WHO's global recommendations on physical activity for health.[6,7] This translates into 1.4 billion adults not benefitting from improved health through sufficient regular physical activity and it is especially concerning that there has been little change in global self-reported levels of insufficient (or 'low') physical activity since 2001 (28.5%).[8]

Levels of physical inactivity vary greatly across countries (e.g. 5.5% in Uganda, 67.0 % in Kuwait) and World Bank income groups. In 2016, the prevalence of physical inactivity was more than twice as high in high-income countries (HICs) (36.8%) than in low-income countries (LICs) (16.2%). Across all income groups, women were less active than men.[6]

Levels of physical activity decrease with socio-economic development and changing patterns in urbanization, including leisure, transportation and occupation.[9] However, these relationships are not straightforward. Differences in levels of physical activity are also explained by significant inequities in opportunities for physical activity. For example, girls, women, older adults, people of low socio-economic position, people with disabilities and chronic diseases, and marginalized populations, often have less access to safe, accessible, affordable and appropriate spaces and places in which to be physically active.[10]

Table 25.1 WHO recommendations on physical activity for children and adolescents, and adults[23]

Population group	Levels of sufficient physical activity and related recommendations
Children and adolescents, 5–17 years.	At least an average of 60 min. per day of moderate to vigorous intensity, mostly aerobic, physical activity, across the week. Vigorous-intensity aerobic activities, as well as those that strengthen muscle and bone, should be incorporated ≥3 days a week.
Adult, 18–64 years.	At least 150–300 min. of moderate-intensity aerobic physical activity; or ≥ 75–150 min. of vigorous-intensity aerobic physical activity; or an equivalent combination of moderate- and vigorous-intensity activity throughout the week for substantial health benefits. Muscle-strengthening activities at a moderate or greater intensity that involve all major muscle groups on ≥2 days a week, as these provide additional health benefits. Adults may increase moderate-intensity aerobic physical activity to >300 min.; or do >150 min. of vigorous-intensity aerobic physical activity; or an equivalent combination of moderate- and vigorous-intensity activity throughout the week for additional health benefits.
Adults 65 years and older.	At least 150–300 min. of moderate-intensity aerobic physical activity; or ≥75–150 min. of vigorous-intensity aerobic physical activity; or an equivalent combination of moderate- and vigorous-intensity activity throughout the week, for substantial health benefits. Muscle-strengthening activities at a moderate or greater intensity that involve all major muscle groups on ≥2 days a week, as these provide additional health benefits. Varied multicomponent physical activity that emphasizes functional balance and strength training at moderate or greater intensity, on ≥3 days a week, to enhance functional capacity and to prevent falls. Adults may increase moderate-intensity aerobic physical activity to more than 300 min; or do >150 min. of vigorous-intensity aerobic physical activity; or an equivalent combination of moderate- and vigorous-intensity activity throughout the week for additional health benefits.

Disease burden

The proportion of all deaths attributable to physical inactivity has increased over the last 30 years, across all World Bank groups except HICs, although age-standardized mortality rates have reduced over this same period, and this is especially so in HICs (Table 25.2, IHME). In 2019, IHME estimated that among all deaths due to low physical activity, 77% were attributable to CVD, 15% to diabetes mellitus and 8% to cancer. As with all modifiable risk factors, attributable risk depends on the cut-offs defined for optimal levels of a risk factor and the shape of the relation between a risk factor (i.e. physical activity) and outcomes (e.g. whether the relation of physical activity with health

Table 25.2 Mortality attributable to low physical activity (IHME)

	Global		HICs		Upper MICs		Lower MICs		LICs	
	1990	2019	1990	2019	1990	2019	1990	2019	1990	2019
Proportion of all deaths (%)	1.0	1.5	2.3	1.9	1.0	1.8	0.5	1.2	0.2	0.3
Age-standardized mortality rates (per 100,000)	15	11	15	8	15	13	15	14	9	9

outcomes is linear or has a plateau).[11] Overall, 3–5 million deaths globally could be averted every year by reducing levels of physical inactivity.[12,13]

Socio-economic impact

Physical inactivity was estimated to cost healthcare systems international $ (INT$) 53·8 billion worldwide in 2013 ($ 31·2 billion was paid by the public sector, $ 12·9 billion by the private sector and $ 9·7 billion by households).[14] Estimates from both HICs, as well as low-middle-income countries, indicate that between 1% and 3% of national healthcare expenditures are attributable to physical inactivity.[15] However, these are regarded as underestimates as they do not include costs attributable to musculoskeletal injury, falls, depression, anxiety and other conditions. These costs are distributed unequally and disproportionately across the world: HICs carry a larger proportion of the economic burden; low- and middle-income countries have a larger proportion of the disease burden.

Recommendations at the population level

The WHO Global NCD Action Plan and the WHO Global Action Plan on Physical Activity 2018–2030 (GAPPA)[8] set out the global target of a 15% relative reduction in the prevalence of physical inactivity in adults and adolescents by 2030 (from a 2010 baseline). GAPPA provides 20 recommended policy actions relevant for all countries that are aligned with the WHO best buys and other recommended interventions (see Box 25.2 and Chapter 34 on WHO best buys and recommended interventions).

To implement these actions, whole-of-system approaches are required, with engagement and partnership across government (health, transport, education, sports, information and communication, youth, urban planning, environment, tourism, finance and labour, including city leaders and local government [Chapter 53]) as well as the private sector and civil society (including media, professional bodies, NGOs and communities themselves). An example of a whole-of-system approach is the structural steps taken by many countries to improve active mobility (e.g. by establishing highly connected bike lanes networks and programmes in cities)[16,17,18] which have been accelerated as part of the COVID-19 response.[19]

Given the diversity of ways to be physically active across a range of settings, national responses must address the wide range of factors that facilitate or serve as barriers to physical activity. Some relate more to the individual (e.g. knowledge, work-life balance and personal preferences), while others are broader socioecological issues (e.g. sociocultural norms and values, traditions, as well as economic and physical environments). Further details on the social determinants of NCDs and health through the life-course are provided in chapters 17 and 37.

BOX 25.2 WHO GLOBAL ACTION PLAN ON PHYSICAL ACTIVITY 2018-2030

Objective 1. Create active societies – enhancing knowledge and understanding of, and appreciation for, the multiple benefits of regular physical activity across society.

Four policy actions focus on implementing national public education and behaviour change campaigns and mass participation events which aim to increase knowledge and experience of the multiple benefits of regular physical activity and provide free access to community-based events to encourage participation.

Objective 2. Create active environments – creating and maintaining environments that promote and safeguard access to safe places and spaces, for regular physical activity.

Five policy actions focus on improving access to opportunities and environments for physical activity. This includes delivery of safe, well-maintained infrastructure, for walking and cycling as well as other access to recreational and sports facilities and public open spaces, and strengthening or designing regulations for streets, public facilities (such as schools) to improve access by walking and cycling.

Objective 3. Create active people – creating and promoting access to opportunities and programmes, across multiple settings, to help people engage in regular physical activity as individuals, families and communities.

Six policy actions focus on improving access to appropriate and affordable opportunities for physical activity through community-based programmes and services across multiple settings, that are culturally appropriate for people of all ages and abilities.

Objective 4. Create an active system – creating and strengthening leadership, governance, multisectoral partnerships, workforce capabilities, advocacy and information systems across sectors.

Five policy actions focus on strengthening national leadership, policy and governance, investment and advocacy. These actions support the other three strategic objectives and include the development of national policy, action plans, guidelines and monitoring systems on physical activity; as well as national and sub national coordination and multisectoral engagement. Enhancing research and evaluation, advocacy and data systems are also recommended to support effectively coordinated policy implementation.

Interventions at the individual level

Physical activity assessment and counselling, along with behaviour change support through the use of a brief intervention and including referral systems where appropriate are recommended as part of routine primary health care services and also recommended in the WHO UHC Compendium.[20] The systematic assessment and follow-up on physical activity, as well as reinforcement of the direct benefits to patients' health conditions combined with motivational interviewing techniques, are effective and supported by organizations such as the American Heart Association.[21] Primary care-based interventions that target physical activity alone, or in combination with interventions for other modifiable risk factors such as tobacco use, the harmful use of alcohol, and unhealthy diets, can be effective, including for brief advice, particularly when linked with community opportunities and support.[22]

Monitoring

Prevalence of physical inactivity among adults and adolescents (aged 11–17 years) is used to chart global and country progress towards the 2030 physical activity target. Currently, there are no indicators for those aged <11 years owing to the absence of a global consensus on self-reported or objective measurement instruments or cut points.

The Global Physical Activity Questionnaire, that forms part of STEPS surveys, collects information across three settings (work, travel to and from places and recreation). However, as self-report instruments of behaviours are prone to bias (e.g. recall, social desirability), newer more objective complementary approaches are needed. Sensor technology (e.g. pedometers or accelerometers) is increasingly used and may provide more reliable data in the future. Broader issues around surveillance are described in more detail in chapters 4 and 5.

Global monitoring of countries' implementation of policies described in the WHO Global NCD Action Plan and GAPPA are provided in WHO country progress monitor reports and global status reports on physical activity.[23]

Notes

1 Guidelines on physical activity and sedentary behaviour. WHO, 2020.
2 Paluch ES et al. Daily steps and all-cause mortality: a meta-analysis of 15 international cohorts. *Lancet Public Health* 2022;7:e219–28.
3 Bull F et al. Physical activity for the prevention of cardiometabolic disease. In Prabhakaran D et al. (eds.), *Cardiovascular, respiratory, and related disorders*, 3rd ed. Washington, DC: The International Bank for Reconstruction and Development/The World Bank, 2017.
4 International Society for Physical Activity and Health. *The Bangkok declaration on physical activity for global health and sustainable development*. Bangkok, Thailand, 2016.
5 Guidelines on physical activity, sedentary behaviour and sleep for children under 5 years of age. WHO, 2019.
6 Guthold R et al. Worldwide trends in insufficient physical activity from 2001 to 2016: a pooled analysis of 358 population-based surveys with 1.9 million participants. *Lancet Global Health 2018*;6:e1077–86.
7 Guthold R et al. Global trends in insufficient physical activity among adolescents: a pooled analysis of 298 population-based surveys with 1·6 million participants. *Lancet Child Adolesc Health* 2000;4:23–35.
8 Global action plan on physical activity 2018–2030: more active people for a healthier world. WHO, 2018.
9 Sallis J et al. Progress in physical activity over the Olympic quadrennium. *Lancet* 2016;388:1325–36.
10 Global status report on noncommunicable diseases. WHO, 2014.
11 Mielke GI et al. Shifting the physical inactivity curve worldwide by closing the gender gap. *Sports Med* 2018;48:481–89.
12 Bull FC et al. Physical inactivity. In Ezzati M et al. (eds.), *Comparative quantification of health risks: global and regional burden of disease attributable to selected major risk factors*. WHO, 2004, pp. 729–81.
13 Lee IM et al. Effect of physical inactivity on major non-communicable diseases worldwide: an analysis of burden of disease and life expectancy. *Lancet* 2012;380:219–29.
14 Ding D et al. The economic burden of physical inactivity: a global analysis of major non-communicable diseases. *Lancet* 2016;388:1311–24.
15 Cecchini M, Bull F. Promoting physical inactivity. In McDaid D et al. (eds.), *The economic case for public health action*. WHO, 2015, pp. 101–34.
16 Bike lanes: how cities across the world are responding to the pandemic. *El Pais*, 6 November 2021.
17 Urban design, transport, and health. *Lancet* series with four articles and four comments. *Lancet Global Health*, June 2022.
18 Global Observatory of Healthy and Sustainable Cities. https://www.healthysustainablecities.org/.
19 Jáuregui A et al. Scaling up urban infrastructure for physical activity in the COVID-19 pandemic and beyond. *Lancet* 2021;398:370–72.

20 WHO Universal Health Care Compendium. https://www.who.int/universal-health-coverage/compendium.
21 Lane-Cordova et al. Supporting physical activity in patients and populations during life events and transitions: a scientific statement from the American Heart Association. *Circulation* 2022;145:e117–28.
22 Kettle VE et al. Effectiveness of physical activity interventions delivered or prompted by health professionals in primary care settings: systematic review and meta-analysis of randomised controlled trials. *BMJ* 2022;376:e068465.
23 Global status report on physical activity. WHO, 2022.

26 Harmful use of alcohol and NCDs
Burden, epidemiology and priority interventions

Pascal Bovet, Nick Banatvala, Nicolas Bertholet, Maristela G Monteiro

Harmful use of alcohol causes significant mortality and morbidity globally, including through NCDs. In addition, there is a significant socioeconomic burden from the harmful use of alcohol. A number of interventions, including WHO best buys, aim at reducing alcohol consumption at both the whole population and individual levels.

Disease burden

Alcohol use accounted for 4.31% of all deaths globally in 2019 (up from 3.5% in 1990), with upward proportionate trends in low- and middle-income countries, from lower levels, but a downward trend in high-income countries (HICs), from higher levels (Table 26.1). While the proportion of all deaths due to alcohol is lowest in LICs, the age-standardized mortality rates per 100,000 attributable to alcohol use were highest. This indicates that in spite of a relative lower proportion of deaths compared to other risk factors, the absolute levels are still very high. The reduction in age-standardized mortality rates for alcohol follows the general trend of decreased overall mortality rates in all World Bank income groups between 1990 and 2019.

Alcohol use accounted for approximately 3.7% of all disability-adjusted life years lost (DALYS) globally in 2019 and ranked first among men in the 15–49 age group (IHME). The disease burden attributable to alcohol is consistently higher in men than women, consistent with a higher prevalence in men than in women.

Among all deaths related to alcohol use in 2019 (IHME), 31% were attributable to digestive diseases, 20% to cancer, 18% to cardiovascular disease (CVD), 12% to respiratory infections and tuberculosis, 7% to substance use disorders, 6% to self-harm and interpersonal violence, 3% to unintentional injuries and 3% to transport injuries.

Trends in alcohol use

In recent years, the global consumption of alcohol (in terms of 'pure alcohol' or ethanol) per capita (among those aged ≥15 years) per year has increased, e.g.

DOI: 10.4324/9781003306689-29

Table 26.1 Mortality attributable to alcohol use (IHME)

	Global		HICs		Upper MICs		Lower MICs		LICs	
	1990	2019	1990	2019	1990	2019	1990	2019	1990	2019
Proportion of all deaths (%)	3.5	4.3	5.7	5.1	4.6	5.2	2.0	3.4	2.1	3.0
Age-standardized mortality rates (per 100,000)	39	30	40	27	42	31	29	28	62	42

from 5.9 l ethanol in 1990 to 6.5 l in 2017, and is forecast to reach 7.6 l in 2030.[1] The average consumption of alcohol per capita substantially increased in low- and middle-income countries (from lower levels) but decreased in HICs (from higher levels, e.g. currently >10 l per capita and per year among men in many countries). Of note, a large proportion of the total alcohol consumption in the population arises from large alcohol consumption among fairly small proportions of the population (e.g. 50–75% of the total alcohol sold is consumed by the small proportion of heaviest drinkers in the OECD countries),[2,3] with substantial proportions of abstainers, particularly among women, and with different consumption patterns across countries and cultural norms. WHO regularly provides consumption reports.[4]

Substantial consumption of alcohol arises from unrecorded alcohol products that are not accounted for by official government systems and/or market studies. This includes informally produced products (fermented, distilled, small-scale alcohol production), illicit alcohol smuggled across borders or produced illegally to avoid taxes and tariffs, or ethanol-based products that are not officially intended for human consumption (mouthwash, medical tinctures, windshield washer fluid, hand sanitizer, pharmaceutical alcohol, antifreeze, cleaning fluids, among others). *Ethanol* in all alcoholic beverages, whether commercial or not, is the ingredient responsible for most of the harm from alcohol products. However, unrecorded alcohol may also contain contaminants such as methanol and heavy metals that are harmful. For example, methanol can result in blindness and death, even in relatively small doses.

Social and economic impact

In addition to its direct impact on many health conditions (as mentioned above),[5] alcohol use also has a large negative socioeconomic impact on individuals, families and communities, including domestic and sexual violence, homicide, victimization, risky behaviour and criminal activity.[6] The economic costs related to alcohol use have been estimated to amount, for example, to $ 249 billion in the USA in 2010, or about $ 2.05 per drink, with three-quarters of it due to heavy episodic drinking.[7]

Standard unit of an alcoholic drink

Different alcoholic beverages have different concentrations of 'pure alcohol' (i.e. ethanol), typically ranging from 3–8% alcohol by volume (ABV) for beers, 11–14% ABV for wines and 40–55% ABV for spirits. The alcohol content of a standard drink is defined differently across countries, e.g. 8 g (10 ml) of pure alcohol in the UK and 14 grams (18 ml) in the US, but 10 g (13 ml) in many other countries). A 10 g standard alcohol unit corresponds, approximately, to a 100 ml glass of wine (at 12% ABV), a 333 ml bottle/can of beer (at 5% ABV) or a 44 ml shot of spirit (at 40% ABV).

Heavy episodic drinking

WHO defines heavy episodic drinking as the consumption of ≥60 grams of pure alcohol on ≥1 occasion in the past 30 days. This equates to approximately one-sixth of a bottle of spirits of 40% ABV, just under two-thirds of a 750 ml bottle of wine of 13% ABV, or 2.5 l of a beer of 5% ABV. Worldwide almost one billion drinkers are heavy episodic drinkers.[4]

Alcohol, cardiovascular disease and threshold

Globally, alcohol use is an important cause of CVD (e.g. ischaemic heart disease, stroke, hypertension). Heavy episodic drinking also increases the risk of heart arrhythmia, including sudden death. There is much debate in the scientific literature about the effects of low levels of alcohol consumption associated with lower mortality from ischaemic heart disease (IHD) in many observational studies.[8,9] The possibility of a confounding effect is reinforced by the observation that no cardiovascular protection has been found in bias-free Mendelian randomization studies (an approach that helps understand the relationship between exposures and outcomes, particularly where randomized controlled trials are not feasible).[10,11] It must be noted that the association between alcohol use and many alcohol-related outcomes (e.g. liver disease, several cancers, injuries) is linearly associated with alcohol use, which emphasizes that there is no safe threshold for alcohol consumption.[12]

Effective interventions to reduce alcohol consumption and the related NCD burden

Several cost-effective interventions to reduce alcohol consumption in the population are recommended in the WHO Global NCD Action Plan, the WHO Global strategy to reduce harmful use of alcohol, the WHO SAFER initiative and the new WHO Global Alcohol Action Plan. They are all related to the regulation and control of the availability of alcohol (physical, social and economic). Analyses in OECD countries show that health gains can be particularly large for tax increases and brief interventions in primary care targeting high-risk drinkers.[2]

Risky vs harmful use. Hazardous use (or risky use) refers to alcohol consumption viewed from a risk factor perspective (independent of any current harm but with the potential to cause harm to self and others) while harmful use and dependence refer to health conditions with diagnostic codes under the umbrella of 'alcohol use disorders' in various diagnostic classification systems (Diagnostic and Statistical Manual of Mental Disorders – DSM, International Classification of Diseases – ICD). At the individual level, the risks related to alcohol use disorders are broadly classified as low, moderate or high risk, through a combination of levels of consumption, reported harms and the role of drinking in the person's life.[13] Harmful alcohol use is defined more broadly by WHO (both in the Global strategy to reduce the harmful use of alcohol and the Global NCD Action Plan) as "drinking that causes detrimental health and social consequences for the drinker, the people around the drinker and society at large, as well as patterns of drinking that are associated with increased risk of adverse health outcomes". Interventions at the population level aim first at reducing overall alcohol consumption, while interventions at the individual level also aim at identifying and managing risk reduction and alcohol use disorders.

Recommended WHO interventions (★ denotes a **WHO best buy intervention**):

- Increase excise taxes on alcoholic beverages.★ This requires an effective system for tax administration and should be combined with efforts to prevent tax avoidance and tax evasion.
- Enact and enforce bans or comprehensive restrictions on alcohol marketing.★ This requires the capacity for implementing and enforcing regulations and legislation.
- Enact and enforce restrictions on the physical availability of retailed alcohol (via reduced hours of sale).★ As part of this, formal controls on sale need to be complemented by actions addressing illicit or informally produced alcohol.
- Enact and enforce drink-driving laws and test blood alcohol concentration limits via random sobriety checkpoints.
- Provide brief psychosocial intervention for persons with hazardous and harmful alcohol use (requires trained providers at all levels of health care).
- Carry out regular reviews of prices in relation to the level of inflation.
- Establish minimum unit prices for alcohol where applicable.
- Enact and enforce an appropriate minimum age for the purchase or consumption of alcoholic beverages and reduce the density of retail outlets.
- Restrict or ban promotions of alcoholic beverages in connection with sponsorships and activities targeting young people.

- Provide prevention, treatment and care for alcohol use disorders and comorbid conditions in health and social services.
- Provide consumer information about, and label, alcoholic beverages to indicate, the harm related to alcohol.

The **SAFER package**, launched by WHO in 2018, promotes the following:

Strengthening restrictions on alcohol availability

Enact and enforce restrictions on the commercial or public availability of alcohol through laws, policies, and programmes to reduce the harmful use of alcohol, particularly to prevent easy access to alcohol by young people and other vulnerable and high-risk groups.

Advancing and enforce drink-driving countermeasures

Enact and enforce strong drink-driving laws and low blood alcohol concentration (BAC) limits via sobriety checkpoints and random breath testing.

Facilitating access to screening, brief interventions and treatment

Health professionals have an important role in helping people to reduce or stop their drinking to reduce health risks and health services should provide effective interventions for those in need of help and their families.

Enforcing bans or comprehensive restrictions on alcohol advertising, sponsorship and promotion

Bans or comprehensive restrictions on alcohol advertising, sponsorship and promotion are impactful and cost-effective measures, including through reducing exposure to them on social media, particularly to help protect children, adolescents and abstainers from the pressure to start consuming alcohol.

Raising prices on alcohol through excise taxes and pricing policies

Alcohol taxation and pricing policies are among the most effective and cost-effective alcohol control measures. An increase in excise taxes on alcoholic beverages is a proven measure to reduce the harmful use of alcohol, and it provides governments revenue to offset the economic costs of the harmful use of alcohol.

Special considerations related to reducing alcohol intake in the population

The fact that low and infrequent alcohol consumption does not necessarily result in significantly increased harm for adults adds to the challenge of encouraging legislators and policymakers to tackle the harmful use of alcohol.

However, arguments to develop and enforce public health policy can be strengthened by emphasizing the importance of protecting minors, protecting people from harms caused by drinkers, the negative economic impact of alcohol consumption on governments[14] and other regulatory measures to better control the alcohol market, given that alcohol is not an ordinary commodity (e.g. the addictive nature of alcohol for many users and the large health and social consequences of harmful alcohol use).

Stringent fiscal and regulatory measures to tackle the harmful use of alcohol are fiercely opposed by the alcohol industry. It is therefore important that the alcohol industry is not involved in the development of public health policy and that strong coalitions of stakeholders are built to combat interference from the alcohol industry. Governments can also develop transparent consultative processes of policy development and approval that enable the separation of commercial from public health interests. Working across sectors would help balance such interests as well.

Chapters in this book on law, fiscal measures, private sector, private–public partnerships, whole-of-government action and scaling up behaviour change describe these issues in more detail.

Monitoring

Alcohol use in the population can be assessed in different ways, including population surveys (e.g. STEPS and similar surveys in adults and GSHS and similar surveys in adolescents; see Chapter 5 on surveillance tools) which enable to estimate, based on questions, the prevalence of abstainers, drinkers, former drinkers, the pattern of alcohol use (e.g. frequency of heavy episodic occasions) and alcohol use disorders. Electronic or telephone-based surveys can also be useful. Estimates can be presented according to various socioeconomic variables. As surveys rely on self-reported data, estimates may not be reliable (quantity is particularly underestimated), including in countries where alcohol consumption is not tolerated socially or prohibited by law. Annual alcohol per capita consumption (APC) is considered the most accurate and precise indicator of alcohol exposure in the population but cannot be easily calculated from population surveys. APC includes both recorded and unrecorded consumption adjusted for tourist consumption, using several sources, including sales data provided by governments and economic operators.

Relevant global targets and indicators for alcohol control

By 2030, at least 20% relative reduction (in comparison with 2010) in the harmful use of alcohol.	• Total alcohol per capita consumption is defined as the estimated total (recorded plus unrecorded) alcohol per capita (aged 15 years and older) consumption within a calendar year in litres of pure alcohol, adjusted for tourist consumption. • Age-standardized prevalence of heavy episodic drinking. • Age-standardized alcohol-attributable deaths. • Age-standardized alcohol-attributable DALYs.

A number of additional targets are formulated in relation to the implementation of high-impact policy options and interventions.[15]

The authors gratefully acknowledge the valuable inputs and critical review provided by Dag Rekve, WHO, Geneva.

Notes

1. Manthey J et al. Global alcohol exposure between 1990 and 2017 and forecasts until 2030: a modelling study. *Lancet* 2019;393:2493–502.
2. Sassi F et al. Health and economic impacts of key alcohol policy action. In *Tackling harmful alcohol use economics and public health policy*, F Sassi (ed.), OECD, 2015.
3. Watts M. America's heaviest drinkers consume almost 60% of all alcohol sold. *Newsweek*, 24 July 2020.
4. Global status report on alcohol and health 2018, WHO.
5. Rehm J et al. The relationship between different dimensions of alcohol use and the burden of disease-an update. *Addiction* 2017;112:968–1001.
6. Rehm J. The risks associated with alcohol use and alcoholism. *Alcohol Res Health* 2011;34:135–43.
7. Excessive drinking is draining the U.S. Economy, CDC. https://www.cdc.gov/alcohol/features/excessive-drinking.html.
8. Roerecke M, Rehm J. The cardioprotective association of average alcohol consumption and ischaemic heart disease: a systematic review and meta-analysis. *Addiction* 2012;107:1246–60.
9. Wood AM et al. Risk thresholds for alcohol consumption: combined analysis of individual-participant data for 599 912 current drinkers in 83 prospective studies. *Lancet* 2018;391:1513–23.
10. Rosoff DB et al. Evaluating the relationship between alcohol consumption, tobacco use, and cardiovascular disease: a multivariable Mendelian randomization study. *PLoS Med* 2020;17:e1003410.
11. Biddinger KJ et al. Association of habitual alcohol intake with risk of cardiovascular disease. *JAMA Network Open* 2022;5:e223849.
12. GBD 2016 Alcohol Collaborators. Alcohol use and burden for 195 countries and territories, 1990–2016: a systematic analysis for the global burden of disease study 2016. *Lancet* 2018;392:1015–35.
13. Saitz R. Unhealthy alcohol use. *NEJM* 2005;352:596–607.
14. Parry IWH et al. Fiscal and externality rationales for alcohol taxes. Resources for the Future. Washington, 2016.
15. Political declaration of the third high-level meeting of the General Assembly on the prevention and control of non-communicable diseases. WHO Executive Board, 2022.

27 Air pollution and NCDs

Burden, epidemiology and priority interventions

Julia Fussell, Sophie Gumy, Hualiang Lin, Mala Rao

The WHO Global Action Plan highlights the importance of outdoor and household air pollution in the prevention and control of NCDs. In 2018, the UN General Assembly included air pollution as the fifth leading risk factor for NCDs. Air pollution is responsible for over five million premature deaths from NCDs each year,[1] on par with tobacco smoking. Improving air quality not only reduces the burden of NCDs but also supports a range of broader health and development objectives.

> **BOX 27.1   AIR POLLUTION AND CLIMATE CHANGE: COMMONLY USED TERMS**
>
> **Outdoor (or ambient) air pollution**: a mix of particulate matter (PM) and gases that varies in both type and quantity according to location as a result of sources, population density, topography and weather. PM, ground-level ozone (O_3), nitrogen dioxide (NO_2), sulphur dioxide (SO_2) and carbon monoxide (CO) are the air pollutants that are most widely studied for their health impacts.
>
> **Household air pollution**: a mix of PM and irritant gases released by inefficient combustion of fuels (e.g. wood, charcoal, kerosene) in the homes for cooking, lighting and heating.
>
> **Particulate matter:** described as PM_{10}, $PM_{2.5}$ and $PM_{0.1}$ (or ultrafine) with particle sizes of <10, <2.5 and <0.1 μm diameter respectively. Human-made sources include emissions from motor vehicles, coal-burning power plants, industrial activities and indoor activities involving combustion. Natural sources include desert dust storms, wildfires and volcanic eruptions. The smaller the PMs, the deeper they (and their chemical components described below) penetrate the lungs (and to the bloodstream and other organs), and the more hazardous it is to health.

DOI: 10.4324/9781003306689-30

O$_3$: unlike natural stratospheric ozone, which protects against the sun's ultraviolet radiation, ground-level ozone is formed when sunlight reacts with nitrogen oxides and volatile organic compounds. Exposure to ozone reduces lung function, causes respiratory symptoms and worsens lung diseases.

NO$_2$: emitted from the burning of fossil fuels (oil, gas and coal). Exposure to NO$_2$ can worsen or even contribute to the development of lung diseases.

SO$_2$: predominantly emitted from the burning of sulphur-containing fossil fuels. SO$_2$ irritates the lining of the nose, throat and airways and can make breathing difficult.

Carbon monoxide (CO): produced when fuels such as gas, oil, coal and wood do not burn fully. Exposure to concentrations in closed spaces (e.g. poorly ventilated homes) can be fatal.

Carbon dioxide (CO$_2$): an important heat-trapping (greenhouse) gas, which is released through the combustion of fuels.

Short-lived climate pollutants: include black carbon, methane, ground-level ozone and hydrofluorocarbons. They remain in the atmosphere for a much shorter period than CO$_2$, yet their potential to warm the atmosphere can be many times greater.

WHO Air Quality Guidelines (AQGs): are recommendations for national, regional and city governments to protect public health by reducing air pollution. Developed in 1987 and updated in 2021, they include recommended levels and interim targets for PM$_{10}$ and PM$_{2.5}$, O$_3$, NO$_2$, SO$_2$ and CO.[1]

Disease burden

The burden of disease attributable to air pollution falls unevenly across the world, highlighting both disparities in exposure and responses to addressing air pollution.[2] However, currently, no country reports average national PM$_{2.5}$ levels below those recommended by WHO (5 µg/m^3).[3] Whilst air quality has improved in many high-income countries (HICs) over the past decades overall, progress has been slower in low- and middle-income countries owing to large-scale urbanization, economic development and insufficient response to air pollution. The globalized production and movement of goods also contribute to higher emissions and poorer air quality standards in low- and middle-income

Table 27.1 Mortality attributable to air pollution (IHME)

	Global 1990	Global 2019	HICs 1990	HICs 2019	Upper MICs 1990	Upper MICs 2019	Lower MICs 1990	Lower MICs 2019	LICs 1990	LICs 2019
Proportion (%) of all deaths due to:										
All air pollution	13.9	11.8	6.3	3.3	16.9	12.5	15.1	15.0	13.8	13.9
Ambient particulate matter	4.4	7.3	5.6	3.0	6.1	9.9	3.3	8.3	0.9	2.5
Household air pollution from solid fuels	9.3	4.1	0.4	0.1	10.4	2.2	11.7	6.2	12.8	11.3
Age-standardized mortality rates (per 100,000) due to:										
All air pollution	156	86	42	15	188	79	228	146	287	189
Ambient particular matter	53	53	47	14	68	62	54	81	22	37
Household air pollution from solid fuels	100	30	3.0	0.3	115	14	171	59	264	149

countries compared with HICs.[4,5] There are studies which highlight a link between environmental and social inequalities within and between countries, with areas with poorer air quality also being characterized by social deprivation, in general.[6] In the UK, air pollution is high in cities, and especially in areas near major transport corridors, which are associated with an over-representation of socio-economically disadvantaged and ethnic minority residents.[7]

In 2019, 11.8% of all deaths worldwide (6.7 million) were attributable to air pollution (Table 27.1, data from IHME), with the highest rates in low- and middle-income countries. However, there has been a reduction in age-standardized mortality rates attributable to air pollution in the last 30 years in all regions, which in part reflects some progress in public health measures to reduce emissions of exposure to PMs. Mortality from air pollution is attributable predominantly to ambient PM and household air pollution in lower-income countries. In addition, 365,000 deaths were attributable to ozone in 2019 globally.

In 2019, mortality from ambient and household air pollution was attributable to cardiovascular disease (55%), chronic respiratory diseases (17%), respiratory infections and tuberculosis (12%), cancer (6%), maternal and neonatal disorders (6%) and diabetes (4%) (IHME). This corresponds to approximately 40% of all deaths from chronic obstructive pulmonary diseases (COPD), 26% from stroke, and approximately 20% of all deaths from diabetes, ischaemic heart disease and lung cancer.[8] While most of these deaths are from long-term exposure to air pollution, short-term exposure over a few days or weeks can trigger exacerbations (and deaths) from asthma, COPD and heart attacks.[9,10] Adverse effects of air pollution can be observed at very low concentrations with no observable threshold below which exposure can be considered safe.[11]

Economic impact

Premature deaths due to air pollution cost the global economy about US$ 225 billion in lost labour income and more than US$ 5 trillion in welfare losses in 2013.[12] The latter is about the size of the GDP of India, Canada and Mexico combined for the same year.

Public health interventions

Interventions to reduce air pollution are effective at the sectoral, household and individual levels. Guidance, policy recommendations and tools for creating healthier environments and improving health (including air pollution and NCDs) are available.[13]

Sectoral interventions

Addressing air pollution requires actions in many sectors (Box 27.2).[14,15]

BOX 27.2 EXAMPLES OF SECTORAL INTERVENTIONS TO REDUCE AIR POLLUTION

Energy and industry

- Use of low-emissions fuels.
- Use of renewable combustion-free sources (e.g. solar, wind, hydropower, geothermal) and cleaner technologies to reduce smokestack emissions.
- Improve management of urban and agricultural waste (e.g. capture of methane gas as an alternative to incineration for use as biogas).
- Strengthen emission control for waste combustion where incineration is unavoidable.

Transport and urban planning[16]

- Promote and incentivise clean, efficient and expanded urban transit (i.e. buses and trains), car share schemes and low-emission zones, and better environments for walking and cycling (which along with noise reduction has co-benefits for the prevention of NCDs).
- Transition to low-emission private, public and commercial road vehicles (i.e. electricity, hydrogen), with sustainable energy supplies.
- Improve planning to optimize green space and ensure that new buildings: (i) are close to essential amenities to reduce motorized

travel; and (ii) factor in air pollution sources, especially those (e.g. nurseries, schools, care facilities) designed for vulnerable populations.
- Reduce building emissions by incorporating energy efficiency measures (e.g. insulation, heat pumps) and encourage construction methods and materials that have lower levels of emissions.
- Monitor concentrations of air pollutants in order to close/divert traffic when levels are high.

Food and agriculture[17]

- Ban the open burning of agricultural residues.
- Reduce mineral fertilizer application.
- Improve manure management.
- Encourage a shift away from animal-based diets, which contribute to poor air quality owing to the release of air pollutants from manure, fertilizer use and tillage of land when growing the crops – primarily corn, hay and soybeans – that animals eat.[18]

Disincentivize the use of oil and petroleum products

- Use fiscal measures, such as taxation.
- Educational campaigns.

Health sector

- Provide leadership by being an exemplar in the areas above.
- Educate the public and advocate for action from other sectors.

Interventions at the household level

Measures to reduce air pollution at the household level include:

- Access to affordable and less polluting fuels (e.g. liquefied petroleum gas [LPG] and renewables) and technologies (e.g. improved cook stoves) for cooking, heating and lighting.
- Provision of chimneys or other ventilation changes (e.g. opening windows).
- Movement of the traditional indoor cooking hearth to one that is well ventilated, which usually means outdoors.
- Motivating changes in behaviour (e.g. removal of children from the cooking area, frequent household ventilation, wearing more clothes to allow a reduction in indoor heating).

Interventions at the individual level

Emission reductions also require changes in individual behaviour (ensuring that public policy provides the necessary support for this so that the responsibility to lower emissions is not shifted entirely to the individual), such as a decision to use public transport and active travel rather than private motor vehicle use as well as dietary and leisure activities. Personal interventions to mitigate the effects of air pollution include:[19]

- Use of apps that provide real-time information on air quality before travelling to work or school.
- Using less polluted streets for walking or cycling, travelling before or after rush hour.

The effectiveness of indoor air filtration systems and air-filtering masks remains unproven.

Climate change

There are complex relationships and interactions between air pollution, climate change and human health.[20,21] The burning of fossil fuels is not only a major cause of CO_2 emissions, the main contributor to global warming, but also of $PM_{2.5}$, nitrogen oxides, volatile organic compounds, CO and SO_2, all of which affect the climate and air quality and contribute to chronic cardiorespiratory diseases. Increased levels of ambient ultraviolet radiation also result in skin cancer.

Strategies to reduce air pollutants, therefore, contribute to global warming mitigation. Compared with the long-term impacts of greenhouse gases (CO_2, NO_2, methane and ozone), which have long atmospheric lifetimes, PM is short-lived, so reductions can result in rapid improvements in air quality. Many of the interventions described above for air pollution are important for tackling the public health effects of climate change.

Climate change itself may adversely affect air quality in a number of ways. Consequently, policies and management strategies to address air pollution have to account for the fact that increased temperatures make it more difficult to reach targets for the reduction of certain air pollutants. Well-designed climate change policies in sectors such as energy, transportation, agriculture, land and forestry and construction provide win-win opportunities for climate change mitigation, improving air quality and reducing NCDs.[22,23] The importance of working across sectors is described further in Chapter 53 on whole-of-government action.

Global and regional partnerships and initiatives

Examples include:

- The Convention on Long-Range Transboundary Air Pollution: includes over 50 Parties (countries) that work together to identify specific measures to reduce emissions.

- The Climate and Clean Air Coalition (CCAC): a voluntary partnership of governments, intergovernmental organizations, businesses, scientific institutions and civil society organizations committed to improving air quality and protecting the climate by reducing short-lived climate pollutants.
- The Breathe Life campaign: a network of UN system agencies and cities, regions and countries that provides a platform to share best practices, accelerate solutions and educate people about the relationships between air pollution, health and climate change.
- Health and Energy Platform of Action: consists of WHO, UN Development Programme, UN Department of Economic and Social Affairs, World Bank, International Renewable Energy Agency and a number of other stakeholders, with the aim of strengthening cooperation between health and energy sectors.
- C40 (a network of city mayors focusing on action to confront climate change) and ICLEI (a global network of local and regional governments that promotes sustainable development).

Monitoring

Monitoring concentrations of and exposure to (and main sources of) air pollution is important to promote the actions described above and monitor the impact of interventions.

Examples of relevant SDG indicators are shown below.

SDG Indicator	Measurement
3.9.1. Mortality rate attributed to household and ambient air pollution.	Attributable deaths due to PM for five cause-specific diseases: COPD, lung cancer, ischaemic heart disease, stroke and acute lower respiratory infections.
7.1.2. Proportion of the population with primary reliance on clean fuels and technology for cooking.	Modelled estimates based on household survey and census data.
11.6.2. Annual mean levels of PM in cities (population-weighted).	Modelled estimates based on ground measurements and satellite data.

Notes

1 WHO global air quality guidelines. Particulate matter ($PM_{2.5}$ and PM_{10}), ozone, nitrogen dioxide, sulfur dioxide and carbon monoxide. WHO, 2021.
2 Landrigan PJ et al. The Lancet Commission on pollution and health. *Lancet* 2018;391:462–512.
3 *How does your air measure up against the WHO air quality guidelines? A state of global air special analysis.* Boston, MA: Health Effects Institute, 2022.
4 Zhang Q et al. Transboundary health impacts of transported global air pollution and international trade. *Nature* 2017;543:705–709.

5 Stafoggia M et al. Long-term exposure to low ambient air pollution concentrations and mortality among 28 million people: results from seven large European cohorts within the ELAPSE project. *Lancet Planet Health* 2022;6:e9–18.
6 Hajat A, Hsia C, O'Neill MS. Socioeconomic disparities and air pollution exposure: a global review. *Curr Environ Health Rep* 2015;2:440–50.
7 Fecht D et al. Associations between air pollution and socioeconomic characteristics, ethnicity and age profile of neighbourhoods in England and the Netherlands. *Environmental Pollution*. 2015;198:201–10.
8 State of Global Air 2020. *A global report card on air pollution exposures and their impacts on human health*. Boston, MA: Health Effects Institute, 2020.
9 Thurston GD et al. A joint ERS/ATS policy statement: what constitutes an adverse health effect of air pollution? An analytical framework. *Eur Respir J* 2017;49:1600419.
10 Chen R et al. Hourly air pollutants and acute coronary syndrome onset in 1.29 million patients. *Circulation* 2022;145:1749–60.
11 Brunekreef B et al. Mortality and morbidity effects of long-term exposure to low-level $PM_{2.5}$, black carbon, NO_2 and O_3: an analysis of European cohorts - elapse project: effects of low-level air pollution. Research report 208. Health Effects Institute, Boston, 2021.
12 *The cost of air pollution: strengthening the economic case for action*. Washington, DC: The World Bank, 2016.
13 Compendium of WHO and other UN guidance on health and environment - 2022 update. WHO, 2022.
14 Kaufman JD et al. Guidance to reduce the cardiovascular burden of ambient air pollutants: a policy statement from the American Heart Association. *Circulation* 2020;142:e432–47.
15 WHO global strategy on health, environment and climate change: the transformation needed to improve lives and well-being sustainably through healthy environments. WHO, 2020.
16 Integrating health in urban and territorial planning: a sourcebook. WHO, 2020.
17 Measures to address air pollution from agricultural sources. International Institute for Applied Systems Analysis (IIASA), 2017.
18 Domingo NGG et al. Air quality–related health damages of food. *Proc Natl Acad Sci* 2021;118:e2013637118.
19 Personal interventions and risk communication on air pollution. WHO, 2020.
20 Air pollution and climate change. Two sides of the same coin. United Nations Environmental Programme, 2019.
21 Friel S et al. Climate change, noncommunicable diseases, and development: the relationships and common policy opportunities *Ann Rev Public Health* 2011;32:133–47.
22 Human health, global environmental change and transformative action: the case for health co-benefits. Institute for Advanced Sustainability Studies, Potsdam, Germany, 2018.
23 Air pollution and climate change – links between greenhouse gases climate change and air quality. Institute for Advanced Sustainability Studies, Potsdam, Germany, 2022.

28 Infectious diseases and NCDs

Nick Banatvala, Emily B Wong, Giuseppe Troisi, Antoine Flahault

This chapter outlines the relationship between NCDs and infectious disease conditions. Infectious conditions cause substantial NCD burden, and, inversely, those with NCDs can be at higher risk of acquiring infection. It is therefore to some extent a rather artificial construct to classify diseases as noncommunicable or transmissible as many NCDs are now known to be partly or even entirely caused by transmissible bacteria, viruses or other micro-organisms. It is important that public health responses to NCDs and infectious conditions are integrated as part of universal health coverage in order to maximize efficiencies and the effectiveness of resources.

Epidemiology

Globally, the overall proportion of the NCD burden attributable to infectious causes has been estimated to be approximately 8% of global NCD disability-adjusted life years (DALYs), and estimates of this burden are likely to increase as evidence that can be used for quantification expands.[1] There are significant geographic variations for this burden which are driven by differences in rates of specific infectious conditions and the related NCD outcomes (e.g. the age-standardized NCD rates attributable to infection being highest in Oceania and central sub-Saharan Africa and lowest in Australia and New Zealand). Examples of infectious agents that cause or are associated with NCDs are shown in Box 28.1.

BOX 28.1 EXAMPLES OF INFECTIOUS AGENTS THAT CAUSE OR ARE ASSOCIATED WITH NCDs

Viruses

- Coxsackie virus and mumps: diabetes.
- Cytomegalovirus: atherosclerosis and ischaemic heart disease.
- Epstein-Barr virus (EBV): Burkitt's lymphoma, nasopharyngeal cancer.

DOI: 10.4324/9781003306689-31

- Hepatitis B and C viruses: liver cancer (and liver cirrhosis).
- Herpes virus: Kaposi's sarcoma, cervical cancer.
- Human papillomavirus (HPV): cervical, laryngeal, penile, vulva, and anal cancers.
- Human T-lymphotropic virus type-1 (HTLV-1): adult T-cell leukaemia.

Fungi

- *Aspergillus*: asthma.

Bacteria

- Alterations in the diversity of microbiota ('dysbiotic microbiota'): obesity, cardiovascular disease (CVD), lung diseases, cancer.
- *Chlamydia trachomatis*: atherosclerosis and ischemic heart disease.
- *Helicobacter pylori*: gastric cancer.
- *Streptococcus pyogenes* (Group A): rheumatic heart disease.

Protozoa (i.e. one cell with a nucleus)

- *Trypanosoma cruzi*: Chagas heart disease (American trypanosomiasis).
- Flatworms, e.g. *Schistosoma haematobium*: bladder cancer.

Although HIV does not itself cause cancer, HIV infection renders patients vulnerable to developing malignancies, especially those transmitted by oncogenic viruses. Estimates suggest that infectious diseases are responsible for a significantly larger proportion of cancer cases than many risk factors such as smoking, alcohol and unhealthy diet combined.[2]

Increasingly, variations in the microbiota composition (i.e. the around 100 trillion micro-organisms living in the body, mostly bacteria in the gut) and microbiome (their genomes) are also being associated with obesity, diabetes, immunological disorders, cancers and cardiovascular diseases.[3,4] The NCD burden attributable to infectious causes is therefore likely to increase still further with increased understanding of the role of the microbiota in the pathogenesis of NCDs.

The influence of social determinants on rates of many infectious diseases (e.g. HIV, tuberculosis (TB), human papillomavirus, viral hepatitis infections) is well described.[5] Tackling the underlying determinants of infectious disease is therefore also an important part of the response to NCDs (Chapter 17 on social determinants of NCDs).

Determinants and mechanisms of NCD outcomes following infection[6]

NCD outcomes following infection are determined by an interaction between the infectious agent (e.g. type of infection, the infecting dose, the strain involved, and the virulence of the infecting agent), the host (e.g. age, sex, genetics, immune response and nutritional status), and the environment (e.g. smoking, air pollution). Mechanisms include inflammation, hypersensitivity and autoimmunity, and cellular transformation (with mechanisms of infectious carcinogenesis including oncogene activation), loss of tumour suppressor ability, epithelial metaplasia and immunosuppression. HIV has been associated with an increased risk of developing CVD, partly because HIV-related inflammation is a mediator of atherosclerosis and because antiviral HIV medicines increase blood cholesterol (and cholesterol-lowering medicines may be needed).[7]

NCDs and their risk factors increase susceptibility to infectious diseases

NCDs and their risk factors are associated with worse outcomes for many infectious diseases. For example:

- Active TB is twice as likely in smokers vs non-smokers[8] and three times more likely among people who drink >50 ml of alcohol (vs less) per day.[9]
- Harmful use of alcohol is associated with a delay in seeking TB or HIV care and lower adherence to prevention and treatment.[10]
- TB and other acute stages of other infectious diseases have been associated with a transient increase in blood sugar levels, which may need glucose-lowering treatment.[11]
- Those with NCDs are at greater risk of more severe infection from a number of respiratory viruses, including influenza and COVID-19.

HIV, TB and malaria

The importance of the linkages between NCDs and HIV, TB and malaria has been recognized by the Global Fund in their framework for financing clinical management of co-infections and co-morbidities.[12] A large number of hospital admissions for people living with HIV/AIDS are related to NCDs.[13] The Global Fund co-infections and co-morbidities policy prioritizes the scale-up of existing interventions that: (i) extend life expectancy, (ii) prevent and/or reduce mortality and morbidity of people living with HIV, TB or malaria and (iii) those that prevent or treat co-infections and co-morbidities that have a disproportionate impact on people living with HIV, TB and malaria. This includes NCDs and their risk factors. The Global AIDS Strategy 2021–2026 emphasizes the importance of tackling NCDs as part of the HIV response, with a target that 90% of people living with HIV have access to integrated or linked services for HIV treatment as well as for CVD, cervical cancer, diabetes diagnosis and treatment, including counselling on healthy lifestyle, smoking cessation advice and physical activity.[14]

COVID-19

The COVID-19 pandemic has had a significant impact on people with NCDs and on health care delivery for NCDs.[15] Those with NCDs and NCD risk factors have increased susceptibility to COVID-19 infection and increased likelihood of worse outcomes, including in younger people.[16] Since almost one-quarter of the world's population is estimated to have an underlying condition that increases their vulnerability to COVID-19, and most of these conditions are NCDs, this has enormous public health significance.[17] Age is the first determinant for severe COVID-19 outcomes, mainly due to the increased prevalence of NCDs with age. The term 'syndemic' has been used to describe how communities are experiencing COVID-19 and NCDs as a co-occurring, synergistic pandemic that is interacting with and increasing social and economic inequalities.[18] Furthermore, the pandemic has posed a particular threat to migrants and people in fragile and humanitarian settings with chronically weak health systems, disrupted supply chains for medicines and basic supplies for COVID-19 and/or NCDs, overcrowded space and shelter and insufficient hygiene and sanitation facilities.

COVID-19 and NCDs interact in a number of ways, including a large impact on health care systems:

- NCDs and their metabolic, behavioural and environmental risk factors, including being overweight and obese, are associated with greater susceptibility to COVID-19 infection and increased risk of severe disease and death from COVID-19.[19]
- The pandemic has severely disrupted diagnostic, treatment, rehabilitation and palliation services for people at risk of NCDs or living with NCDs, and there will be significant backlogs for investigating, treating and caring for people living with or at risk of NCDs.[20]
- The pandemic and measures taken in response (e.g. lockdowns) are, for some people, increasing certain behavioural risk factors for NCDs, such as physical inactivity, tobacco use, unhealthy diet and harmful use of alcohol.
- Pressure on health services is likely to increase in the long term once they are restored because of possible increases in cardiovascular, metabolic (e.g. diabetes) and respiratory complications among COVID-19 survivors.
- The public and political attention paid to the pandemic has, in many places, resulted in difficulty in maintaining population preventive interventions for tobacco use, harmful use of alcohol, unhealthy diet and physical inactivity.

The role of vaccinations and treatment

The WHO Global Action Plan includes a number of best buys and other recommended interventions with regard to the prevention and treatment of infectious diseases and their impact on NCDs. They include those for:

CVD

- Primary prevention of rheumatic fever and rheumatic heart diseases by increasing appropriate treatment of streptococcal pharyngitis at the primary care level.
- Secondary prevention of rheumatic fever and rheumatic heart disease by developing a register of patients who receive regular prophylactic penicillin.

Cancer

- Vaccination against HPV (two doses) of 9–14-year-old girls.
- HPV test every five years linked with timely treatment of pre-cancerous lesions among women aged 30–49 years.
- Prevention of liver cancer through hepatitis B virus immunization.

Other important interventions, although not included in the WHO Global NCD Action Plan, include:

- Antibiotic treatment of *H. pylori* infection.
- Anthelmintic treatment for schistosomiasis and *Trypanosoma cruzi*.
- Prioritising those with NCDs for COVID-19 vaccination and other vaccines (e.g. influenza, pneumococcus).

Chronic respiratory disease

- Influenza vaccination for patients with chronic obstructive pulmonary disease (with most countries offering seasonal vaccination extending vaccination to all older age groups, and all those with CVD, diabetes, the obese and those with weakened immune systems, such as those with malignancies or on steroids or chemotherapy).

Other important interventions include:

- Vaccination against COVID-19 (four doses) in people aged over 60 years or vulnerable segments of the population.
- SARS-CoV-2 PCR testing in symptomatic vulnerable and elderly patients, allowing the administering of antiviral drugs or monoclonal antibodies to reduce the risk of severe outcomes and deaths.

Broader health system response

The chronicity and evolution and life courses of many infectious diseases, such as viral hepatitis, TB and HIV infection, mean there is substantial opportunity for developing and strengthening health systems that meet the needs of those with long-term conditions, whether they are infectious diseases or NCDs. Integrating communicable diseases and NCDs is therefore critical to maximizing both effective and efficient health system responses. The second high-level meeting on NCDs in 2014 (Chapter 31) included a commitment to promote the inclusion of NCD prevention and control within communicable diseases programmes.[21] Examples of actions that can be taken include:

- Using existing HIV, TB and vaccination infrastructures to ensure that those being seen in the clinic for the prevention, treatment or follow-up of infection should, where appropriate, have their BP, blood cholesterol and blood sugar levels measured, as well as being given counselling on healthy behaviours to reduce their exposure to NCD risk factors.
- Including guidance on alcohol consumption for those with TB and other infections to improve TB treatment outcomes and decrease alcohol consumption.
- Ensuring that infectious disease care providers provide brief counselling to smokers as part of routine care, which can lead up to smoking cessation in a substantial proportion of them.[22] Each of these interventions would lead to a material improvement in TB outcomes.

The relationships between NCDs and communicable diseases should be included in training programmes for all health care workers in all settings and guidance on NCDs should include communicable diseases and vice versa.

Monitoring

Where possible, surveillance and monitoring and evaluation systems should include indicators of both NCDs and infectious diseases. The NCD Global Monitoring Framework includes the following:

- Availability, as appropriate, of cost-effective and affordable vaccines against HPV, according to national programmes and policies.
- Vaccination coverage against hepatitis B virus is monitored by the number of third doses of hepatitis B vaccine administered to infants.
- Proportion of women aged 30–49 years screened for cervical cancer at least once and for lower or higher age groups according to national programmes or policies.

Monitoring can also include, as appropriate, indicators on availability and/or coverage of other vaccines (COVID-19, influenza), proportions of patients with TB,

HIV and other infectious conditions who are diagnosed and treated for hypertension, diabetes, high blood cholesterol (e.g. among patients with HIV).

Notes

1. Coates MM. Burden of non-communicable diseases from infectious causes in 2017: a modelling study. *Lancet Glob Health* 2020;8:e1489–98.
2. Parkin DM et al. Cancer in Africa 2018: the role of infections. *Int J Cancer* 2019;146:2089–103.
3. Finlay BB et al. Are noncommunicable diseases communicable? *Science* 2020;367: 250–51.
4. Valdes AM et al. Role of the gut microbiota in nutrition and health. *BMJ* 2018;361:k2179.
5. Hargreaves JR et al. The social determinants of tuberculosis: from evidence to action. *Am J Public Health* 2011;101:654–62.
6. Ogoina D, Onyemelukwe GC. The role of infections in the emergence of non-communicable diseases (NCDs): compelling needs for novel strategies in the developing world. *J Infect Public Health* 2009;2:14–29.
7. Gutierrez J. HIV infection as vascular risk: a systematic review of the literature and meta-analysis. *PLoS ONE* 2017;12:e0176686.
8. Hassmiller KM. The association between smoking and tuberculosis. *Salud Publica Mex* 2006;48 Suppl 1:S201–16.
9. Lönnroth K et al. Tuberculosis control and elimination 2010–50: cure, care, and social development. *Lancet* 2010;375:1814–29.
10. Rehm J et al. The association between alcohol use, alcohol use disorders and tuberculosis (TB): a systematic review. *BMC Public Health* 2009;9:450.
11. Boillat-Blanco N et al. Transient hyperglycemia in patients with tuberculosis in Tanzania: implications for diabetes screening algorithms. *J Infect Dis* 2016;213:1163–72.
12. Global Fund support for coinfections and co-morbidities. Global Fund, GF/B33/11, 2015.
13. Crowell TA et al. Hospitalization rates and reasons among HIV elite controllers and persons with medically controlled HIV Infection. *J Infect Dis* 2014;211:1692–702.
14. End Inequalities. End AIDS. Global AIDS Strategy 2021–2026. UNAIDS, 2021.
15. Chang AY et al. The impact of novel coronavirus COVID-19 on noncommunicable disease patients and health systems: a review. *J Intern Med* 2021;289:450–62.
16. Responding to non-communicable diseases during and beyond the COVID-19 pandemic: State of the evidence on COVID-19 and non-communicable diseases: a rapid review. WHO and UNDP, 2020.
17. Clark A et al. Global, regional, and national estimates of the population at increased risk of severe COVID-19 due to underlying health conditions in 2020: a modelling study. *Lancet Global Health* 2020;8:e1003–17.
18. Yadav UN et al. A syndemic perspective on the management of non-communicable diseases amid the covid-19 pandemic in low- and middle-income countries. *Front Public Health*, 25 September 2020.
19. Wise J. Covid-19: highest death rates seen in countries with most overweight populations. *BMJ* 2021;372:n623.
20. The impact of the COVID-19 pandemic on noncommunicable disease resources and services: results of a rapid assessment. WHO, 2020.
21. Outcome document of the high-level meeting of the General Assembly on the comprehensive review and assessment of the progress achieved in the prevention and control of non-communicable diseases. United Nations General Assembly, A/RES/68/300, 2014.
22. Stead LF et al. Physician advice for smoking cessation. *Cochrane Database Syst Rev* 2013;5:CD000165.

29 Genetics and NCDs

*Murielle Bochud, Ambroise Wonkam,
Pascal Bovet, Vincent Mooser*

The risk of acquiring (or being protected from) NCDs arises from the complex interplay between the environment that an individual lives in (e.g. work and living conditions), patterns of behaviour (e.g. tobacco use, diet, physical activity) and genetic makeup. Unlike physical and behavioural characteristics, an individual's germline genetic makeup does not change over time, which implies that it can be analyzed once in a person's lifetime. Advances in sequencing technologies and IT, associated with a dramatic drop in costs over the last few decades have resulted in sequencing of the first complete human genome in 2001. This spectacular achievement has prompted large efforts which have led to the elucidation at the molecular level of many NCDs and improved risk prediction, as well as better diagnosis and treatment.[1] These discoveries have now implications for developing preventive or treatment strategies tailored to the individual (personalized or precision medicine).[2,3]

BOX 29.1 COMMONLY USED TERMS IN GENETICS

Genomics. The study of the genome of a human or another organism (e.g. bacteria of the gut). Almost every cell of the human body contains a complete copy of the genome. The genome contains all the information needed for a person to develop and grow. The human genome consists of about 3 billion base pairs, with more than 99% of those bases being identically shared across people, and includes ~21,000 protein-coding genes and ~20'000 non-coding genes. Both coding and non-coding genes can be involved in human diseases.

Gene. A DNA sequence that controls the expression of a single protein.

Gene modifications and variants. Most DNA modifications are rapidly repaired but some of them persist and are transmitted across generations. A single nucleotide polymorphism (SNP, pronounced 'snip') refers to a substitution of one single nucleotide (building block of the DNA)

DOI: 10.4324/9781003306689-32

at a specific position in the genome. The vast majority of genetic variants do not lead to diseases. Germline variants are present in sperm, eggs and their progenitor cells and are therefore heritable, while somatic variants occur in other cell types (including tumour cells) and are not inheritable.

Epigenome. Chemical modifications that can affect genetic regions and influence gene expression by turning genes on or off, thereby controlling the production of proteins in cells and tissues during the lifetime of a person in response to environmental exposures or disease processes. Much of the epigenome is reset when parents pass their genomes to their offspring.[4]

Genetics to understand NCD aetiology

All diseases have a genetic component. The contribution of genetics *vs* environment varies between diseases. *Monogenic* diseases are due to one single faulty gene and are rare. Around 7,000 primarily monogenic diseases are known, including familial hypercholesterolemia, cystic fibrosis, sickle cell anaemia, Huntington's disease, polycystic kidney disease or haemophilia A. Common diseases usually result from the cumulative effect of numerous genetic variants with small effects. They are called *polygenic diseases* and include type-2 diabetes (T2D), obesity, ischaemic heart disease (IHD) and several cancers. Common variants can be detected using genotyping and analyzed through genome-wide association studies (GWAS).[5]

Genetics to support the molecular diagnosis of NCDs

For a variety of rare diseases, having a molecular diagnosis greatly helps in shortening the time to definite diagnosis (i.e. 'diagnosis odyssey') and in defining the optimal healthcare, prevention and treatment, as well as family planning. As an example, the presence of deleterious mutations within the gene encoding the LDL-cholesterol receptor (which controls the clearance of LDL particles from the bloodstream) establishes the diagnosis of familial hypercholesterolemia (FH), which is responsible for early-onset IHD. Similarly, assessing mutations in the *BRCA1* or *BRCA2* genes helps diagnose selected breast cancer cases or identify individuals at high risk of developing this condition. Detection of such mutations has implications for preventive measures, diagnosis and treatment.

Genetics to predict the risk of NCDs

Family history is easy, but an often underused tool to point to understand patterns of hereditary conditions in an individual or family. A strong family history may suggest an underlying genetic cause, its mode of inheritance and related genetic risk, but equally a common exposure to external causes or environment among those affected. Genetic tests can confirm the genetic link to a disease where resources allow. A genetic predisposition (or genetic susceptibility) results in an increased likelihood of developing a particular disease as a result of a person's genetic makeup. *Polygenic risk scores* (PRS, i.e. genetic scores based on thousands, often hundreds of thousands, of variants associated with a specific disease) have been constructed for a variety of NCDs, including IHD, T2D, obesity and several cancers.[6] For example, individuals who have a PRS within the upper decile are exposed to a two-fold increased risk of developing CVD compared to people within the other nine deciles, *independent* of the effect of other conventional risk factors.[7] Similarly, a PRS was found to have the same high and independent impact as an unhealthy diet for T2D risk.[8] Beyond well-defined Mendelian risk for single gene disorders, PRS for complex diseases might be increasingly considered, in the near future, as useful tools to assess risk in complement to conventional risk factors, particularly for CVD (for which treatment is often based on total CVD risk),[9] but also for diabetes and cancer, to guide risk reduction counselling and treatment. As genetic makeup is already present at birth, early risk prediction of NCDs is feasible at a very early age;[10] still, a number of ethical issues need to be considered before embarking upon using this approach.

Genetics to support NCD prevention

The identification of a monogenic condition or a high PRS for an NCD provides the opportunity for early prevention, aiming at delaying the onset of this NCD, reducing its severity and extending years of life without disability, cascade retrospective testing in families and genetic counselling for reproductive options. For example, a person who knows having an increased genetic risk for a particular disease may engage more actively in a healthier lifestyle to mitigate the increased risk,[11,12,13] although the public health utility and cost-effectiveness of this effect need to be assessed further. Preventive mastectomy starting at the age of 25–30 years is an option for carriers of selected *BRCA1/2* variants, as these individuals have a lifetime risk of developing invasive breast cancer as high as 60–85%.[14] Careful counselling is required ahead of undergoing such genetic tests for patients, as well as for their relatives.

Genetics to optimize NCD treatment

Genes encoding proteins involved in the absorption, metabolism, distribution and excretion (ADME) of drugs are called 'pharmacogenes'. The purpose of pharmacogenetics is to understand how genetic variation affects treatment outcomes, with the intent of guiding therapy. Currently, >30 pharmacogenes have been identified that may be useful to adjust treatment (e.g. to adjust the dose of usual medications or to prescribe drugs that act on particular genetic pathways, such as *CYP2D6, CYP3A5, G6PD*). There are important differences in the frequencies of variants between ethnogeographic groups,[15] which means that treatment approaches need to be tailored for different populations. It is estimated that genomic variation can account for 20–95% of therapeutic effects.

Examples of public health and clinical implications of genetics in relation to NCDs are summarized in Table 29.1.

Genetics to cure NCDs

The increased knowledge of causes of single genes disorders or factors that affect their severity, paired with the development of gene editing and gene therapy technology, has opened new prospects for curative treatment for genetic conditions. For example, a highly successful gene-editing strategy for treating individuals with sickle cell disease is the induction of foetal haemoglobin through the manipulation of a gene that controls its production (e.g. *BCL11A*).[16]

Databases and technological advances in genomics

As costs of analyzing genomic variants have decreased dramatically in recent years (e.g. <US$ 500 for whole genome sequencing or <US$ 50 for genotyping hundreds of thousands of common variants), information on the links between genetic data and diseases has accumulated exponentially. Many online population-based genetic databases are widely available, enabling us to aggregate and harmonize genomic variation (e.g. gnomAD), assess genotype-phenotype relationships (e.g. OMIM, GWAS catalogue), examine the functional and clinical relevance of genetic variants (e.g. ClinVar, ClinGen) or assess tissue-specific expression (i.e. how a gene defect translates into altered RNA and subsequent proteins) and epigenomics. Initiatives are also developed in low- and middle-income countries.[17,18] These genetic databases have greatly accelerated the transfer of knowledge from the laboratory into the clinical setting. Tools to analyze large-scale genetic data have also evolved, including machine learning and artificial intelligence (AI). For example, the open-access UK Biobank has generated >90 million testable genetic variants that can be explored for their associations with numerous phenotypes, including linkages with routinely collected data in health medical records.[19]

The molecular mechanisms of several diseases are being uncovered thanks to sharing data from transnational collaborative large-scale population-based cohorts that collect whole genome sequencing and other omics data. An implication of these rapid advances in medical genetics is that it may become possible to fairly inexpensively perform systematic genome sequencing at birth or an early age among all or groups of individuals, for early identification of risk of certain NCDs (and other diseases). Beyond enabling targeted prevention and diagnosis for persons who undergo such tests, data from large genetic databases

Table 29.1 Examples of public health and clinical implications of genetics in relation to NCDs

	Domain	Examples	Current applications	Future applications
Understand NCD aetiology.	Analyses of genetic variants across the genome in large populations for research.	Identification of rare coding variants responsible for monogenic forms of NCDs and common variants contributing to polygenic forms of NCDs (e.g. 240 regions in the genome are associated with T2D).	Essential to understand disease mechanisms at the molecular level and to identify and validate new drug targets.	Develop new therapeutics. Develop new diagnostic tests.
Establish molecular diagnosis of an NCD.	Specific genetic analyses in the clinic.	FH (e.g. *LDLR, PCSK9, APOB*), breast cancer (e.g. *BRCA*), diabetes (e.g. *GCK, HNF1A*). Familial adenomatous polyposis (e.g. *AFAP, HNPCC*).	Molecular diagnosis in familial/atypical forms of selected NCDs.	Systematic genome sequencing at birth.
Predict risk of an NCD.	Family history.	Breast cancer, FH.	May point to familial forms of NCDs and to indication for genetic analyses.	Systematic genome sequencing at birth or early ages.
	Analyses of selected genes.	FH (e.g. *LDLR, APOB, PCSK9*), breast cancer (e.g. *BRCA*), colon cancer (e.g. *AFAP, HNPCC*).	Test relatives in cascade screening for clinically actionable mutations.	Systematic genome/candidate genes sequencing in people diagnosed with NCD to identify those with a monogenic form (e.g. MODY, FH).
	Polygenic risk scores.	IHD, T2D, obesity, breast or colon cancer.	None yet.	Systematic analysis of PRS for NCDs in everybody or otherwise high-risk individuals for targeted prevention.

NCD prevention.	Analysis of common and rare genetic variants.	*BRCA* for breast cancer; *LDLR*, *APOB*, *PCSK9* for FH; *AFAP*, *HNPCC* for colon cancer.	Preventive mastectomy in carriers of specific mutations. Intensive lipid-lowering therapy in FH. Early screening of cancer.	Cutting/replacing gene(s) (e.g. CRISPR). Vaccination (tobacco smoking, dyslipidaemia, hypertension).
Optimize NCD treatment.	Genetic analysis of pharmacogenes (genes that modify the impact of medicines).	*CYP3A5* (alters the metabolism of drugs, e.g. nifedipine). *BRCA* (implying specific immunotherapy), etc.	Helps titrate medicines and/or select specific medicines or assess adverse drug reactions and drug interactions.	Systematic analysis of pharmacogenes, embedded in electronic medical records and prescriptions.

CRISPR: a genetic engineering technique in molecular biology by which the genomes of living organisms can be modified.

will advance knowledge on disease diagnosis and classification, the development of new diagnostic tests and new treatments. For example, a systematic analysis of a patient's pharmacogenes, embedded through algorithms or AI procedures in patients' electronic medical records, could help guide prescriptions for some patients with an NCD.

Implications of integrating genomics into healthcare

As benefits from genomics are increasingly demonstrated, the demand for integrating genomic medicine into routine healthcare (for NCDs and other diseases) will increase – and health systems will need to adapt accordingly, including: (i) develop appropriate facilities for data processing, storage and analysis; (ii) train personnel accordingly; (iii) develop regulatory frameworks including standards around ethics and informed consent ('genethics'); (iv) data sharing, community engagement, protection of privacy (where and how information is stored and used); (v) develop protocols (e.g. which tests should be done in which circumstances); (vi) establish adequate quality control (e.g. analytics, how results are communicated to individuals); (viii) train health professionals and educate the public ('genome literacy'); (viii) provide guidance to appraise and set directions on how to use genomics in healthcare (e.g. board made of experts from different areas, such as ethicists, civil society, etc.); and (ix) ensure universal access.

Implications for individuals

While genomics and its application for clinical medicine and public health are still in their infancy, a number of tests are already used for NCDs in some countries, as part of 'personalized' or 'precision' medicine and this area will continue to develop. The implications of genetic testing are very significant and need to be considered carefully with appropriate counselling both before and after testing.[20]

Nowadays, people can easily get information on their genome (based on hundreds of thousands of genetic markers on many traits, including risks of NCDs and other diseases) through a variety of direct-to-consumer genetic testing kits (using a swab of saliva) marketed and sold directory to consumers without the involvement of a healthcare provider (including on the internet, e.g. 23andMe), often at a low cost (e.g. <US$ 100). While some interpretation is provided by these providers about the significance of an individual's results, such testing raises a number of complex issues about what people, their families and wider society will feel and do once the results are known.

However, despite advances in genetic technologies and exponential drops in costs, inequalities in healthcare systems, deficits in the genetic research workforce and a lack of access to research funding have prevented knowledge produced by genomic research from truly informing and improving the global public good, particularly in Africa and other low resource settings.

Nevertheless, research into African genomic variations is a scientific imperative for all populations because African genomes, more than any other population, harbour millions of uncaptured variants accumulated over 300,000 years of modern humans' evolutionary history.[21] Moreover, investigating all world populations will contribute to making the outcomes of genetic medicine truly equitable.

Notes

1   Claussnitzer M et al. A brief history of human disease genetics. *Nature* 2020;577;179–89.
2   Genomics beyond health – report overview. UK Government Office for Science, Foresight, UK, 2022.
3   Bilkey GA et al. Optimizing precision medicine for public health. *Front Public Health* 2019;7:42.
4   Zheng Y et al. Association of cardiovascular health through young adulthood with genome-wide DNA methylation patterns in midlife: the CARDIA study. *Circulation* 2022;146:94–109.
5   Sun BB et al. Genetic associations of protein-coding variants in human disease. *Nature* 2022;603:95–102.
6   Khera AV et al. Polygenic prediction of weight and obesity trajectories from birth to adulthood. *Cell* 2019;177:587–96.
7   Khera AV et al. Genome-wide polygenic scores for common diseases identify individuals with risk equivalent to monogenic mutations. *Nat Genet* 2018;50:1219–24.
8   Merino J et al. Polygenic scores, diet quality, and type-2 diabetes risk: an observational study among 35,759 adults from 3 US cohorts. *PLoS Med* 2022;19:e1003972.
9   Brigden T et al. *Implementing polygenic scores for cardiovascular disease into NHS health checks*. University of Cambridge, UK: PHG Foundation, 2021.
10 Richardson TG et al. Harnessing whole genome polygenic risk scores to stratify individuals based on cardiometabolic risk factors and biomarkers at age 10 in the lifecourse – brief report. *Arterioscler Thromb Vasc Biol* 2022;42:362–65.
11 Hollands GJ et al. The impact of communicating genetic risks of disease on risk-reducing health behaviour: systematic review with meta-analysis. *BMJ* 2016;352:i1102.
12 Rutten-Jacobs LC et al. Genetic risk, incident stroke, and the benefits of adhering to a healthy lifestyle: cohort study of 306'473 UK Biobank participants. *BMJ* 2018;363:k4168.
13 Widén E et al. How communicating polygenic and clinical risk for atherosclerotic cardiovascular disease impacts health behavior: an observational follow-up study. *Circ Genom Precis Med* 2022;15:e003459.
14 Ludwig KK et al. Risk reduction and survival benefit of prophylactic surgery in BRCA mutation carriers, a systematic review. *Am J Surg* 2016;212:660–69.
15 Zhou Y, Lauschke VL. Population pharmacogenomics: an update on ethnogeographic differences and opportunities for precision public health. *Hum Genet* 2022;141:1113–36.
16 Esrick EB et al. Post-transcriptional genetic silencing of BCL11A to treat sickle cell disease. *NEJM* 2021;384:205–15.
17 Patrinos GP et al. Roadmap for establishing large-scale genomic medicine initiatives in low- and middle-income countries. *Am J Hum Genet* 2020;107:589–95.
18 Wonkam A. Sequence three million genomes across Africa. *Nature* 2021;590:209–11.
19 Bycroft C. The UK Biobank resource with deep phenotyping and genomic data. *Nature* 2018;562:203–09.
20 Institute of Medicine. *Integrating large-scale genomic information into clinical practice*. Washington, DC: National Academies Press, 2012.
21 Wonkam A et al. Five priorities of African genomics research: the next frontier. *Annu Rev Genomics Hum Genet* 2022;23:499–521.

Part 4

Global policy for NCD prevention and control

30 The WHO Global Strategy for the Prevention and Control of NCDs 2000

Nick Banatvala, George Alleyne

NCDs emerged as the main causes of mortality and morbidity in industrialized countries in the twentieth century and by the end of the century were the major cause of mortality and morbidity in most countries in the world.

Studies, such as the United States Framingham Heart Study,[1] that started in 1948, the UK Whitehall studies of the 1960 and 1970s,[2] WHO Multinational MONItoring of Trends and Determinants in CArdiovascular Disease (MONICA) Project in 21 countries, that began in the 1980s[3] and several other major studies provided powerful data on the aetiology, incidence and trends of NCDs and their metabolic risk factors (including hypertension, overweight/obesity, high cholesterol and high blood glucose) and behavioural risk factors (such as tobacco use, unhealthy diet and physical inactivity).

These studies formed the evidence base for the early community-based public health programmes to combat NCDs, of which the North Karelia Project in Finland is one of the best known.[4]

From its creation in 1948, WHO anticipated there would be changes in disease patterns as developing countries became industrialized and urbanized, moving away from infectious diseases to diseases associated with aging and lifestyle. WHO governing body resolutions and action plans initially focused on individual diseases, such as cardiovascular disease and cancer.[5] In the 1990s efforts were made to recognize the commonality of the risk factors of four major diseases, cardiovascular disease, cancer, chronic obstructive pulmonary disease and diabetes and to develop a common approach for their prevention and control.

In 2000, the World Health Assembly (WHA) endorsed the WHO Global Strategy for the Prevention and Control of NCDs (WHO Global Strategy) which focused on the four diseases above, along with three common modifiable behavioural risk factors: tobacco use, unhealthy diet and physical inactivity, that are all causally linked to these four diseases.[6] Harmful use of alcohol was subsequently included as a fourth risk factor, leading to the so-called '4x4 strategy', which has the potential to prevent a large proportion of NCDs in the population if fully implemented.

The goal of the WHO Global Strategy was to reduce the toll of morbidity, disability and premature mortality from NCDs. The strategy highlighted that action to prevent these diseases should focus on reducing the levels of risk

DOI: 10.4324/9781003306689-34

factors at the whole population level (largely based on multisectoral interventions) and that interventions at the level of the family and community (largely conducted at the primary healthcare level) were essential to reduce risk factors of NCDs and control patients with clinical NCDs at the individual level, also recognizing that the causal risk factors of NCDs are deeply entrenched in the social and cultural framework of the society.

The three objectives of the WHO Global Strategy are consistent with comprehensive approaches to address health conditions of public health importance: (i) to map the epidemic in order to understand the burden of NCDs and their determinants and trends in order to guide policy and programming; (ii) to reduce the level of exposure of individuals and populations to the above risk factors and their determinants; and (iii) to strengthen healthcare for people with NCDs through cost-effective interventions.

The WHO Global Strategy urged WHO's Member States to: (i) develop government-led multisectoral policy frameworks (that promote community action) for NCDs; (ii) establish programmes for NCD prevention and control; (iii) scale up prevention, treatment and care, ensuring that their healthcare systems are providing equitable access to cost-effective interventions; and (iv) share their experiences in order to build the capacity to develop, implement and evaluate NCD prevention and control programmes.

While many high-income countries had developed comprehensive NCD strategies prior to 2000, the WHO Global Strategy and other initiatives such as the Collaborative Action for Risk Factor Reduction and Effective Management of NCDs (CARMEN) network in the Americas[7] provided a strong impetus for low- and middle-income countries to start to develop their own strategies and programmes for the prevention and control of NCDs. As such, the WHO Global Strategy provided the key elements for the 2008–2013 Global NCD Action Plan, and its successor, the 2013–2030 Global NCD Action Plan (Chapter 32), and was an important milestone in furthering the development of global, national, political and technical efforts to address NCDs.

Notes

1. Mahmood S et al. The Framingham Heart Study and the epidemiology of cardiovascular disease: a historical perspective. *Lancet* 2013;383:999–1008.
2. Blackburn H. The origins and early evolution of epidemiologic research in cardiovascular diseases: a tabular record of cohort and case-control studies and preventive trials initiated from 1946 to 1976. *Am J Epidemiol* 2019;188:1–8.
3. Luepker RV. WHO MONICA project: what have we learned and where to go from there? *Public Health Rev* 2012;33:373–96.
4. Puska P. Successful prevention of non-communicable diseases: 25 year experiences with North Karelia Project in Finland. *Public Health Med* 2002;4:5–7.
5. Schwartz LN et al. The origins of the 4 × 4 framework for noncommunicable disease at the World Health Organization. *SSM Popul Health* 2021;13:100731.
6. WHA53.17 global strategy for the prevention and control of noncommunicable diseases. WHO, 2000.
7. CARMEN. Pan American Health Organization. https://www.paho.org/carmen/index-en.html.

31 United Nations high-level meetings on NCD prevention and control

Nick Banatvala, Werner Obermeyer, George Alleyne

High-level meetings in 2011, 2014 and 2018, with a meeting mandated for 2025

There have been three high-level meetings on NCDs at the United Nations General Assembly (UNGA) – 2011, 2014 and 2018. A fourth meeting will take place in 2025. These meetings recognize the crucial roles of whole-of-government and whole-of-society approaches for preventing and controlling NCDs, i.e. that NCDs are not an issue that the health sector can tackle on its own and that NCDs have an impact on socio-economic development beyond health.

The 2011 High-level Meeting on NCDs was the second time in history that the United Nations General Assembly met on a 'health' issue (the first being the Declaration of Commitment on HIV/AIDS in 2001), and this resulted in the adoption of the resolution, Political Declaration of the High-Level Meeting of the General Assembly on the Prevention and Control of NCDs.[1]

The Political Declaration highlighted four main NCDs (cardiovascular disease, cancers, diabetes and chronic respiratory diseases) and four common main risk factors (tobacco use, unhealthy use of alcohol, unhealthy diet and physical inactivity), the so-called 4 × 4 agenda. The Political Declaration emphasized that an organized and bold response to reduce these four NCDs, along with sound scientific and politically acceptable means, can have a major impact not only on public health but also on socio-economic development.

Through the 2011 Political Declaration, Heads of State and Government committed to actions in five areas: (i) reducing exposure to risk factors in the population and creating health-promoting environments; (ii) strengthening national policies and health systems to better manage these NCDs among individuals at risk or with NCDs; (iii) international cooperation, including developing collaborative partnerships; (iv) research and development; and (v) monitoring and evaluation (particularly through regular surveys of risk factors in the population).

The second high-level meeting in 2014 resulted in an outcome document that took stock of progress since 2011 and reaffirmed leadership at the highest levels of government with a set of national and international commitments and actions as part of intensifying efforts towards a world free of the avoidable burden of NCDs.[2] This meeting also emphasized the importance of national ownership and the need to integrate NCDs into existing national health programmes (e.g. HIV/AIDS, tuberculosis, reproductive health) and avoid a siloed approach to NCDs.

The third high-level meeting in 2018 again reaffirmed political commitment to accelerate the implementation of the 2011 Political Declaration and the 2014 outcome document.[3] The 2018 Political Declaration expanded the NCD agenda to include mental health and air pollution – (moving the NCD agenda from 4 × 4 to 5 × 5). The 2018 Political Declaration once again highlighted a set of actions for countries and their partners, including the commitment to implement a set of cost-effective, affordable and evidence-based interventions and good practices,[4] including designing/updating national strategies and plans of action for NCDs and accelerating the implementation of the WHO Framework Convention on Tobacco Control.[5]

The General Assembly is the only charter body of the UN which is truly universal. As such its resolutions, when adopted by consensus, reflect the political will of all Member States. Ahead of the 2018 high-level meeting, the UN Secretary-General issued a report that reviewed progress since the 2014 meeting. This report made clear that action to realize the commitments made in 2011 and 2014 had been inadequate and that the current level of progress had been insufficient to meet Sustainable Development Goal (SDG) Target 3.4 (by 2030 reduce by one-third pre-mature mortality from NCDs through prevention and treatment, and promote mental health and wellbeing). The report made clear that *'the world has yet to fulfil its promise of implementing measures to reduce the risk of dying prematurely from NCDs through prevention and treatment'*.[6]

Progress indicators

WHO reported in 2015, 2017, 2020 and 2022[7] on the progress that each Member State had made against commitments made at the UN high-level meetings on NCDs. These progress reports provide information on whether a Member State has: (i) set time-bound targets to reduce NCD deaths; (ii) developed all-of-government policies to address NCDs; (iii) implemented key tobacco demand-reduction measures, measures to reduce the harmful use of alcohol and unhealthy diets and promote physical activity; and (iv) implemented selected measures for strengthening health systems related to NCDs through primary health care. The indicators to measure progress are summarized in Box 31.1, with a more comprehensive table provided in Chapter 35 on global accountability.

BOX 31.1   PROGRESS INDICATORS (SIMPLIFIED)

1 National time-bound targets set.
2 A functioning system for generating reliable cause-specific mortality data on a routine basis in place.

3   A STEPS survey or a similar comprehensive health examination survey conducted every five years.
4   An operational multisectoral national strategy/action plan in place that integrates NCDs and their risk factors.
5   Implementation of a set of WHO Framework on Tobacco Control demand-reduction measures.
6   Implementation of measures to reduce the harmful use of alcohol.
7   Implementation of measures to reduce unhealthy diets.
8   At least one recent national public awareness/mass media campaign to encourage physical activity.
9   Evidence-based national guidelines/protocols/standards for the management of NCDs through a primary care approach.
10 Provision of drug therapy, including glycaemic control, and counselling for those at high risk of heart attacks and strokes.

High-level meetings have also emphasized the importance of countries having full ownership of global targets and indicators, as well as having the capacity to measure progress.

Other high-level meetings relevant to NCDs

In 2019, the UN General Assembly adopted a political declaration on universal health coverage (UHC).[8] In this resolution, Heads of State and Government highlighted the importance of addressing NCDs as part of UHC, in particular committing to legislative, regulatory and fiscal measures to reduce NCD risk. The political declaration noted that price and tax measures can be effective not only in promoting healthy behaviours and thus reducing healthcare costs, but also providing a potential source of revenue for governments (Chapter 41).

In 2020 the UN General Assembly adopted a resolution on a comprehensive and coordinated response to the COVID-19 pandemic.[9] The resolution encouraged Member States to strengthen their responses to NCDs as part of UHC, emphasizing that people living with NCDs are at a higher risk of developing severe COVID-19 symptoms and are among the most impacted by the pandemic.

The UN High-Level Political Forum on Sustainable Development (HLPF) is the main UN platform on sustainable development and has a central role in the follow-up and review of the 2030 Agenda for Sustainable Development and the SDGs at the global level. It meets annually under the auspices of the UN Economic and Social Council, and NCDs are included in a number of events during the eight-day forum.[10] As part of countries' commitment to hold themselves accountable for progress towards the SDGs, over 300 voluntary national reviews have been conducted since 2018.

Table 31.1 Challenges to the implementation of WHO best buys and other recommended interventions for the prevention and control of NCDs

Challenge	Obstacles
Political choices.	• Insufficient action to integrate the prevention and control of NCD agenda into broader development priorities. • Inadequate capacity to develop policy coherence (and trade-offs) across economic, trade, and public health (including NCDs) objectives.
Health systems.	• Lack of access to affordable, safe, effective and good-quality essential medicines and vaccines for NCDs. • Insufficiently roll out of evidence-based inventions across primary health care. WHO best buys and other recommended interventions remain insufficiently integrated into national universal health coverage programmes. • Health systems in the poorest developing countries still lack the capacity to integrate WHO best buys and other recommended interventions into primary health care, referral services, human resources and monitoring systems. • Limited progress towards target 3.8 of the SDGs on achieving universal health coverage, with insufficient investment in health systems.
National capacities.	• Most low-income and lower-middle-income countries have no policy backbone or advanced technical expertise for the prevention and control of NCDs. • Most countries still have insufficient capacity to establish and manage complex cross-sectoral partnerships for the prevention and control of NCDs. • There remains limited capacity in most low- and lower-middle-income countries to develop and implement programmes to increase the price and introduce tax-related measures on tobacco, alcohol and sugar-sweetened beverages. • Most countries still lack the capacity to find common ground between policymakers and private sector entities when it comes to NCDs prevention and control and then convert consensus into public health policy and programming.
International finance.	• Prevention and control of NCDs is still not a priority in bilateral development cooperation, with demands and needs from many countries unmet.
Industry interference.	• Industry interference continues to be an issue in implementing WHO best buys and other recommended interventions, including the taxation of tobacco, alcohol and sugar-sweetened beverages. • Multinationals with vested interests routinely interfere with health policymaking at national and supranational levels in countries. • Countries hosting headquarters of multinationals that have the largest market share in exporting cigarettes, alcoholic beverages and sugar-sweetened beverages to low- and middle-income countries continue to rely on those multinationals to 'responsibly market' their health-harming products in other countries.

Adapted and simplified from A/72/662. Progress on the prevention and control of non-communicable diseases. UN Secretary General, 2017.

Impact of these meetings

The high-level meetings and their resolutions reflect the intention of Member States to do progressively more to address NCDs. Their efforts have been positive in the sense of raising the issue above the sectoral concerns of health. There has been progress but the results at the country level have been varied and in general have not matched the majestic rhetoric of the declarations. A 2017 report by the UN Secretary-General demonstrated that these meetings and their declarations/outcome documents have not yet managed to unblock many of the challenges required to scale up action to tackle NCDs (Table 31.1). A missing ingredient is perhaps the lack of a sufficiently strong civil society voice calling for accountability for the commitments made when for example compared to the way that civil society advocated for action on AIDS, TB and malaria. It is hoped that the decision to convene another meeting in 2025 will provide a greater spur to sourcing and allotting the necessary resources to fulfil the commitments made.

Notes

1 Political declaration of the high-level meeting of the general assembly on the prevention and control of non-communicable diseases. United Nations General Assembly, A/66/L.1, 2011.
2 Outcome document of the high-level meeting of the general assembly on the comprehensive review and assessment of the progress achieved in the prevention and control of non-communicable diseases. United Nations General Assembly, A/RES/68/300, 2014.
3 Political declaration of the third high-level meeting of the general assembly on the prevention and control of non-communicable diseases. Time to deliver: accelerating our response to address non-communicable diseases for the health and well-being of present and future generations. United Nations General Assembly, A/RES/73/2, 2018.
4 Tackling NCDs: best buys and other recommended interventions for the prevention and control of noncommunicable diseases. WHO, 2017.
5 WHO Framework Convention on Tobacco Control. WHO, 2003.
6 Progress on the prevention and control of non-communicable diseases. UN Secretary General, A/72/662, 2017.
7 Noncommunicable diseases progress monitor 2022. WHO, 2022.
8 Political declaration of the high-level meeting on universal health coverage. United Nations General Assembly, A/RES/74/2, 2019.
9 Comprehensive and coordinated response to the coronavirus disease (COVID-19) pandemic. United Nations General Assembly, A/74/L.92, 2020.
10 United Nations: high level political forum on sustainable development. https://sustainabledevelopment.un.org/hlpf; high level political forum on sustainable development; sustainable development knowledge platform; voluntary national reviews https://sustainabledevelopment.un.org/vnrs/#VNRDatabase.

32 The WHO Global Action Plan for the Prevention and Control of NCDs 2013–2030

Nick Banatvala, Svetlana Akselrod, Pascal Bovet, Shanthi Mendis

The WHO Global NCD Action Plan 2013–2030 (NCD GAP)[1] was developed in response to commitments made by Heads of State and Government in the Political Declaration at the first high-level meeting on NCDs at the UN General Assembly in 2011.[2] It is a successor to the WHO Global NCD Action Plan 2008–2013, which in turn stemmed from the WHO Global NCD Strategy 2000 (Chapter 30).[3] The NCD GAP was originally developed for 2013–2020 but in 2019 was extended to 2030[4] to align with the 2030 Sustainable Development Agenda.

The NCD GAP recognizes that four main NCDs (cardiovascular disease [CVD], cancer, chronic respiratory disease [CRD] and diabetes) are the main causes of mortality (including premature mortality i.e. deaths under the age of 70 years) and disease burden in the world (Chapter 1). These diseases are also largely preventable or can be delayed to later life by reducing a set of shared risk factors, namely tobacco use, unhealthy diet, physical inactivity and harmful use of alcohol, although of course not all the four main risk factors are associated in equal measure with each of the four diseases (sometimes referred as the 4 x 4 approach). With regard to mental health, WHO adopted the Comprehensive Mental Health Action Plan in 2013:[5] mental health is therefore not part of the NCD GAP.

The NCD GAP focuses on the four major NCDs and their risk factors in order to emphasize common causes and highlights potential synergies in prevention and control. In 2018, air pollution was included as a fifth risk factor for the four main NCDs above.[6] The NCD GAP focuses on actions to prevent these NCDs at the population level, including multisectoral action to address social and commercial, including fiscal, legislative and regulatory measures. The NCD GAP also sets out actions that strengthen health systems to detect, diagnose and treat people with NCDs as well as those at greater risk of NCDs due to raised intermediate NCD risk factors (e.g. raised blood pressure, blood glucose, cholesterol, or increased body mass index) in order to reduce their risk of developing NCDs. The NCD GAP also provides actions to improve surveillance as well as the monitoring and evaluation of policies and programmes. The NCD GAP is based on scientific evidence and national and international experience accumulated over many years.

The WHO Secretariat provides reports to the World Health Assembly (WHA) on progress against the NCD GAP annually and has provided reports to the UN General Assembly in 2014, 2018 and will also do so in 2025. The UN Economic and Social Council (ECOSOC) is responsible for the ongoing monitoring and reviewing of progress on the 2030 Agenda, including the NCD-related SDG targets, in particular through the ECOSOC High-Level Political Forum (HLPF). Countries at national and sub-national levels are also encouraged by ECOSOC to undertake voluntary national reviews of progress at national and sub-national levels to HLPFs.[7]

Objectives

The NCD GAP has six objectives to accelerate action on NCD prevention and control. These are presented in a simplified form in Box 32.1.

BOX 32.1 THE SIX OBJECTIVES OF THE NCD GAP

1. *Advocacy*: to garner greater attention and cooperation for NCDs globally, regionally and nationally.
2. *Governance and partnerships*: to strengthen national capacity, leadership, governance, multisectoral action and partnerships for NCDs.
3. *Population-level prevention*: to reduce exposure to NCD risk factors and create health-promoting environments.
4. *Health system response*: to strengthen primary health care and promote universal health coverage in order to diagnose, manage and care for persons with NCDs and at risk of NCDs.
5. *Research and development*: to increase national capacity for high-quality research and development on NCDs.
6. *Monitoring and evaluation*: to monitor trends and determinants of NCDs, as well as the public health and health system response, and evaluate progress.

Underlying principles

The NCD GAP relies on a set of nine overarching principles and approaches: (i) human rights approach; (ii) equity-based approach; (iii) national action, international cooperation and solidarity; (iv) multisectoral action; (v) life-course approach; (vi) empowerment of people and communities; (vii) evidence-based strategies; (viii) universal health coverage; and (ix) management of real, perceived or potential conflicts of interest.

Evidence-based effective and feasible interventions

For Objectives 3 and 4 of the NCD GAP, a set of feasible and affordable interventions are described for each of the four diseases and the four risk factors. They were updated in 2017 and consist of:[8]

- 16 best buys: specific interventions with a cost-effective ratio <I$ 100/DALY in low- and middle-income countries.
- 21 effective interventions: specific interventions with a cost-effective ratio >I$ 100.
- 36 other recommended interventions: interventions where cost-effective analysis is not available.

The WHO best buys, effective interventions and other recommended interventions are set out in full in Chapter 34 on best buys and are also described in more detail in many of the other chapters in this compendium. They are currently being revised once again ahead of the WHA in 2023.

Policy options and enabling actions

The NCD GAP also includes:

- 15 overarching/enabling actions to support the delivery of Objectives 3 and 4.
- 19 policy options to support Objectives 1, 2, 5 and 6.

Examples of policy options and enabling actions are:

- Strengthening leadership and political commitment (e.g. to address the harmful use of alcohol).
- Implementing broader strategic approaches (e.g. for the health system: training health workers, strengthening capacity and expanding the use of digital technologies to increase health service access).
- Prioritizing and increasing budgetary allocations.
- Establishing and/or strengthening a comprehensive NCD surveillance system.
- Strengthening research capacity.
- Implementing other relevant guidance (e.g. the Global strategy on diet, physical activity, WHO recommendations on the marketing of foods and non-alcoholic beverages to children, etc.).

Strategies, guidance, guidelines and toolkits have been developed (and continue to be developed) by WHO and other agencies to support countries across the six NCD GAP objectives. Many of these are described in chapters throughout the compendium.

Targets and indicators

The NCD GAP includes:

- 25 indicators. These include two for *outcomes* (one for mortality and one for morbidity), 15 for modifiable *risk factors* (behavioural and biological), and eight for *national systems response.*
- Nine global voluntary targets. These include one for mortality, four for behavioural risk factors, two for biological risk factors and two for national systems response.

The full list of these nine targets and 25 indicators and further details are shown in Table 35.1 in the chapter on global accountability.

Evaluation

An independent mid-point evaluation of the NCD GAP was undertaken in 2020 and the report was reviewed at the 2021 WHA.[9] The evaluation indicates that while there had been progress across all NCD GAP objectives, action needed to be scaled up considerably if the targets are to be met. A final evaluation is planned after 2030.

How the NCD GAP should be used

The NCD GAP emphasizes the primary role and responsibility of governments in responding to the challenge of NCDs and the important role of international cooperation in supporting national efforts.

Each objective has: (i) specific policy options for WHO Member States; (ii) actions for the WHO Secretariat; and (iii) proposed actions for international partners and the private sector. This latter group covers: (a) international development agencies; (b) intergovernmental organizations, including the UN system; (c) foundations; (d) nongovernmental organizations; and (e) relevant private sector entities.

More details on these stakeholders and how they need to work together are provided in Section 6 of the compendium. Table 32.1 provides examples of actions across the three different groups for one of the NCD GAP objectives.

Most importantly, the NCD GAP can be used by governments and development agencies to develop their own NCD action strategies, plans and policies and national targets as well as those for more detailed ones, for example for individual risk factors or health systems specific improvement.

Implementation road map 2023–2030

In 2022, the WHA adopted an implementation roadmap for 2023–2030 for the NCD GAP to accelerate action to meet global and national NCD targets.[10]

Table 32.1 Examples of actions described in the WHO Global NCD Action Plan under Objective 1: raising the priority of NCDs in global, regional and national agendas through international cooperation and advocacy (simplified)

Policy options for Member States	Actions for the WHO Secretariat	Proposed actions for international partners and the private sector
• Generate actionable evidence and disseminate information about the effectiveness of interventions or policies. • Integrate the prevention and control of NCDs into national health-planning processes and broader development agendas. • Forge multisectoral partnerships among governmental agencies, intergovernmental organizations, nongovernmental organizations, civil society and the private sector.	• Facilitate coordination, collaboration and cooperation among the main stakeholders including Member States, UN funds, programmes and agencies, civil society and the private sector. • Offer technical assistance and strengthen global, regional and national capacity to raise public awareness about the links between NCDs and sustainable development. • Provision of policy advice and dialogue to increase revenues for prevention and control of NCDs through domestic resource mobilization, and improve budgetary allocations particularly for strengthening of primary health care systems. • Promote and facilitate international and intercountry collaboration for the exchange of best practices.	• Encouraging the continued inclusion of NCDs in development agendas and initiatives. • Strengthening advocacy to sustain the interest of Heads of State and Government in the implementation of the commitments of the Political Declaration. • Support national efforts for prevention and control of NCDs, through the exchange of information on best practices and dissemination of research findings in the areas of health promotion, legislation, regulation, monitoring and evaluation and health systems strengthening. • Promote the development and dissemination of appropriate, affordable and sustainable transfer of technology.

The roadmap has three strategic directions for implementing the NCD GAP: They are to: (i) accelerate national responses on the basis of epidemiology, risk factors, taking into account barriers and enablers; (ii) prioritize and scale up the implementation of the most impactful and feasible interventions in the national context; and (iii) ensuring timely, reliable and sustained national data on NCD risk factors, diseases and mortality to drive forward action and to strengthen accountability. The road map injects a new level of urgency into the NCD GAP, taking into account new developments since the publication of the NCD GAP in 2013. The road map includes the following actions for

WHO: (i) updating the set of best buys and other interventions; (ii) developing an NCD data portal to provide a visual summary of all NCD indicators; and (iii) develop heat maps for countries to identify specific NCDs and their contribution to the premature mortality.

Notes

1 Global action plan for the prevention and control of noncommunicable diseases 2013–2020. WHO, 2013.
2 Political declaration of the high-level meeting of the general assembly on the prevention and control of non-communicable diseases. United Nations General Assembly, 2011.
3 Global strategy for the prevention and control of noncommunicable diseases. WHO, 2000.
4 Implementation of the 2030 agenda for sustainable development. Report by the Director-General. United Nations, 2019.
5 Comprehensive mental health action plan 2013–2030. WHO, 2013 (updated 2019).
6 Political declaration of the third high-level meeting of the general assembly on the prevention and control of non-communicable diseases. United Nations, 2018.
7 Voluntary national reviews. United Nations, Dept of Economic and Social Affairs, Sustainable Affairs Development Knowledge Platform. https://sustainabledevelopment.un.org/vnrs/
8 Tackling NCDs: best buys and other recommended interventions for the prevention and control of noncommunicable diseases. WHO, 2017.
9 Mid-point evaluation of the implementation of WHO global action plan for the prevention and control of noncommunicable diseases 2013–2020 (Volume 1: Report). WHO, 2020.
10 Draft implementation road map 2023–2030 for the global action plan for the prevention and control of noncommunicable diseases 2013–2030. WHO, A75/10 Add.8, 2022.

33 The WHO Framework Convention on Tobacco Control and Protocol to Eliminate Illicit Trade in Tobacco Products

Douglas William Bettcher, Juliette McHardy, Pascal Bovet, Adriana Blanco Marquizo

The WHO Framework Convention on Tobacco Control (WHO FCTC) was adopted by WHO Member States in 2003 and came into force in 2005.[1] The WHO FCTC was developed in response to the globalization of the tobacco epidemic and its large negative socioeconomic impacts, as demonstrated by the World Bank and others in the 1990s, as well as significant advocacy from civil society. It is the first public health treaty negotiated under the auspices of WHO and has become one of the most rapidly and widely embraced treaties in UN history with more than 180 Parties.

The WHO FCTC seeks 'to protect present and future generations from the devastating health, social, environmental and economic consequences of tobacco consumption and exposure to tobacco smoke' by obliging countries to enact a set of universal and comprehensive provisions for limiting its use. The treaty is a powerful, evidence-based, politically endorsed, multilateral and comprehensive tool to spearhead national action for tobacco control in the context of the powerful transnational nature of the tobacco industry, e.g. for addressing global issues such as smuggling or leakage of tobacco advertisement between countries. Of note, a treaty is a legal instrument that requires much stronger action as compared to nonbinding 'declarations' or 'codes of conduct' with Parties bound to implement WHO FCTC's provisions.

The treaty's provisions include rules that govern the production, sale, distribution, advertising and taxation of tobacco, among others. Parties are encouraged to implement more stringent measures than the treaty requires. The treaty requires that a Party shall implement all the treaty's measures (i.e. no cherry-picking is allowed).

The WHO FCTC is governed by the Conference of the Parties (COP), which meets every two years to review the implementation of the Convention and make decisions to promote its effective implementation, which may involve adopting protocols, guidelines, annexes and amendments to the Convention. The COP is open to Parties and Observers.

To support the implementation of the WHO FCTC, a number of guidelines and policy options have been adopted by the COP.[2,3] These guidelines are agreed to by Parties to the Convention on specific and established

DOI: 10.4324/9781003306689-37

evidence-based measures for the implementation of key provisions that represent statements of best-practice and immense practical value. Because they are adopted by the Parties to the treaty, these guidelines also have legal significance and have been successfully relied on to justify State interpretations of the WHO FCTC and defend related tobacco control measures when challenged.[4] Also in its eighth Session, the COP adopted a strategy providing the priorities for the implementation of the WHO FCTC from 2019 to 2025, including the work of the Parties and the Geneva-based Convention Secretariat.[5]

The WHO FCTC includes a number of measures to reduce the demand and supply of tobacco and its products (Table 33.1).

Table 33.1 Measures to reduce the demand for and supply of tobacco

Measures to reduce the demand for tobacco	
Implementing tax and price policies and prohibiting or restricting sales to and/or importations by international travellers of tax and duty-free tobacco products.	Article 6
Protection from exposure to tobacco smoke in indoor workplaces, public transport, indoor public places and, as appropriate, other public places.	Article 8
Testing and measuring the contents and emissions of tobacco products, and for the regulation of these contents and emissions.	Article 9
Ensuring manufacturers and importers of tobacco products disclose information about the contents and emissions of tobacco products and parties to make public information about the toxic constituents of the tobacco products and their emissions.	Article 10
Health warnings are included on the packaging and labelling of tobacco products in the country's language and are 50% or more of the display areas (but shall be no less than 30%), ideally with pictures. Packaging and labelling need to be approved by the national authority and should not be misleading or deceptive.	Article 11
Promoting education, communication, training and public awareness.	Article 12
A comprehensive ban on all forms of tobacco advertising, promotion and sponsorship (often referred to as TAPS).	Article 13
Implementing cessation programmes for people with tobacco dependence.	Article 14
Measures to reduce the supply of tobacco	
Action to eliminate illicit trade in tobacco products, including smuggling, illicit manufacturing and counterfeiting – a provision further articulated in the Protocol to Eliminate Illicit Trade in Tobacco Products, see below.	Article 15
Prohibiting the sales of tobacco products (or provision or free products) to minors, requiring evidence of age be provided at sale, making them inaccessible, whether via vending machine or store shelves, without proof of age, and prohibiting their sale in small packets or as individual sticks.	Article 16
Supporting economically viable alternative activities for tobacco workers, growers and, if required, individual sellers.	Article 17

Article 5.3 of the WHO FCTC obliges Parties to protect tobacco control policies from commercial and other vested tobacco industry interests – insulating all policymakers and regulators from tobacco industry influence and making all interactions with the industry transparent. While tobacco industry interference remains among the most significant obstacles to the WHO FCTC's implementation, evidence suggests that national initiatives enshrining the independence and transparency of tobacco control policymaking have often preceded and accompanied effective tobacco control. Other measures include the protection of the environment and the health of persons in relation to the environment in respect of tobacco cultivation and manufacture (Article 18), and research, surveillance, reporting and exchange of information (Articles 20–22).

The Convention Secretariat provides technical support to countries in implementing the treaty's obligations, including through the FCTC 2030 project.[6] WHO and other development partners also provide technical support, including through the WHO MPOWER package, a set of six cost-effective and high-impact measures that help countries reduce demand for tobacco (Chapter 18).

The Protocol to Eliminate Illicit Trade in Tobacco Products

Illicit trade poses a serious threat to public health because it increases access to – often cheaper – tobacco products, thus fuelling the tobacco epidemic and undermining tobacco control policies, such as graphic health warnings or plain packaging. It also causes substantial losses in government revenues, and at the same time contributes to the funding of international criminal activities. The Protocol to Eliminate Illicit Trade in Tobacco Products (Protocol) which entered into force in 2018 is intended to eliminate all forms of illicit trade in tobacco products. As of 2021, it has been ratified by more than 60 countries. Among the Protocol's Sections (which include supply chain control, offences and international cooperation), the Parties are expected to take forward a set of obligations including establishing a tracking and tracing system for tobacco products and implementing effective controls on all tobacco product manufacturing and transactions in tax-free zones. The Protocol is governed through biennial Meetings of the Parties (MOP) that occur immediately following COP sessions. More information on the Protocol is available on the WHO FCTC website.[7] The Convention Secretariat also serves as the Secretariat to the Protocol.

Novel and emerging tobacco products and nicotine products

With the growing success of tobacco control efforts and declining cigarette sales in high-income countries, the tobacco and other industries have devised new products that can be posed as 'less harmful' with consequences for the applicability of existing regulations and appeal to both current and non-users.

The first major grouping, *heated tobacco products* (HTPs) began to appear in the 1980s but only achieved any substantial use in the mid-2010s. HTPs are specially engineered tobacco product inserts that, when placed inside custom-designed heating units, produce inhalable aerosols containing nicotine and other chemicals. As tobacco products, they are subject to the provisions of the WHO FCTC despite industry arguments that they should receive different treatment.[8]

By contrast, the second major grouping, *electronic nicotine delivery systems* (ENDS), do not contain tobacco and instead vaporize a solution composed of numerous substances, including nicotine and flavouring chemicals. Although the long-term health effects of inhaling these substances are still unknown, there is evidence of potential adverse health effects as well concerning population health impacts in the form of nicotine uptake among youth.

Although minor as a share of the overall global market for tobacco products and nicotine products, these novel nicotine and tobacco products have threatened to hijack discussions on tobacco control policy and the tobacco industry has sought to create and exploit an appearance of discord to undermine impetus toward implementing evidence-based tobacco control measures. This can, in particular, be seen in the industry's contention that ENDS and HTPs can form part of a harm reduction strategy, such as that used to reduce harm from the use of injectable drugs, with mass advertising and widespread commercial availability claimed as necessary. In reality, HTPs are tobacco products that need to be regulated as such, and science-based evidence, rather than industry-driven marketing strategies, needs to guide the regulation of ENDS. Any public health approach to tobacco harm reduction must be led by this evidence and organized around the fundamental principle of opposition to industry involvement in line with Article 5.3.

The problems associated with ENDS are regularly discussed at the COP. The current position of the COP is as follows: (i) allowing such products to penetrate national markets without regulating them could threaten the implementation of tobacco control strategies and undermine the denormalization of tobacco use upheld by the Convention; (ii) ENDS' health claims should be prohibited until they are scientifically proven; (iii) Parties should consider prohibiting or otherwise regulating ENDS (including as tobacco products, medicinal products, consumer products, or other categories); (iv) Parties should apply regulatory measures to prohibit or restrict the manufacture, importation, distribution, presentation, sale and use of ENDS; and (v) HTPs are recognized as tobacco products, subject to all relevant provisions of the WHO FCTC and the relevant domestic legislation and controls.[9] The COP will next review ENDS and HTPs in 2023.

UN Interagency Taskforce on NCDs

The Convention Secretariat and WHO have together worked to ensure support for and adherence to the WHO FCTC across the international system with marked success in the treaty's explicit incorporation within both target 3.A of the UN Sustainable Development Goals (SDGs) and the outcomes of the UN General Assembly's three high-level meetings on NCDs. To give substance to this high-level recognition, cooperation for tobacco control was institutionalized in the UN Inter-Agency Taskforce on the Prevention and Control of NCDs (Chapter 58). Led by WHO and comprising over 40 intergovernmental organizations, the Taskforce has paid particular attention to the WHO FCTC. This can be seen in its creation and monitoring of a policy on preventing tobacco industry interference within the UN system that was adopted by the UN Economic and Social Council. The Taskforce's thematic group on tobacco control, chaired by the Convention Secretariat, ensures a concerted focus on all aspects of WHO FCTC's implementation within the UN system and prevents the UN agencies from working at a cross-purpose from one another.

Implications of the WHO FCTC and the Protocol for policymakers and practitioners

These institutions and organizations together constitute a powerful set of tools for accelerating tobacco control, promoting health and saving lives. Although there has been substantial progress – with the proportion of the global population benefiting from at least one cost-effective and high impact WHO tobacco control policy quadrupling between 2007 and 2021 – there are still over eight million tobacco-use-related deaths each year.[10] An estimated 100 million deaths could have been averted between 2009 and 2017 if just three main WHO FCTC obligations (increased tax, ban on TAPS and smoking ban in enclosed premises) had been implemented strictly since 2009.[11] In the absence of further effort to implement the evidence-based and highly cost-effective WHO FCTC, we will fail to prevent an estimated one-billion people's deaths over the course of the 21st century – with the great majority of this tragic loss of life occurring in low- and middle-income countries.[12]

Because of the global tobacco epidemic's devastating impact on social and economic wellbeing, as well as the sustainability of universal health coverage, implementing the WHO FCTC is key to sustainable development. Because of this it was included as a specific component of the broader 2030 Agenda for Sustainable Development.[13] The annual economic cost of the global burden of smoking-related diseases, including lost productivity and health care exceeds US$ 1.4 trillion, with a third of this manifesting in more than US400 billion in additional healthcare costs.[14] At the same time, cigarettes are the single greatest source of litter worldwide and tobacco farming is responsible for various forms of severe environmental degradation due to soil depletion and deforestation.[15]

The ongoing COVID-19 pandemic's human, social and economic toll has also been exacerbated by the tobacco epidemic, with current tobacco users exposed to a higher risk of infection and severe disease progression, while people living with NCDs, a significant proportion of which are tobacco-related, have been more vulnerable to severe COVID-19 and suffered from disruptions to treatment caused by the public health responses to this infectious disease (Chapter 28). This deadly interplay between the COVID-19 pandemic and the global tobacco epidemic reveals how the tobacco industry's globalization of this directly harmful product has also rendered our health systems more vulnerable to communicable diseases with consequences that are evident today and will be faced again unless action is taken.

Accordingly, to preserve human and planetary health, improve social and economic wellbeing, and prepare for the next pandemic, countries need to urgently accelerate their implementation and enforcement of the WHO FCTC provisions with reference to both COP guidance and WHO's MPOWER technical package. Policymakers, health and finance sector officials, public health professionals and civil society organizations all have an active part to play in ensuring their countries are Parties to both the WHO FCTC and the Protocol and, if so, adhering to the legal obligations assumed through ambitious adoption and implementation of its provisions. In addition to this core set of obligations, it is also incumbent on these actors to militate in favour of countries fulfilling supportive responsibilities such as sharing lessons, reporting on progress and promoting global implementation with technical assistance and critically needed financing.

Notes

1 WHO Framework Convention on Tobacco Control. WHO, 2005.
2 WHO FCTC. Guidelines, and policy options and recommendations for implementation of the WHO FCTC. https://fctc.who.int/who-fctc/overview/treaty-instruments.
3 Policy options and recommendations. Articles 17 and 18. WHO FCTC, 2013.
4 Zhou S, Liberman J. The global tobacco epidemic and the WHO Framework Convention on Tobacco Control—the contributions of the WHO's first convention to global health law and governance. In Burci GL, Toebes B (eds.), *Research handbook on global health law*. Cheltenham, UK: Edward Elgar Publishing, 2018.
5 Global strategy to accelerate tobacco control: advancing sustainable development through the implementation of the WHO FCTC 2019–2025. WHO, 2019.
6 FCTC 2030. WHO FCTC. https://www.who.int/fctc/implementation/fctc2030/en/.
7 Protocol to eliminate illicit trade in tobacco products. WHO FCTC, 2013.
8 Conference of the parties to the WHO framework convention on tobacco control. Decision FCTC/COP8/8(22) Novel and emerging tobacco products. WHO, 2018.
9 WHO FCTC. The Convention Secretariat calls parties to remain vigilant towards novel and emerging nicotine and tobacco products. https://fctc.who.int/newsroom/news/item/12-09-2019-the-convention-secretariat-calls-parties-to-remain-vigilant-towards-novel-and-emerging-nicotine-and-tobacco-products.
10 Peruga A et al. Tobacco control policies in the 21st century: achievements and open challenges. *Mol Oncol* 2021;15:744–52.
11 Flor LS et al. The effects of tobacco control policies on global smoking prevalence. *Nat Med* 2021;27:239–43.
12 Drope J et al. *The tobacco atlas*, 6th ed. American Cancer Society and Vital Strategies, Atlanta, USA, 2018.
13 SDG Target 3.a is to strengthen the implementation of the WHO FCTC in all countries, as appropriate, SDG indicator 3.a.1 is age-standardized prevalence of current tobacco use among persons aged 15 years and older.
14 Goodchild M et al. Global economic cost of smoking-attributable diseases. *Tobacco Control* 2018;27:58–64.
15 An assessment of tobacco's global environmental foot print across its entire supply chain, and policy strategies to reduce it. WHO FCTC Global Studies Series. WHO, 2018.

34 Best buys and other recommended interventions for NCD prevention and control

Nick Banatvala, Pascal Bovet, Wanrudee Isaranuwatchai, Melanie Y Bertram

When the WHO Global NCD Action Plan was first published in 2013, it included a menu of policy options and cost-effective and recommended interventions for cardiovascular disease (CVD), diabetes, cancer and chronic respiratory disease, and for reducing tobacco use, harmful use of alcohol, unhealthy diet and physical inactivity.

In 2017, these were updated to form a suite of WHO best buys and other recommended interventions (Table 34.1).[1] They consist of 88 interventions divided into:

- *Best buys*, which are considered highly cost-effective and feasible for implementation in most settings. These are interventions where a WHO CHOICE analysis [2,3,4] found an average cost-effectiveness ratio (ACER) of ≤100 international dollars per disability-adjusted life year (DALY) averted in low- and lower-middle-income countries. The CHOICE (CHOosing Interventions that are Cost-Effective) initiative was developed in 1998 to provide policymakers with evidence for deciding on interventions and programmes that maximize health for the available resources.
- *Other effective interventions* for which WHO CHOICE analysis produced an ACER >100 international dollars per DALY averted.
- *Other recommended interventions* that have been shown to be effective but for which no cost-effective analysis (CEA) was conducted.

The need for best buys

WHO best buys and recommended interventions have been selected for their feasibility for implementation in almost all settings as well as their cost-effectiveness. They promote action across the life-course. The interventions span from prevention at the population and individual level to treatment and care, with the recognition that early intervention reduces the costs of treatment in the long term. The best buys help policymakers focus investment and action on those interventions that have a high impact at an affordable cost rather than being overwhelmed with a myriad of policy options and interventions.

DOI: 10.4324/9781003306689-38

Table 34.1 WHO best buys (interventions with ACER ≤100 international dollars per DALY averted), recommended interventions (those with CEA estimates available but ACER >100), and other recommended interventions (those without CEA estimates)

Reducing tobacco use

Best buys
- Increase excise taxes and prices on tobacco products.
- Implement plain/standardized packaging and/or large graphic health warnings on all tobacco packages.
- Enact and enforce comprehensive bans on tobacco advertising, promotion and sponsorship.
- Eliminate exposure to second-hand tobacco smoke in all indoor workplaces, public places, public transport.
- Implement effective mass media campaigns that educate the public about the harms of smoking/tobacco use and second-hand smoke.

Effective interventions
- Provide cost-covered, effective and population-wide support (including brief advice, national toll-free quit line services) for tobacco cessation to all those who want to quit.

Other recommended interventions
- Implement measures to minimize illicit trade in tobacco products.
- Ban cross-border advertising, including using modern means of communication.
- Provide mobile phone-based tobacco cessation services for all those who want to quit.

Reducing the harm from alcohol

Best buys
- Increase excise taxes on alcoholic beverages.
- Enact and enforce bans or comprehensive restrictions on exposure to alcohol advertising (across multiple types of media).
- Enact and enforce restrictions on the physical availability of retailed alcohol (via reduced hours of sale).

Effective interventions
- Enact and enforce drink-driving laws and blood alcohol concentration limits via sobriety checkpoints.
- Provide brief psychosocial intervention for persons with hazardous and harmful alcohol use.

Other recommended interventions
- Carry out regular reviews of prices in relation to the level of inflation and income.
- Establish minimum prices for alcohol where applicable.
- Enact and enforce an appropriate minimum age for the purchase or consumption of alcoholic beverages and reduce the density of retail outlets.
- Restrict or ban promotion of alcoholic beverages in connection with sponsorships and activities targeting young people.
- Provide prevention, treatment and care for alcohol use disorders and comorbid conditions in health and social services.
- Provide consumer information about, and label, alcoholic beverages to indicate, the harm related to alcohol.

(*Continued*)

Table 34.1 (Continued)

Reducing unhealthy diet

Best buys
- Reduce salt intake through the reformulation of food products to contain less salt and the setting of target levels for the amount of salt in foods and meals.
- Reduce salt intake through the establishment of a supportive environment in public institutions such as hospitals, schools, workplaces and nursing homes, to enable lower sodium options to be provided.
- Reduce salt intake through a behaviour change communication and mass media campaign.
- Reduce salt intake through the implementation of front-of-pack labelling.

Effective interventions
- Eliminate industrial trans-fats through the development of legislation to ban their use in the food chain.
- Reduce sugar consumption through effective taxation on sugar-sweetened beverages.

Other recommended interventions
- Promote and support exclusive breastfeeding for the first six months of life.
- Implement subsidies to increase the intake of fruits and vegetables.
- Replace trans-fats and saturated fats with unsaturated fats through reformulation, labelling, fiscal policies or agricultural policies.
- Limiting portion and package size to reduce energy intake and the risk from being overweight/obese.
- Implement nutrition education and counselling in different settings (e.g. in preschools, schools, workplaces and hospitals) to increase the intake of fruits and vegetables.
- Implement nutrition labelling to reduce total energy intake (kcal), sugars, sodium and fats and vegetables.
- Implement mass media campaigns on healthy diets, including social marketing to reduce the intake of total fat, saturated fats, sugars and salt, and promote the intake of fruits.

Reducing physical inactivity

Best buys
- Implement community-wide public education and awareness campaign for physical activity which includes a mass media campaign combined with other community-based education, motivational and environmental programmes aimed at supporting behavioural change of physical activity levels.

Effectivess interventions
- Provide physical activity counselling and referral as part of routine primary health care services through the use of a brief intervention.

Other recommended interventions
- Ensure that macro-level urban design incorporates the core elements of residential density, connected street networks that include pavements/sidewalks, easy access to a diversity of destinations and access to public transport.
- Implement a whole-of-school programme that includes quality physical education, availability of adequate facilities and programmes to support physical activity for all children.
- Provide convenient and safe access to quality public open space and adequate infrastructure to support walking and cycling.
- Implement multi-component workplace physical activity programmes.
- Promotion of physical activity through organized sports groups and clubs, programmes and events.

(Continued)

Table 34.1 (Continued)

Managing cardiovascular disease and diabetes

Best buys
- Drug therapy (including glycaemic control for diabetes and control of hypertension using a total risk approach) and counselling to individuals who have had a heart attack or stroke and to persons with high risk (≥ 30 percent) of a fatal and non-fatal cardiovascular event in the next ten years.
- Drug therapy (including glycaemic control for diabetes and control of hypertension using a total risk approach) and counselling to individuals who have had a heart attack or stroke and to persons with moderate to high risk (≥ 20 percent) of a fatal and non-fatal cardiovascular event in the next ten years.

Effective interventions
- Treatment of new cases of acute myocardial infarction with either: acetylsalicylic acid, or acetylsalicylic acid and clopidogrel, or thrombolysis, or primary percutaneous coronary interventions (PCI).
- Treatment of new cases of acute myocardial infarction with aspirin, initially treated in a hospital setting with follow-up carried out through primary health care facilities at a 95 percent coverage rate.
- Treatment of new cases of acute myocardial infarction with aspirin and thrombolysis, initially treated in a hospital setting with follow-up carried out through primary health care facilities at a 95 percent coverage rate.
- Treatment of new cases of myocardial infarction with primary percutaneous coronary interventions (PCI), aspirin and clopidogrel, initially treated in a hospital setting with follow-up carried out through primary health care facilities at a 95 percent coverage rate.
- Treatment of acute ischaemic stroke with intravenous thrombolytic therapy.
- Primary prevention of rheumatic fever and rheumatic heart diseases by increasing appropriate treatment of streptococcal pharyngitis at the primary care level.
- Secondary prevention of rheumatic fever and rheumatic heart disease by developing a register of patients who receive regular prophylactic penicillin.

Other recommended interventions
- Treatment of congestive cardiac failure with angiotensin-converting-enzyme inhibitor, beta blocker and diuretic.
- Cardiac rehabilitation post myocardial infarction.
- Anticoagulation for medium-and high-risk non-valvular atrial fibrillation and mitral stenosis with atrial fibrillation.
- Low-dose acetylsalicylic acid for ischaemic stroke.
- Care of acute stroke and rehabilitation in stroke units.

Managing diabetes

Best buys
- None

Effective interventions
- Preventive foot care for people with diabetes (including educational programmes, access to appropriate footwear, multidisciplinary clinics).
- Diabetic retinopathy screening for all diabetes patients and laser photocoagulation for the prevention of blindness.
- Effective glycaemic control for people with diabetes, along with standard home glucose monitoring for people treated with insulin to reduce diabetes complications.

(*Continued*)

Table 34.1 (Continued)

Other recommended interventions
- Lifestyle interventions to prevent diabetes.
- Influenza vaccination for patients with diabetes.
- Preconception care among women of reproductive age who have diabetes including patient education and intensive glucose management.
- Screening of people with diabetes for proteinuria and treatment with angiotensin-converting enzyme inhibitors for the prevention and delay of renal disease.

Managing cancer

Best buys
- Vaccination against human papillomavirus (two doses) of 9–13-year-old girls.
- Prevention of cervical cancer by screening women aged 30–49 years, either through:
  - Visual inspection with acetic acid linked with timely treatment of pre-cancerous lesions.
  - Pap smear (cervical cytology) every 3–5 years linked with timely treatment of pre-cancerous lesions.
  - Human papillomavirus testing every five years linked with timely treatment of pre-cancerous lesions.

Effective interventions
- Screening with mammography (once every two years for women aged 50–69 years) linked with timely diagnosis and treatment of breast cancer.
- Treatment of colorectal cancer stages I and II with surgery +/- chemotherapy and radiotherapy.
- Basic palliative care for cancer: home-based and hospital care with a multidisciplinary team and access to opiates and essential supportive medicines.

Other recommended interventions
- Prevention of liver cancer through hepatitis B immunization.
- Oral cancer screening in high-risk groups (for example, tobacco users, betel-nut chewers) linked with timely treatment.
- Population-based colorectal cancer screening, including through a faecal occult blood test, as appropriate, at age >50 years, linked with timely treatment.

Managing chronic respiratory diseases

Effective interventions
- Symptom relief for patients with asthma with inhaled salbutamol.
- Symptom relief for patients with chronic obstructive pulmonary disease with inhaled salbutamol.
- Treatment of asthma using low-dose inhaled beclometasone and short-acting beta agonist.

Other recommended interventions
- Access to improved stoves and cleaner fuels to reduce indoor air pollution.
- Cost-effective interventions to prevent occupational lung diseases, for example, from exposure to silica, asbestos.
- Influenza vaccination for patients with chronic obstructive pulmonary disease.

The importance of non-financial considerations

While cost-effectiveness analysis is an important tool, it has limitations and should not be used as the sole basis for decision-making. When selecting interventions, consideration should also be given to other criteria through a transparent and fair decision-making process. Other criteria often included are effectiveness, affordability, implementation capacity and feasibility. In addition, national health priorities, impact on health equity and other local considerations should be made. Finally, cost-effectiveness estimates for individual interventions should be considered within the context of the need to implement a combination of population-wide policy interventions and individual interventions.

The importance of context

Much of the evidence base for the development of WHO best buys relies on effectiveness data from high-income countries,[5] and it is assumed that this level of effectiveness can be achieved elsewhere. However, it is important to recognize that cost-effectiveness ratios may be different in countries from other regions with their different disease profiles, population characteristics, economic structures, health systems platforms and other distinctive local characteristics.[6,7] WHO best buys were developed by taking global evidence on their effectiveness and developing country-specific models to estimate cost-effectiveness in a representative sample of countries, allowing the drawing of general conclusions. However, simply taking cost-effectiveness estimates from the literature and assuming they apply in other settings is not possible. Cost-effectiveness will vary across countries due to various factors such as disease profiles, population characteristics, health systems and local characteristics. However, the ranking in cost-effectiveness between the three types of interventions (e.g. best buys being more cost-effective than recommended interventions) could potentially be similar in all regions, which emphasizes the need to prioritize interventions with the highest cost-effectiveness ratio in all regions.

The importance of supporting enabling actions

The implementation of the WHO best buys and recommended interventions need to be supported by 'enabling actions', for example:

- Leadership (e.g. strengthening leadership and commitment to address the harmful use of alcohol).
- Strengthening of the capacity of government to develop, implement and monitor regulatory and legislative actions to address behavioural risk factors.
- Broader strategic approaches (e.g. training health workers, strengthening health system capacity and expanding the use of digital technologies to increase health service access).

- Other relevant guidance that provides details on selected processes for implementation (e.g. WHO recommendations on the marketing of foods and non-alcoholic beverages to children).

How to use the WHO best buys and other recommended interventions

Countries should select from the list of best buys and other recommended interventions based on their national context, taking into account: (i) which interventions will bring the highest return on investment in national responses to the overall implementation of the 2030 Agenda for Sustainable Development; (ii) priority government sectors that need to be engaged (in particular health, trade, commerce and finance); and (iii) concrete coordinated sectoral commitments based on co-benefits for inclusion in national SDG responses.

When considering the different interventions, emphasis should be given to both economic and non-economic criteria, as both will affect the implementation and impact of interventions. Among other recommended interventions, a lack of a cost-effectiveness analysis (based on data in some countries and/or in a particular setting) should not necessarily be a sufficient reason not to implement an intervention, and vice versa, as there may be many explanations why such an analysis cannot be carried out (e.g. concerns around equity and feasibility). In addition, the implementation of interventions depends upon epidemiological, cultural and/or political factors in the setting concerned.

Updating the WHO best buys

An updated set of best buys and recommended interventions is currently being developed for consideration by the World Health Assembly in 2023.

Notes

1. Tackling NCDs: best buys and other recommended interventions for the prevention and control of noncommunicable diseases. WHO, 2017.
2. New cost-effectiveness updates from WHO-CHOICE. WHO, 2021 (web site).
3. Bertram MY et al. Methods for the economic evaluation of health care interventions for priority setting in the health system: an update from WHO CHOICE. *Int J Health Policy Manag* 2021;10:673–77.
4. Bertram MY. Cost-effectiveness of population level and individual level interventions to combat non-communicable disease in Eastern Sub-Saharan Africa and South East Asia: a WHO-CHOICE analysis. *Int J Health Policy Manag* 2021;10:724–33.
5. Allen LN et al. Evaluation of research on interventions aligned to WHO best buys for NCDs in low-income and lower-middle-income countries: a systematic review from 1990 to 2015. *BMJ Global Health* 2018;3:e000535.
6. Isaranuwatchai W et al. Prevention of NCDs: best buys, wasted buys, and contestable buys. *BMJ* 2020;368:m141.
7. *Non-communicable disease prevention: best buys, wasted buys and contestable buys.* Eds. Isaranuwatchai W et al. Cambridge: Open Book Publishers, 2019.

35 Accountability for NCD prevention and control

Nick Banatvala, Melanie Cowan, Manju Rani, Leanne Riley

Accountability for the prevention and control of noncommunicable diseases (NCDs) is important to drive progress and provide the foundation for advocacy, raising awareness, reinforcing political commitment and promoting action at global, regional and country levels. Global accountability for NCDs includes: (i) the WHO global monitoring framework; (ii) a set of progress indicators for charting progress in policy, programming and governance against the commitments of the UN high-level meetings on NCDs; and (iii) Sustainable Development Goal (SDG) targets and indicators.

The NCD Global Monitoring Framework

In 2013, the World Health Assembly (WHA) adopted the WHO NCD Global Monitoring Framework (GMF) to track global, regional and national progress in addressing the burden of NCDs. The GMF consists of 25 indicators (one for mortality, one for morbidity, 15 related to key NCD risk factors, and eight for national system responses). Nine of these indicators have time-bound targets across three domains: outcomes (morbidity and mortality), risk factors (behavioural and biological) and national system response in line with the WHO Global NCD Action Plan. Table 35.1 provides a description of these indicators and targets, including several updates that have been made since their original adoption. The targets were decided based on the level of achievement considered feasible over the timeframe based on the historical performance of the top tenth percentile of countries. The targets were seen as ambitious but attainable. When achieved, they will represent major progress in NCD risk factors prevention and control. Countries are encouraged to use these global targets as a guide to set national targets in their national multisectoral action plans, which can be more or less ambitious based on the national situation.

WHO will report to the WHA and the UN General Assembly on progress towards the nine global targets in 2025 and 2030 by periodically calculating comparable global, regional and national estimates where sufficient data are available from countries. Countries are thus encouraged to not only set national targets but track progress against these indicators through an institutionalized

Table 35.1 WHO NCD Global Monitoring Framework

Framework element	Target for 2025 with a 2010 baseline unless stated otherwise	Indicator
Outcomes	1. A one-third relative reduction in mortality from CVD, cancer, diabetes, or CRD (by 2030 against a 2015 baseline –aligned to SDG target 3.4.1).*	1. Unconditional probability of dying between the ages of 30 and 70 from CVD, cancer, diabetes or chronic respiratory diseases.
Additional indicators		2. Cancer incidence, by type of cancer, per 100 000 population.
Behavioural risk factors		
Harmful use of alcohol.	2. A 20% relative reduction in the harmful use of alcohol, as appropriate, within the national context. (by 2030).*	3. Total (recorded and unrecorded) alcohol per capita (aged 15+ years old) consumption within a calendar year in litres of pure alcohol, as appropriate, within the national context. 4. Prevalence of heavy episodic drinking among adolescents and adults, as appropriate, within the national context.† 5. Alcohol-related morbidity and mortality among adolescents and adults, as appropriate, within the national context.
Physical inactivity.	3. A 15% relative reduction in the prevalence of insufficient physical activity (by 2030).*	6. Prevalence of insufficiently physically active adolescents (<60 minutes of moderate to vigorous intensity activity daily). 7. Prevalence of insufficiently physically active persons aged 18+ years (<150 minutes of moderate-intensity activity per week, or equivalent).†
Salt/sodium intake.	4. A 30% relative reduction in mean population intake of salt/sodium.	8. Mean population intake of salt (sodium chloride) per day in grams in persons aged 18+ years.
Tobacco use.	5. A 30% relative reduction in the prevalence of current tobacco use.	9. Prevalence of current tobacco use among adolescents. 10. Prevalence of current tobacco use among persons aged 18+ years.†

(Continued)

Table 35.1 (Continued)

Framework element	Target for 2025 with a 2010 baseline unless stated otherwise	Indicator
Biological risk factors		
Raised blood pressure (BP).	6. A 25% relative reduction in the prevalence of raised BP or contain the prevalence of raised BP, according to national circumstances.	11. Prevalence of raised BP among persons aged 18+ years (systolic/diastolic BP ≥140/90 mmHg).
Diabetes and obesity.	7. Halt the rise in diabetes and obesity.	12. Prevalence of raised blood glucose/ diabetes among persons aged 18+ years (defined as fasting plasma glucose concentration ≥ 7.0 mmol/l (126 mg/dl) or on medication for raised blood glucose).†
		13. Prevalence of overweight and obese adolescents (according to WHO growth reference for school-aged children and adolescents).
		14. Prevalence of overweight and obesity in persons aged 18+ years (BMI ≥25 kg/m² and ≥30 kg/m², respectively).†
Additional indicators.		15. Mean proportion of total energy intake from saturated fatty acids in persons aged 18+ years.†
		16. Prevalence of persons (aged 18+ years) consuming <5 total servings (400 grams) of fruit and vegetables per day.†
		17. Prevalence of raised total cholesterol in persons aged 18+ years (total cholesterol ≥5.0 mmol/l or 190 mg/dl); and mean total cholesterol concentration.†
National systems response		
Drug therapy to prevent heart attacks and stroke.	8. At least 50% of eligible people receive drug therapy and counselling (including glycaemic control) to prevent heart attacks and strokes.	18. Proportion of eligible persons (aged ≥40 years with a ten-year CVD risk ≥20%, including those with existing CVD) receiving drug therapy and counselling (including glycaemic control) to prevent heart attacks and strokes.★

(*Continued*)

Table 35.1 (Continued)

Framework element	Target for 2025 with a 2010 baseline unless stated otherwise	Indicator
Essential NCD medicines and basic technologies to treat major NCDs.	9. An 80% availability of affordable basic technologies and essential medicines, including generics required to treat major NCDs in both public and private facilities.	19. Availability and affordability of quality, safe and efficacious essential NCD medicines, including generics, and basic technologies in both public and private facilities.
Additional indicators.		20. Access to palliative care assessed by morphine equivalent.
		21. Adoption of national policies that limit saturated fatty acids and virtually eliminate partially hydrogenated vegetable oils in the food supply, as appropriate, within the national context and national programmes.
		22. Availability, as appropriate, of cost-effective and affordable vaccines against human papillomavirus, according to national programmes and policies.
		23. Policies to reduce the impact on children of marketing of foods and non-alcoholic beverages high in saturated fats, trans fatty acids, free sugars or salt.
		24. Vaccination against hepatitis B virus is monitored by number of third doses of hepatitis B vaccine administered to infants.
		25. Proportion of women aged 30–49 years screened for cervical cancer at least once and for lower or higher age groups according to national programmes or policies.

★Targets updated since 2013, †age-standardized.

national NCD surveillance system as part of the overall health information system. Currently around 56% of countries have set targets on mortality along with at least one other target.

Further details on the GMF are available elsewhere.[1]

NCD Progress Monitor

In addition to tracking progress on the specific health-related metrics outlined in the GMF, WHO is also mandated to track country progress on the implementation of a wide range of recommended actions to address the burden of NCDs. As agreed in 2015, WHO reported to the UN General Assembly in 2017 on the progress achieved in the implementation of commitments included in the 2011 UN Political Declaration and the 2014 UN Outcome Document on NCDs.[2] Slightly updated in 2017, the NCD progress monitor included a series of 19 indicators against which WHO will measure progress (Box 35.1).

These indicators cover a range of data-related activities (e.g. risk factor surveillance), policy options addressing NCDs and their risk factors, as well as health service capabilities to address NCDs. Many of the indicators directly measure whether or not countries have implemented one or more of the WHO best buys. Since 2017, WHO has continued to report regularly on country progress on these indicators in a series of Progress Monitor reports using data provided by countries to WHO.[3]

BOX 35.1 PROGRESS INDICATORS (SIMPLIFIED)

1. National time-bound targets set.
2. A functioning system for generating reliable cause-specific mortality data on a routine basis in place.
3. A STEPS survey or a similar comprehensive health examination survey conducted every five years.
4. An operational multisectoral national strategy/action plan in place that integrates NCDs and their risk factors.
5. Implementation of a set of WHO FCTC tobacco demand-reduction measures:
   a. Reduction in the affordability by increasing excise taxes and prices on tobacco products.
   b. Elimination of exposure to second-hand tobacco smoke in all indoor workplaces, public places and public transport.
   c. Implementation of plain/standardized packaging and/or large graphic health warnings on all tobacco packages.
   d. Enacting and enforcing comprehensive bans on tobacco advertising, promotion and sponsorship.
   e. Implementing effective mass media campaigns that educate the public about the harms of smoking/tobacco use and second-hand smoke.
6. Implementation of measures to reduce the harmful use of alcohol:
   a. Enacting and enforcing restrictions on the hours of sale.
   b. Enacting and enforcing bans or comprehensive restrictions on exposure to advertising.
   c. Increasing excise taxes on alcoholic beverages.

7 Implementation of measures to reduce unhealthy diets:
   a. National policies to reduce population salt/sodium consumption in place.
   b. National policies that limit saturated fatty acids and virtually eliminate industrially produced trans fatty acids in the food supply in place.
   c. Enacting WHO recommendations on the marketing of foods and non-alcoholic beverages to children.
   d. Legislation/regulations on the International Code of Marketing of Breast-milk Substitutes implemented.
8 At least one recent national public awareness/mass media campaign to encourage physical activity.
9 Evidence-based national guidelines/protocols/standards for the management of NCDs through a primary care approach.
10 Provision of drug therapy, including glycaemic control, and counselling for those at high risk of heart attacks and strokes.

Sustainable Development Goals

In 2015, the SDGs were adopted by the UN, which comprise a broad set of indicators and targets spanning social, economic and environmental issues organized under 17 goals. Goal 3 is to ensure healthy lives and promote well-being for all at all ages and includes NCD-specific and NCD-related targets (Box 35.2).

BOX 35.2   NCD SDG TARGETS AND EXAMPLES OF NCD-RELATED SDG TARGETS

3.4 By 2030, reduce by one-third premature mortality from NCDs through prevention and treatment and promote mental health and well-being.
3.5 Strengthen the prevention and treatment of substance abuse, including narcotic drug abuse and harmful use of alcohol.
3.8 Achieve universal health coverage, including financial risk protection, access to quality essential healthcare services and access to safe, effective, quality and affordable essential medicines and vaccines for all.
3.9 By 2030, substantially reduce the number of deaths and illnesses from hazardous chemicals and air, water and soil pollution and contamination.

> 3.B Support the research and development of vaccines and medicines for the communicable and NCDs that primarily affect developing countries, provide access to affordable essential medicines and vaccines, in accordance with the Doha Declaration on the TRIPS Agreement and Public Health, which affirms the right of developing countries to use to the full the provisions in the Agreement on Trade Related Aspects of Intellectual Property Rights regarding flexibilities to protect public health, and, in particular, provide access to medicines for all.
> 3.C Substantially increase health financing and the recruitment, development, training and retention of the health workforce in developing countries, especially in least developed countries and small island developing States.

The UN Department of Economic and Social Affairs (UNDESA) leads the reporting on progress towards meeting the SDG targets. Resources from UNDESA's statistical division include annual SDG reports, an SDG Global Database that allows access to data on more than 210 SDG indicators by indicator category, country, region or period, and also provides information on methods used for data collection and analysis, and an extensive SDG Monitoring and Reporting Toolkit to support countries.[4]

The UN High-level Political Forum on Sustainable Development (HLPF) is the main UN platform on sustainable development and has a central role in the follow-up and review of the 2030 Agenda for Sustainable Development and the SDGs at the global level. It meets annually under the auspices of the UN Economic and Social Council, and NCDs are included in a number of events during the forum.[5] As part of countries' commitment to hold themselves accountable for progress towards the SDGs, over 300 voluntary national reviews have been conducted since 2018. Guidance for countries on how to undertake these reviews is available.[6]

Notes

1 NCD global monitoring framework. WHO (website).
2 How WHO will report in 2017 to the United Nations General Assembly on the progress achieved in the implementation of commitments included in the 2011 UN Political Declaration and 2014 UN Outcome Document on NCDs. WHO, 2015.
3 Noncommunicable diseases progress monitor 2022. WHO, 2022.
4 Welcome to the sustainable development goal indicators website. UNDESA. https://unstats.un.org/sdgs.
5 United Nations: high level political forum on sustainable development. https://sustainabledevelopment.un.org/hlpf; high level political forum on sustainable development; sustainable development knowledge platform; voluntary national reviews. https://sustainabledevelopment.un.org/vnrs/#VNRDatabase.
6 Handbook for the preparation of voluntary national reviews - the 2021 Edition. UNDESA, 2022.

Part 5

Cross cutting issues around NCD prevention and control

36 Population and individual approaches for NCD prevention and control

Pascal Bovet, Nick Banatvala, Kay-Tee Khaw, K Srinath Reddy

Interventions to prevent and control NCDs, including WHO best buys and other recommended interventions, can be categorized into those at the population and individual levels. These two approaches are largely based on the work of Geoffrey Rose, who introduced the concept of 'sick individuals' and 'sick populations' into the public health literature and thus the need for different strategies for the prevention and control of health problems.[1]

Level of action of population-wide versus high-risk individual-level interventions. Population-wide interventions aim at controlling the determinants of NCD incidence in the whole population and they usually require action in multiple sectors beyond the health sector. In contrast, high-risk interventions aim at identifying susceptible high-risk individuals and offering them individual protection. They mainly engage in action at the health care level and require a well-functioning health system. The main characteristics of population-based and high-risk strategies for the prevention and control of diseases are shown in Table 36.1.

Prevention paradox. From an epidemiologic perspective, the largest proportion of NCD events in a population, particularly cardiovascular disease (CVD), arises from individuals with only moderately increased risk factor levels. This is because the majority of individuals in a population have slightly elevated or intermediate levels of risk factors while only a minority have highly elevated risk factor levels. For example, the majority of stroke cases are among those with only moderately elevated blood pressure (BP) rather than the smaller number of individuals with high/very high BP. This is known as the 'prevention paradox' and emphasizes the power of interventions aimed at reducing risk factors in the whole population, thereby addressing the underlying causes of these diseases (i.e. primary prevention of NCDs). However, high-risk interventions remain critically important for prevention, i.e. to protect susceptible individuals (i.e. those at increased risk of NCD or with an NCD).

Selected issues related to population strategies for NCDs

While several of the chapters in the compendium focus on population strategies to reduce NCD risk factors in more detail, key issues for population strategies include:

1. *The importance of interventions that require minimal action from individuals*

Table 36.1 Main characteristics of population-based and high-risk strategies for the prevention and control of diseases

	Population (public health) strategies	Individual-based (high-risk) strategies
Target ('unit').	Whole population.	Individuals at risk.
Objective.	Create environments that are conducive to the adoption of healthy behaviours by all individuals. Seek to produce small changes in highly prevalent risk factors ('good for all'). Try to tackle the causes of the causes ('whole of society', 'health in all policy' approaches).	Seek to make large changes in risk factors/diseases in a few individuals at high risk ('good for some'). Aim at protecting susceptible individuals.
Mechanism.	Shift the whole risk factor curve in the population downwards (to lower values).	Identify individuals at risk (including those with NCDs) through screening and treatment.
Impact: benefit for individuals.	Small.	Large (if patients are cooperative; adherence is the main challenge).
Impact: benefit for the population.	Large.	Small (but can be large if a large proportion of the population at risk is detected and treated).

(Continued)

Table 36.1 (Continued)

	Population (public health) strategies	Individual-based (high-risk) strategies
Sectors from which the interventions arise.	Mainly sectors outside of the health sector.	Mainly the health care sector.
Uptake of interventions by different social groups.	Generally no or little social differential. Can have an amplified impact on the poor (e.g. tobacco/alcohol tax).	Often lower uptake by the poor and/or uneducated (a major issue for efficiency and social equity).
Need to identify targeted individuals.	No (unless an intervention targets special population subgroups).	Yes (screening; requires the willingness of individuals to undergo testing/treatment).
Cooperation by individuals is needed.	No or little (e.g. taxes on tobacco and alcohol; reformulation of foods; modification of environment).	Always.
Level of action in the disease process.	Tackle the underlying causes (↓ incidence).	Do not necessarily address the causes (particularly when the causes are unknown). Delays disease development (↓ case-fatality).
Acceptability.	Often opposed by economic interests.	Often well accepted by individuals ('patients').
Cost for society.	Can be low and/or generate revenue (e.g. alcohol/tobacco/sugar excise taxes).	High or very high, cost-effective use of resources (e.g. haemodialysis or cancer treatment that is often very expensive but life-saving for the affected individuals).
Payer.	Often public (as part of agendas of sectors other than health).	A mix of government, insurance and/or out-of-pocket.
Accountability.	Different sectors, often outside of health, are often subject to decisions by parliaments at national/regional levels.	Health systems, ministry of health.
Evidence of impact.	Can be challenging to assess as evidence most often cannot rely on controlled randomized trials (and observed effects can be biased by confounding factors).	Can rely on strong methods, including randomized controlled clinical trials.

(Adapted from Rose G. Sick individuals and sick populations. *Int J Epidemiol* 1985;14:32–8)

Many people have difficulty engaging in long-term behavioural change to reduce their exposure to NCD risk factors (Chapter 47). Reasons include that NCD risk factors are often asymptomatic for many years and that a large time interval can occur until an NCD actually occurs (e.g. cancer, heart attack). This emphasizes the importance of population-based strategies which can reduce exposure to risk factors in the whole population without requiring behaviour change at the individual level, e.g. by changing the environment in which people live (e.g. clean air) or by altering some external conditions (e.g. reformulation of foods, chapter 23). Similarly, fiscal, legislative and regulatory policies are helpful in making it easier for people to adopt healthy behaviours.

2. *Simultaneous impact on multiple NCD risk factors*

When exposure to risk factors decreases in the whole population, through a supportive environment that encourages and enables the adoption of healthy behaviours such as a balanced diet and regular physical activity, several NCD risk factors are simultaneously improved. The population distributions of body-mass index, blood pressure, blood sugar, blood lipids and inflammatory markers will move in a healthy leftward direction. A healthy diet alone can reduce many of these outcomes, as can physical activity alone. Even the non-consumption of tobacco products achieves many of these goals. Health promotion, through policies that catalyse and sustain the stimulus for healthy behaviours at the population level, can greatly influence multiple risk factors and NCDs simultaneously through common pathways.

3. *Inter-generational benefits*

Measures which are implemented to create a health-promoting environment, to support the population strategy, will not only benefit the current generations but will have carry-over benefits for future generations. A tobacco-free society, a reduction in air pollution, food and agriculture systems that promote healthy diets, and a built environment that enables safe and pleasurable physical activity can be enduring legacies that will reduce the risk of NCDs in future generations, starting with those who are very young at present. Their lifetime exposure to NCD-promoting risk factors will greatly decrease as a result. Fewer persons will then need a high-risk individual strategy for NCD risk reduction.

4. *The benefits beyond health (win–win strategies)*

A number of interventions that are of benefit to NCD prevention and control can also result in benefits beyond health (win–win). For example, bus/cycle lanes in cities, which promote active commuting (hence increasing physical activity for many individuals) are also important interventions to reduce road traffic congestion, decrease time spent commuting and for reducing CO_2 emissions. Similarly, taxes on items that can be harmful to health, such as alcohol, tobacco or sugar, generate revenue for the government (which can be used in part to fund health promotion programmes, health care or broader socioeconomic development). Interventions that benefit several sectors are generally supported by a broader range of sectors and stakeholders, which enables a stronger case to be made for sustainable funding and implementation. Public health policymakers and practitioners, therefore, need to identify, as often as possible, opportunities for these win-win interventions and then work with other sectors to develop and implement them. This 'health in all policies' approach requires an understanding of the language and culture of sectors beyond health; the incentives, opportunities and barriers for those working in non-health sectors; and a recognition that not all interventions need to be framed primarily around health to benefit NCDs. This underlies the importance of multisectoral committees for the prevention of NCDs at national and more local levels to stimulate, facilitate, coordinate and monitor such win–win interventions.

Examples of population strategies

Policies to increase/decrease access to healthy/unhealthy products
- Alter the content of foods and beverages (e.g. salt, trans-fats, saturated fats, sugar in selected foods).
- Limit marketing of unhealthy foods.
- Ban smoking in enclosed and other selected premises.

Policies to improve active mobility
- Limit the role of private vehicles and favour the use of public transport to promote walking/cycling.
- Promote healthy cities, e.g. structures such as green spaces and walkways to promote physical activity for all.

Economic/fiscal policies to increase/reduce the demand/supply of healthy/unhealthy items
- Differential taxes/subsidies on healthy fruits/vegetables vs unhealthy energy-dense foods.
- Excise taxes on tobacco, alcohol, sugar drinks.

Initiatives at the community level[2]
- Most effective when multifaceted, involving the community and culturally acceptable.
- Dose and duration of the interventions should be large enough and sustained over time.

Educational programmes
- Increasing population awareness of NCDs and their risk factors through the media and in different settings (e.g. schools, workplaces).

The examples above correspond to several WHO best buys and recommended interventions described throughout this compendium.[3]

Selected issues related to high-risk strategies for NCDs

While several of the chapters in the compendium focus on high-risk strategies to reduce NCD risk factors in more detail, some key issues for high-risk strategies include:

1. ***High-risk individual-level strategies are generally well supported by individuals and health professionals***

This is because they can result in large and appreciable changes at a patient level. However, when it comes to NCDs, many conditions such as hypertension are asymptomatic and therefore long-term adherence is a significant challenge. Overtreatment is also an issue. It is important that the management of NCD conditions is based on evidence-based principles and that good governance, adequate regulatory frames, and continued monitoring are set up to ensure that the management of NCDs is not driven by the commercial interests of pharmaceutical and private health care industries.[4]

2. ***The importance of using approaches based on total risk rather than single risk factors***

This is an approach used especially for CVD, where clinical management can be better tailored based on an individual's total (absolute) risk,[5,6] which takes into account the combined effect of several risk factors and clinical conditions, as well as the underlying residual risk in a population. The use of risk prediction scores allows the identification of a relatively small proportion of a population who are at greatest risk of subsequent fatal and/or non-fatal events. Hence, risk scores enable minimizing the number of individuals who need to be treated (NNT) in order to avoid one event and thus minimizing total health care costs for health providers.[7] For example, a person with a high level of one particular risk factor (e.g. high BP) may not need medication when the total risk of CVD is low but may need BP-lowering medication even if BP is not elevated when the total risk of subsequent CVD is high (this is discussed in Chapter 7 on CVD and in Chapter 8 on hypertension). While the total risk approach applies largely to CVD, it has also been applied to type-2 diabetes, certain cancers and other NCDs, also using, for example, genetic and other biomarkers or scores. Total risk scores require regular calibration and validation across the population in question (e.g. taking into account changing CVD risk over time).

3. ***Issues around total risk scores***

While well-calibrated total risk scores can reliably predict hard outcomes at the population level (e.g. incidence of myocardial infarction), they are less useful at an individual level (this is again a feature of the 'prevention paradox' where a majority of events in the population occur among those with low or intermediate risk).[8] This is because of the relatively (and perhaps surprisingly) weak associations between conventional risk factors and NCDs (e.g. a relative risk [RR] of 2-5 for most single conventional CVD risk factors or a RR up to 50 or so for combined CVD risk factors), while a reliable prediction of an event at the individual level would require a much stronger association (e.g. a relative risk >200).[9] Research is important to identify new variables such as biological and genetic markers and sub-clinical changes (e.g. coronary artery calcification) to enhance the prediction at the individual level.

Older age is, by far, the strongest risk factor of NCDs, and therefore the most discriminant variable in NCD risk scores (e.g. age alone contributes to up to 80% of the performance of the currently used CVD risk scores).[10] This explains why the management of NCDs based on total risk scores tends to concentrate on older age groups. Many would consider that assessment of NCD risk should also be considered at earlier ages, even if the total risk is not particularly high, in view of the chronic and largely irreversible nature of NCDs (e.g. atherosclerosis and CVD). This may require using scores that predict risk over a longer period (e.g. 30 years vs 10 years).[11] While assessing the risk of CVD at a younger age can have important public health benefits, it also has significant resource implications if individual-level interventions are used.

Population strategies and high-risk individual strategies and WHO best buys and other recommended interventions in the WHO Global NCD Action Plan

Of the approximately 80 WHO best buys and other specific recommended interventions (outlined in Chapter 34 and described in chapters throughout the compendium), 40 can be characterized as population-wide strategies and 33 as high-risk individual-level strategies. Being aware of which intervention is population-based and which is individual high-risk is important to help understand which partners to work with.

Indicators for surveillance

Indicators useful to guide population interventions include population-based surveys in adults and children in order to assess mean levels and prevalence of risk factors in the whole population (e.g. STEPS or similar surveys, Chapter 5), ideally stratified by age, sex, socioeconomic level and other population characteristics. Indicators useful to guide high-risk strategies include surveys at the health care level (e.g. service availability and readiness assessment [SARA] or similar health facility-based surveys assessing the use of services, performance, equipment, etc.) but also population-based surveys (e.g. to assess the level of control of risk factors in the whole population). Data from vital statistics or registers (e.g. cancer), which provide information on rates of diseases in a population, are useful to guide both types of interventions.

Notes

1. Rose G. Sick individuals and sick populations. *Int J Epidemiol* 1985;14:32–8.
2. Soltani S et al. Community-based cardiovascular disease prevention programmes and cardiovascular risk factors: a systematic review and meta-analysis. *Public Health* 2021;200:59–70.
3. Tackling NCDs: best buys and other recommended interventions for the prevention and control of NCDs. WHO, 2017.
4. Clark J. Medicalization of global health 3: the medicalization of the non-communicable diseases agenda. *Global Health Action* 2014;7:24002.
5. Manuel DG et al. Revisiting rose: strategies for reducing coronary heart disease. *BMJ* 2006;18;332:659–62.
6. Bovet P et al. Screening for cardiovascular disease risk and subsequent management in low and middle income countries: challenges and opportunities. *Public Health Rev* 2015;36:13.
7. Ndindjock R et al. Potential impact of single-risk-factor versus total risk management for the prevention of cardiovascular events in Seychelles. *Bull WHO* 2011;89:286–95.
8. Collins GS, Altman DG. An independent and external validation of QRISK2 CVD risk score: a prospective open cohort study. *BMJ* 2010;340:c2442.
9. Wald NJ et al. When can a risk factor be used as a worthwhile screening test? *BMJ* 1999;319:1562–5.
10. Pencina MJ et al. Quantifying importance of major risk factors for coronary heart disease. *Circulation* 2019;139:1603–11.
11. Grundy S et al. Guideline on the management of blood cholesterol: a report of the ACA/AHA task force on clinical practice guidelines. *Circulation* 2019;139:e1082–43.

37 A life-course approach for NCD prevention and control

Julianne Williams, Kremlin Wickramasinghe, Sumudu K Kasturiarachchi, Arnaud Chiolero

NCDs and their risk factors have roots early in life, with complex aetiology involving multilevel socio-environmental, biological and psychological determinants, interacting across all stages of life.[1,2,3] It is therefore important that interventions to reduce the main modifiable risk factors for NCDs (including tobacco and alcohol use, unhealthy diet, and physical inactivity) start in early life and continue throughout life (Figure 37.1). The goal is to minimize the cumulative risk of NCD throughout life.[4,5] Where possible, interventions should be targeted to the relevant stages and settings of life (e.g. schools, workplaces, homes for old people).

Pre-conception, prenatal and perinatal

Different factors in the foetal and perinatal period, including low birth weight, can increase the risk of cardiovascular diseases (CVD) and other chronic diseases in adulthood, and this is often referred to as the 'developmental programming' of health and diseases.[6,7] For instance, tobacco use and alcohol consumption adversely affects the foetus and gestational diabetes is associated with an increased risk of obesity and CVD in the offspring. Further, pregnant women who maintain optimal body weight and have regular physical activity reduce their risk of developing gestational diabetes and hypertension. Maintaining normal levels of glucose during pregnancy can also have long-term benefits in the prevention of NCDs among both mothers and their offspring.

Pregnancy therefore provides a key entry point for the health system to support women (and their families) and perinatal care provides the opportunity for mothers and their families to develop strong relationships with health care professionals that can be continued throughout life.

Women and their families should be encouraged to quit tobacco, avoid alcohol, undertake physical activity, and have a healthy diet, with access to subsidized or free-of-charge food and micronutrient supplements. Body weight, blood pressure, and blood glucose should be monitored in pregnant women.[8]

DOI: 10.4324/9781003306689-42

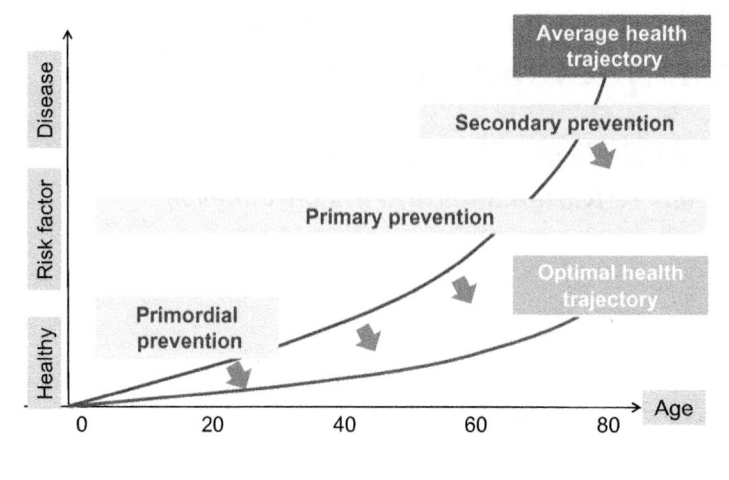

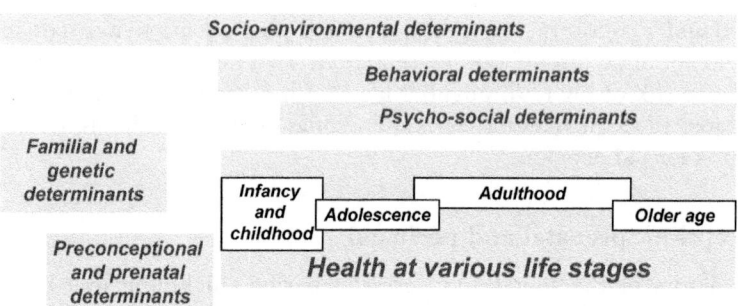

Figure 37.1 Impact of interventions across the life-course to reduce cumulative NCD risk.

Infancy

There is strong evidence that nutrition and environmental determinants of health in infancy shape long-term cardiovascular health and increase the long-term risk of obesity and diabetes.[9]

Breastfeeding has benefits for the short- and longer-term health of both babies and mothers. National labour policies that allow women to have paid maternity leave and workplaces that provide supportive environments for breastfeeding are therefore important. The international code of marketing breastmilk substitutes commits countries to enact legislative and regulatory measures to promote breastfeeding and against the aggressive marketing of commercial milk products.[10] A healthy diet (including exclusive breastfeeding for the first six months of life and continued breastfeeding up to two years and beyond along with a healthy diet in the early years of life) is associated with lower levels of overweight, obesity, diabetes and hypertension in childhood, as well as NCDs in adult life.[2]

Primary health care providers play an important role in working with families to regularly monitor an infant's growth and development, and provide advice for ensuring a healthy diet and physical activity behaviours. Community-based programmes that integrate direct nutrition and physical activity interventions into primary care should be included in efforts to ensure access to universal health care.

Childhood

Schools are important settings for encouraging healthy behaviour among children from all socioeconomic groups. Policies and programmes should be developed to ensure that healthy food is available in school and that the marketing of unhealthy food and drinks within and around schools is restricted or banned. This requires a coordinated response between health, education, commercial and other sectors. The health-promoting school initiative provides guidance, standards and indicators, as well as case studies in order to engage children, teachers and family members to strengthen the capacity of schools to provide healthy settings for living, learning and working.[11]

The school curriculum should for example provide adequate time for physical activity in line with WHO recommendations (i.e. children and adolescents aged 5–17 years should have at least an average of 60 minutes per day of moderate-to-vigorous intensity, mostly aerobic, physical activity, as well as those that strengthen muscle and bone) (see Chapter 25 on physical inactivity). Infrastructure to enable safer cycling and walking to schools is important in contributing to this and building physical activity into the day's routine as well as reducing dependency on vehicles – with additional benefits to the environment.

Education around health-harming behaviours (for example tobacco and alcohol use and unhealthy diet) should start at an early age.[12,13] Where children have already started smoking they should be encouraged to enrol in cessation programmes.[14] Screening for obesity and referring obese children to comprehensive, intensive behavioural interventions to promote improvements in weight status is recommended.[15] There is, however, no solid evidence that screening for high blood pressure or raised blood cholesterol in childhood reduces the risk of NCDs over the long term.[16]

Adolescence and young adulthood

Adolescence is a time when individuals are increasingly exposed to behavioural NCD risk factors – and these often remain for the rest of life. Behaviours are often largely shaped by marketing.[17,18] Policies that restrict the marketing of unhealthy behaviours that target adolescents (for example at school or community, festivals and sporting events) are therefore important. Programmes to support adolescents in making healthy choices and enhancing health literacy should be included in the school curriculum. School-based surveys should be used to assess trends in NCD risk factors among adolescents and young adults, as well as attitudes and behaviours, and information used to guide health policy.

Adulthood

Interventions targeting adults are the subject of a number of chapters in this book. These include the prevention of NCDs, including risk factor reduction, screening programmes, as well as treatment and care for specific NCDs or related conditions.

The workplace provides an important setting for health promotion, improving health literacy, screening for NCDs and their risk factors, and providing a supportive environment for those with NCDs.[19] Examples include promoting the availability of healthy food in cafeterias, banning or restricting tobacco and alcohol use in the workplace, and providing opportunities for physical activity such as promoting active commuting and providing opportunities to be active at work. Those unemployed or socially marginalized often have greater levels of NCDs and may also be more exposed to NCD risk factors. It is therefore important that prevention and control programmes reach these populations.

Older age

Older age is a time of transition from working life to retirement, with changing identities and relationships. Coordination among health and social services is particularly important for NCDs – which are usually long-term conditions – to ensure continuity of care in a way that is both cost-effective and patient-centred. Environments and dedicated programmes need to enable older people, who may be inclined to social isolation and inactivity, to have sufficient opportunities for physical activities and healthy diet (e.g. help with shopping, healthy ready meals), and to be supported in quitting tobacco use and reduce the harmful use of alcohol. In addition, the health and social care system need to be designed to support this age group, including those with NCDs.

Strengthening the evidence base

While the life-course approach provides a useful way of framing interventions across the life-course, for example developing and implementing policies and programmes to reduce risk factors in different age groups and settings such as nurseries, schools, homes, workplaces, nursing homes and health care settings, most of the evidence base around health-promoting and preventive strategies across the life-course is observational. For many interventions especially early in life, there remain few conclusive trials, not least because of the long period of time between interventions at an early age and the development of NCDs in later life. The complex aetiology of most NCDs makes this an even greater challenge.

Monitoring

When it comes to surveillance and monitoring, important issues for the prevention and control of NCDs across the life-course include the need to:

- Conduct NCD risk factor surveys across all age groups and in different settings (e.g. schools, workplaces, nursing homes, marginalized persons).
- Undertake long-term cohort studies to track and understand better the impact of interventions over long periods of time.
- Understand the relationship between biological and environmental mechanisms, as well as public health and health care interventions, and outcomes, both long-term and more immediate, for example, earlier signs of atherosclerosis.

Further details on surveillance and monitoring are provided in Chapters 4 and 5.

Notes

1. Hanson M, Gluckman P. Developmental origins of noncommunicable disease: population and public health implications. *Am J Clin Nutr* 2011;94(Suppl 6):1754S–58S.
2. Gillman MW. Primordial prevention of cardiovascular disease. *Circulation* 2015;131:599–601.
3. Jacobs DR Jr et al. Childhood cardiovascular risk factors and adult cardiovascular events. *NEJM* 2022 387:473–47.
4. Mikkelsen B et al. Life course approach to prevention and control of non-communicable diseases. *BMJ* 2019;364:l257.
5. Kuh D. A life-course approach to healthy ageing: maintaining physical capability. *Proc Nutr Soc* 2014;73:237–48.
6. Barker DJP. *Mothers, babies and health in later life*. Amsterdam, The Netherlands: Elsevier Health Sciences, 1998.
7. Hanson MA, Gluckman PD. Early developmental conditioning of later health and disease: physiology or pathophysiology? *Physiol Rev* 2014; 94:1027–76.
8. Screening for gestational diabetes: US Preventive Services Task Force Recommendation Statement. *JAMA* 2021;326:531–38.
9. Fleming TP et al. Origins of lifetime health around the time of conception: causes and consequences. *Lancet* 2018;391:1842–52.
10. WHO, IBFAN & UNICEF. Marketing of breast-milk substitutes: national implementation of the international code, status report. WHO, 2018.
11. WHO. Health promoting schools. https://www.who.int/health-topics/health-promoting-schools#tab=tab_1.
12. Smoking prevention in schools. Public health guideline [PH23], NICE, 2010.
13. Owens DK et al. Primary care interventions for prevention and cessation of tobacco use in children and adolescents: US Preventive Services Task Force Recommendation Statement. *JAMA* 2020;323:1590–98.
14. Make every school a health promoting school – global standards and indicators. WHO, 2021.
15. Screening for obesity in children and adolescents: US Preventive Services Task Force recommendation statement. *JAMA* 2017;317:2417–26.

16 Screening for high blood pressure in children and adolescents: US Preventive Services Task Force Recommendation Statement. *JAMA* 2020;324:1878–83.
17 Pechmann C et al. Impulsive and self-conscious: adolescents' vulnerability to advertising and promotion. *J Public Policy Mark* 2005;24:202–21.
18 Smith LA, Foxcroft DR. The effect of alcohol advertising, marketing and portrayal on drinking behaviour in young people: systematic review of prospective cohort studies. *BMC Public Health* 2009;9:51.
19 Worksite Health. The community guide: worksite health. https://www.thecommunity-guide.org/topic/worksite-health.

38 Universal health coverage and NCD prevention and control

Nick Banatvala, Kaspar Wyss, Patricia Akweongo, August Kuwawenaruwa, Victor G Rodwin

Universal health coverage (UHC) is a central part of the 2030 Sustainable Development Agenda and the WHO Global NCD Action Plan. Achieving UHC means that all people would have access to the health services they need, when and where they need them, without financial hardship. UHC includes health protection and promotion, as well as disease prevention, treatment, rehabilitation and palliative care, across the life-course.[1]

There will always be trade-offs in allocating resources between each of the UHC dimensions (i.e. population covered, services provided, and direct costs to patients) (Figure 38.1). What levels of coverage can be provided for the population? Or should more services be covered by enlarging the benefits package to include other health services and if so which ones? Or should cost sharing and fees for patients be reduced?

In addressing these questions, it is clear that UHC is more of a political than a technical construct, with governments having to make decisions and trade-offs across: (i) levels of taxation on income, salaries and goods, and levels of public sector financing to improve access to healthcare, promote population health, and more broadly improve social determinants of health (e.g. education,

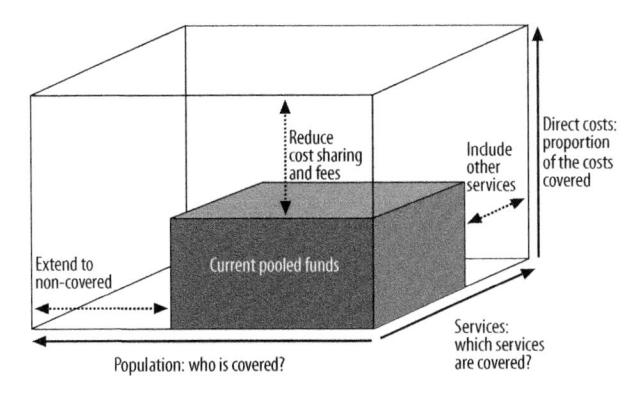

Figure 38.1 The three key dimensions of UHC: population coverage, service coverage and proportion of costs covered. World Health Report. Health systems financing: the path to universal coverage. WHO, 2010.

housing and social care – Chapter 17); (ii) the responsibility of government and the individual in accessing and financing the costs of healthcare, including the acceptable level of household out-of-pocket (OOP) expenditure (e.g. cost-sharing, self-medication and other expenses paid directly by households to the health provider) and the importance attached to preventing people from going into debt and as a result experiencing poverty and/or catastrophic health expenditure; and (iii) issues around levels of healthcare afforded to groups and communities that are marginalized or suffer from discrimination.

UHC poses important governance challenges,[2] including making decisions around health equity, social cohesion, the efficiency of resource allocation and sustainable human and economic development.[3] In this sense, the path to achieving UHC has been viewed as a political struggle and is not value-free.[4] The political importance of UHC was highlighted in 2019 when world leaders committed to ensuring UHC (including for the prevention and control of NCDs) was available in their countries.[5]

An effective health financing system is essential to achieve UHC. This consists of: (i) raising sufficient funding to cover the costs of the health system; (ii) pooling resources to protect people from the financial consequences of ill health; and (iii) purchasing or providing health services to ensure greater efficiency in the allocation of available resources. Most healthcare financing schemes receive transfers from the government, social insurance contributions, voluntary or compulsory prepayments (such as insurance premiums), other domestic revenues, and revenues from abroad (for example, as part of development aid and remittances). Chapter 39 provides more detail on financing for NCDs.

UHC and NCD outcomes

Key issues that those working on NCDs need to address include: (i) inadequate availability of and access to essential services for the prevention and the treatment of NCDs; (ii) inequalities in levels of NCD risk, access to services, and health outcomes; and (iii) the economic burden on national budgets and on individuals (including OOP payments for treatment and care, which can trap households and communities into a cycle of impoverishment and illness). Once accomplished, UHC can result in improved NCD outcomes, greater equity in access to services and enhanced socio-economic development.

As part of UHC, the following principles apply for the four NCDs considered in this compendium

- Comprehensive integrated healthcare across primary, secondary and tertiary care levels (e.g. investigation, treatment and continuum of care for high blood pressure [BP], diabetes, heart attack, stroke, chronic respiratory disease, asthma and cancer).
- Multi-sectoral action to address NCD risk factors (e.g. legislative action to prevent the advertising of tobacco products, taxation of tobacco, alcohol

and sugar-sweetened beverages), as well as decisions on earmarking these taxes for health and the underlying determinants of health.
- Engaging and empowering individuals and communities with their health and healthcare (e.g. food labelling to help promote a healthy diet, increasing health literacy around screening or health checks [e.g. diabetes, hypertension, cancer], and access to self-help groups).
- A life course approach.

Examples of how NCD responses can be improved as part of UHC include: (i) strengthening quality assurance (e.g. provision of quality-assured essential NCD medicines and technologies through improved quality control, procurement practices and regulation); (ii) reorienting health systems for chronic care (e.g. the use of existing service delivery platforms for issues requiring long-term follow-up, such as for HIV/AIDS and tuberculosis to introduce risk assessment, early diagnosis and management of NCDs, and ensuring that staff in these and other platforms are trained to take BP or blood glucose measurements, provide treatment for diabetes patients and provide information on ways of reducing NCD risk factors); (iii) strengthening systems for social care; and (iv) empowering communities, civil society and people living with NCDs (e.g. reducing stigma and discrimination experienced by people living with NCDs); and (v) empowering communities and patient networks to be able to claim their right to health and hold their governments accountable for delivering UHC.[6]

NCDs and UHC priority benefit packages

Average per capita health spending in OECD countries (which are mostly high-income economies) in 2019 (adjusted for differences in purchasing power) is estimated to be approximately USD 4,000 (ranging from almost USD 11,000 in the US to less than USD 2,000 in a number of countries).[7] As a result, most people living in OECD countries have access to a range of services through a publicly defined (even if not publicly funded) benefits package, with OOP spending as a share of final household consumption ranging from 1.3% in Turkey to nearly 5.8% in Switzerland.

However, most countries in the world are not in a position to provide the level of healthcare that the majority of OECD countries can enjoy. Where resources are most limited, prioritizing interventions is even more important. Priorities should be established on the basis of the health of the population (as a whole and for specific groups), interventions that maximize health gain and increase equity, a transparent understanding/assessment of resources available, and the views and preferences of the population.[8] Agreed priorities often come together in the form of an essential UHC priority health benefits package (UHC-PBP) that consists of health services, programmes, intersectoral actions, and fiscal policies that are considered necessary and affordable for a particular population, country or region. However, there is rarely consensus among countries on what constitutes a set of basic benefits beyond the narrowest priority benefit package.

NCD prevention, treatment and care at population and individual levels should be a key component of UHC-PBP in all countries. Tools to support the NCD elements of a UHC-PBP should include the best buys (Chapter 34) as well as a wider set of interventions provided in the interactive WHO UHC Compendium.[9] The web-based Compendium allows users to search for interventions by any NCD (or other disease), risk factor or through keywords, as well as for different stages across the life-course, and increasingly by the technical package (e.g. HEARTS, see Chapter 7).

The current Disease Control Priorities publication (DCP3) includes evidence on cost-effective interventions to address the burden of disease in low-income countries (LICs) and lower-middle-income countries. Each of DCP3's nine volumes defines a package of essential health measures containing both health-sector interventions and intersectoral policies. NCDs are covered in a volume on cardiovascular, respiratory and related disorders, with a second volume on cancer.[10]

Based on DCP3, estimates of minimal financial requirements for a UHC-PBP (including priority interventions for NCDs) have been developed for LICs and lower MICs. Modelled at 80% population coverage, these are USD 79 per capita each year for LICs and USD 130 for lower MICs.[11] Additional investments would require 8% (LICs) and 4% (lower MICs) of gross national income for 2015. DCP3 estimates indicate that a higher priority sub-package, with a reduced number of interventions, would cost approximately half of these amounts. Also, DCP3 estimates that cardiovascular, respiratory and related disorders account for 29% (LICs) and 36% (lower MICs) of the total healthcare cost, while cancer accounts for around 4% of these costs in LICs and 2% in lower MICs.

A series of steps are required to ensure that NCDs are incorporated into a country's UHC-PBP (Box 38.1).

BOX 38.1   STEPS TO ENSURE THAT NCDs ARE INCORPORATED INTO A COUNTRY'S UHC-PBP(ADAPTED FROM 12)

1. Align the NCD strategy with the National Health Sector Plan.
2. Engage relevant stakeholders in the UHC-PBP design process to:
   - Establish a list of priority NCD interventions using existing resources such as the best buys, local evidence and analysis, and tools such as the WHO UHC Compendium, WHO CHOICE (Chapter 34) and DCP3.

   - Estimate current and future costs of NCDs, interventions required and their return on investment (for example through investment cases that are described in Chapter 40).

- Set priorities for NCDs across health and other sectors, as well as communities.

3. Identify opportunities for financing NCD services:
    - Advocacy and development of measures to assess fiscal effort and projections of revenue (including macro-economic and demographic conditions for fiscal potential and health taxes).
    - Review of government funding priorities (fiscal space analysis, links to the investment plan, examination of evidence for efficiency with specific arguments to also develop interventions [e.g. for the prevention of NCDs] in non-health sectors).

4. Enforce implementation:
    - Development of monitoring and evaluation mechanisms to measure progress and to promote health equity.
    - Transparent communication to ensure that communities are aware of their entitlements, and service providers understand their responsibilities.
    - Design of transparent accountability and review processes.

An example of the process and outcomes of incorporating NCDs into Ethiopia's UHC-PBP is described in Box 38.2.[13]

BOX 38.2 REVISION OF THE ESSENTIAL HEALTH SERVICE PACKAGE (EHSP) IN ETHIOPIA

Process

- Over 2000 interventions were identified from the existing EHSP, national publications, WHO CHOICE database, DCP3 and consultations with experts.
- Prioritization criteria were developed based on disease burden, cost-effectiveness, equity, financial protection, budget impact, public acceptability and political feasibility as starting points.
- Expert evaluation of the recommended interventions were undertaken.
- Over 35 meetings were held with stakeholders over the entire process.

Outcomes for NCDs

- NCD interventions were aligned with WHO NCD best buys, with 31% of interventions focusing on cancer, 15% on policy and

> behaviour change communications, 13% on cardiovascular disease and others, including chronic respiratory disease.
> - NCD interventions were characterized as high priority (about 60%), medium priority (about 20%) or low priority (about 20%, which included mostly resource-intensive interventions).
> - The EHSP focused mostly on primary healthcare centres and primary-level hospitals, with nearly 50% of NCD interventions at the primary healthcare level and 20% at the general hospital level.

A review of UHC-PBP in 45 LICs and lower MICs indicates that NCD interventions are increasingly prioritized. Nevertheless, only 2% of total development assistance for health was allocated to NCDs in 2018.[14]

Global partnerships

UHC2030 International Health Partnership.[15] UHC2030 is a global multi-stakeholder partnership for UHC which brings together countries and territories, multilateral organizations and global health initiatives, philanthropic organizations, NGOs (including those working on NCDs) and the private sector. It advocates for increased political commitment to UHC, facilitates accountability and promotes collaborative working on strengthening health systems.

The UHC Partnership.[16] This is one of WHO's largest platforms for international cooperation on UHC and primary healthcare (PHC). It comprises a broad mix of health experts working hand in hand to promote UHC and PHC by fostering policy dialogue on strategic planning and health systems governance, developing health financing strategies and supporting their implementation, and enabling effective development cooperation in countries, including revising and implementing UHC-PBPs.

DCP3 UHC Country Translation Project.[17] This partnership provides technical assistance and capacity building to low- and middle-income countries in revising and implementing national and sub-national UHC-PBPs.

Monitoring progress

Monitoring progress towards the SDG Target 3.8 (to achieve UHC, including financial risk protection, access to quality essential healthcare services and access to safe, effective, quality and affordable essential medicines and vaccines for all) is based, in principle, on all three dimensions of UHC noted at the beginning of this chapter: the extent to which the entire population is covered, the benefits package that is covered and the extent of financial protection attained for patients who access health services. In practice, monitoring to date has focused on the benefits package covered and the extent of financial protection assured.

Financial protection is assessed through the proportion of the population with large household expenditures on healthcare, as a share of total household expenditure or income. Two thresholds are used to define what is meant by 'large': >10% and >25% of total household expenditure or income. Household budget, household income and expenditure, and economic or living standards surveys (including demographic and health surveys) can all provide data for this indicator.

Health service coverage is assessed through 14 tracer indicators in the following categories: (i) NCDs; (ii) infectious diseases; (iii) reproductive, maternal, new-born and child health; and (iv) service capacity and access.[18] Indicators are measured through a range of surveys (household and health facility availability and readiness) and sentinel surveillance systems. There are three tracer indicators for NCDs:

- Prevention of CVD (age-standardized prevalence of non-raised BP among adults aged ≥18 years).
- Management of diabetes (age-standardized mean fasting plasma glucose among adults aged ≥18 years).
- Tobacco control (age-standardized prevalence of adults aged ≥15 years not smoking tobacco in the last 30 days).

The WHO and the World Bank 2017 Global Monitoring Report on UHC noted that at least half of the world's population does not have full coverage of essential health services.[19] The World Bank's 2018 Universal Health Coverage Study reviewed the experience of implementing UHC across 40 countries.[20] This work needs to be expanded to continue the drive for UHC and 'progressive universalism'.[21]

The authors gratefully acknowledge the valuable input and critical review provided by Joe Kutzin, WHO, Geneva.

Notes

1. WHO. Universal health coverage. https://www.who.int/health-topics/universal-health-coverage#tab=tab_1.
2. Greer SJ, Méndez CA. Universal health coverage: a political struggle and governance challenge. *Am J Public Health* 2015;105:S637–9.
3. Global health and foreign policy. A/67/L.36, UN General Assembly, 2012.
4. Machado CV, Silva GA. Political struggles for a universal health system in Brazil: successes and limits in the reduction of inequalities. *Global Health* 2019;15(Suppl 1):77.
5. Political declaration of the high-level meeting on universal health coverage. Resolution A/RES/74/2. UN General Assembly, 2019.
6. Universal health coverage and non-communicable diseases: a mutually reinforcing agenda. NCD Alliance, 2014.
7. Health at a Glance. OECD, 2021.
8. Making fair choices on the path to universal health coverage: final report of the WHO consultative group on equity and universal health coverage. WHO, 2014.
9. UHC Compendium. Health interventions for universal health coverage. WHO, Version 1.2.

10 Debas H et al. (Eds). *Disease control priorities*, 3rd ed. Washington DC: the World Bank, 2015.
11 Watkins DA et al. Resource requirements for essential universal health coverage: a modelling study based on findings from *Disease Control Priorities*, 3rd edition. *Lancet Glob Health* 2020;8:e829–39.
12 Strengthening NCD service delivery through UHC benefit package: technical meeting report. WHO, 2020.
13 Eregata GT et al. Revision of the Ethiopian essential health service package: an explication of the process and methods. *Health Syst Reform* 2020;6:1.
14 Global Burden of Disease Health Financing Collaborator Network. Past, present, and future of global health financing: a review of development assistance, government, out-of-pocket, and other private spending on health for 195 countries, 1995–2050. *Lancet* 2019;393:2233–60.
15 UHC2030. https://www.uhc2030.org/.
16 Universal Health Coverage Partnership. https://www.uhcpartnership.net/about/.
17 The UHC Country Translation Project. DCP3. http://dcp-3.org/translation.
18 SDG Indicators Metadata. United Nations Statistics Division. Last updated 20 December 2021. https://unstats.un.org/sdgs/metadata/files/Metadata-03-08-01.pdf.
19 Tracking universal health coverage: 2017 global monitoring report. WHO and World Bank, 2017.
20 Universal Health Coverage Study Series (UNICO). Going universal: how countries are implementing pro-poor universal health coverage reforms. World Bank (web site: 24 country case studies published in 2017 and 15 additional case studies published in 2018).
21 Cotlear D. An anatomy of progressive universal health coverage reforms in low- and middle-income countries. *World Hosp Health Serv* 2018;54:9–13.

39 Financing and allocating resources for NCD prevention and control

*Nick Banatvala, Victor G Rodwin,
Tseday Zerayacob, Rachel Nugent*

Health financing by which we mean financing to promote health, including healthcare, is a core function of a health system. In addition to making decisions on investing to promote population health and improve healthcare, governments also have to consider spending in other areas, including social protection, education, defence, public order and safety, housing and environment, transportation, agriculture and employment. Health financing is therefore part of the resource allocation process in which advocates for NCDs must find a voice. While there will always be trade-offs in government spending priorities across sectors, this does not mean that public finance is a zero-sum game.

Because NCDs are both a cause and consequence of government policies, there are opportunities to reduce the burden of NCDs in broader financing decisions. For example, spending on education can lead to greater health literacy, a more productive workforce produces stronger economic growth, and public infrastructure investments in green spaces and the built environment can promote physical activity and interaction with nature. Reducing NCD risks through taxing tobacco and unhealthy foods can provide new tax revenue for improving access to disease prevention and health services as part of universal health coverage (UHC) (Chapter 38). Encouraging alternatives to tobacco farming leads to a reduction in tobacco production as well as a reduction in child labour, health risks for farmers and improved opportunities for strengthening food security. A number of chapters in this book, such as those on social determinants of health, the life-course and whole-of-government responses, explain how policies that impact on health are made by ministries beyond health.

Core functions of health financing are: (i) health financing policy, process and governance; (ii) revenue raising; (iii) pooling revenues (the accumulation of prepaid funds on behalf of some or all of the population); (iv) purchasing and provider payment (through strategic allocation of funds to health care providers for health services aimed at some or all of the population); (v) benefits and conditions of access; (vi) public financial management; and (vii) public health functions and programmes.[1,2,3,4]

DOI: 10.4324/9781003306689-44

Countries raise revenue for healthcare through one or a combination of:

- General revenue funds through the fiscal system (e.g. value-added, personal income or excise taxes).
- Compulsory payroll taxes through the social security system (e.g. employer and employee taxes).
- Voluntary or mandatory premiums assessed by various systems of private health insurance (pre-pooling).
- Individual out-of-pocket payments (OOP) that are incurred to receive a service or health product, including medicines. (OOP is a highly regressive and inequitable way of financing healthcare – and this is described in more detail later on).
- Innovative financial instruments, such as social impact bonds and loyalty funds.
- External aid (development assistance).

Whatever combination of methods is used to raise revenues, a stable and predictable flow of funds is important to avoid disruptions in service delivery (e.g. commodity stock-outs), ensure timely payment of salaries and provide a credible basis for contracting with service providers. This can be a challenge, especially when OOPs play a predominant role, but also because budget priorities may shift from year to year as a result of changing economic conditions and politics. A particular challenge for NCDs is that they often require long-term treatment and care.

Transparency and accountability are important objectives for health systems. Patients should have clarity with regard to how much, if anything, they will be expected to pay at the point of use (e.g. some form of user charge), and this is an important part of preventing unofficial payments.[5]

The question of how much should be allocated for the prevention and treatment of NCDs is typically not faced explicitly. Most economists would argue that there is no 'right' amount of spend for the prevention and control of NCDs, or indeed for any other group of diseases or for health in its entirety. Although most economists would argue, in theory, that resource allocation within the health sector should pay greater attention to whether the expenditures generate more benefits than costs (e.g. gain of disability-adjusted life years (DALYs) per $ spent on a particular intervention), countries rarely set budgets in this way. Moreover, in the health sector, many nations do not set explicit budgets, let alone targets, for aggregate healthcare spending. Furthermore, most nations have difficulty disaggregating such budgets by subsector (e.g. hospitals, primary care, pharmaceuticals, medical equipment).

An increasing challenge in health care, particularly for NCDs, is that given progress in genomics, new technologies and pharmaceuticals, even the most wealthy nations will not be able to assure that everyone will be able to receive state-of-the-art diagnosis and treatment for all conditions. Resource allocation decisions must begin with a recognition that difficult choices must be made and if they are not made explicitly with some degree of transparency, then they will be made implicitly. It is essential to promote efficiency and equity in the allocation of limited healthcare resources, no matter how wealthy a nation may be. At the same time, since there will always be new technologies and more possibilities for screening, health promotion and treatment of NCDs, it is important to recognize that healthcare rationing already exists and to consider what we know about costs, benefits, patient preferences, and the importance of public deliberation in making explicit rationing decisions.

It is also important to consider health equity in resource allocation decisions. Equitable health financing is often associated with progressivity, for example, the extent to which households make payments according to their ability-to-pay (ATP). A progressive health financing system is one where high-ATP households pay a higher share of their income than low-ATP households, whether that is through taxes, social and health insurance, or OOP spending. A system is regressive when the poor contribute proportionately more, relative to their income.

There is no one perfect financing model for all countries. Using income taxes (that allows for shares of tax contributions to increase with income) generally enables greater redistribution of resources from the wealthy to the poor. Payroll taxes are typically more regressive, enabling less redistribution from wealthy to poor. Systems of private insurance tend to be voluntary and based on actuarial calculations of risk, except when they are mandatory and universal, as in the case of the Netherlands, Switzerland and Germany (with government subsidies to persons who cannot afford payments of premiums). OOP payments, which account for a disproportionate share of healthcare financing in most LICs and MICs (OOP spending on health care being inversely and strongly associated with country income level) are particularly regressive. Private health insurance can also be regressive if it financially penalizes those with (or at risk of) poor health, particularly for NCDs, which often require long-term treatment and care. Private health insurance is also regressive when the same level of premium is paid by everyone.

Many health systems were financed based on the notion that once levels of child and maternal mortality were reduced and epidemic diseases eliminated, the overall cost of health care would plateau or even fall. This clearly turns out not to be the case: demographic and epidemiological changes have or are in the process of shifting the disease burden from communicable to NCDs in almost all countries. While this may seem to be an impossible conundrum for health financing, opportunities remain to capture part of the 'dividend' from economic growth to increase overall public spending on health, move away from verticalized programming and focus on the most cost-effective interventions, many of which can be delivered through primary care. Even after achieving more efficient resource allocation, many countries will need to increase health financing to meet the challenge of NCDs – and in many cases those countries with the greatest needs for additional resources are the least prepared for the change.[6]

A number of attributes of health financing systems have been described for: (i) health financing policy, process and governance; (ii) revenue raising; (iii) pooling revenues; (iv) purchasing and provider payment; (v) benefits and conditions of access; (vi) public financial management; and (vii) public health functions and programmes. All have relevance for the prevention and control of NCDs. Examples include:[7]

- Moving from fee-for-service and case-based payments towards population-based capitation payments (i.e. the allocation of an annual public fixed budget per unit population) which also takes into account different disease burdens and variations in socioeconomic status.
- Developing incentives for primary care-led outreach, screening, early detection and proactive disease management – especially where specialists and hospitals are remunerated on the basis of volume (although this can lead to overdiagnosis, overtreatment and increased total health expenditures).
- Introducing financial incentives for pay-for-performance, pay-for-coordination, bundled payment (e.g. Diagnosis-Related Groups [DRGs], where the same amount is paid to health providers for treatment of a particular cases mix),[8] or full capitation to integrate prevention, screening, early detection and management for NCDs to maximize health outcomes.
- Ensuring that health financing for NCDs is explicitly linked to other instruments that improve service delivery, including guidelines and protocols, training, performance monitoring with feedback, better information solutions, e.g. task shifting/sharing (Chapter 42 on health systems) and using e-health and m-health[9] (Chapter 49).
- Agreeing on dedicated funds from the health budget to deliver intersectoral activities that will help achieve overall NCD objectives, for instance, improving health literacy around NCD risk factors affecting children and adolescents (physical inactivity, unhealthy diet, tobacco and alcohol use).
- Promoting voluntary or mandatory joint budgeting to leverage funding from multiple sectors, with budget alignment, along with mutually determined NCD targets and outcomes.[10]

Specific challenges for low- and middle-income countries

A significant challenge for low- and middle-income countries is inadequate levels of public financing for health. For instance, in Africa, even though many countries have marginally increased health spending overall, only a small number of countries have reached the commitment they made in 2001 to allocate 15% of their government budgets to health[11] (and this share is <5% in many countries). The prevention and control of NCDs is poorly funded, with LICs allocating about 13% of health expenditure to NCDs, while MICs allocate about 30% of total health spending to NCDs.[12] Governments spend around USD 2 per capita on LICs and USD 46 in MICs on NCDs. While domestic health expenditure is reported by national health accounts through the System of Health Accounts,[13] there is little detail on public sector expenditure by disease. In the absence of adequate amounts of direct public payment for NCDs, countries may have no other option than to rely on insurance, private payment and development assistance. In many cases the lack of such arrangements means there is often very limited access to services. Health insurance is not widely used to pay for NCD services in low- and middle-income countries and even some catastrophic health insurance policies are not achieving that goal. Finally, trans-national and domestic private, for-profit companies and donors also provide health services for NCDs but their focus and magnitude are poorly documented.

As a result, people living with NCDs resort to OOPs to obtain health services. More frequently, inability to pay for services out of pocket means people often cannot access care. Table 39.1 shows a high reliance on OOP, especially in lower-income countries, but likely highest for patients living with NCDs that require treatment and care over many years (e.g. cancer and stroke), compared with conditions that require either treatment and care over the short term (e.g. meningitis) or conditions where development assistance is likely to be more available (e.g. AIDS, tuberculosis and malaria) or highly cost-effective vaccination programmes.

Many of the OOP expenditures (especially for medicines,[14] but also for outpatient visits, diagnostics, hospitalization and transport) worsen poverty. In 2017, about half a billion people were pushed or further pushed into extreme poverty (living with less than PPP$ 1.90 a day) by OOPs and almost one billion people incurred catastrophic health spending because they spent more than 10% of their household budget on health out-of-pocket, which might have disrupted their consumption of necessities.[15] Dedicated studies, using alternative definitions, find very high proportions of low-income patients with NCDs experiencing catastrophic health spending. Rates of catastrophic health expenditure among low-income patients with cardiovascular disease were 92% in Tanzania, 92% in India, and 79% in China. For Chinese patients with stroke, catastrophic OOP affected 71%. Similar levels (68%) were observed among cancer patients in Iran and Vietnam.[16] In a time of rising inflation, higher prices erode the value of real wages and savings, leaving households poorer, with the

Table 39.1 Composition of health spending by funding source in 2019[a]

	LICs (%)	Lower MICs (%)	Upper MICs (%)	HICs (%)
Government transfers	21	34	38	48
Social health insurance contributions	1	7	16	22
External aid	29	12	1	0.1
Voluntary health insurance contributions	2	3	9	5
Out-of-pocket spending	44	40	34	21
Other	3	3	2	4

Note: Other sources are compulsory prepayments to private insurance, domestic nongovernmental organization contributions and health services operated by enterprises for their employees.
Global expenditure on health: public spending on the rise? WHO, 2021 (Figure 1.6).

greatest impact of inflation being on low- and middle-income households.[17] This is of concern for people living with NCDs that have predictable and long-term costs as some of them might have to forego treatment and others, paying out-of-pocket to access or continue their treatment protocol, might be at greater risk of incurring catastrophic and/or impoverishing health spending.

Despite these challenges, there remains significant potential to increase domestic fiscal space for health financing in low- and middle-income countries, for example through improved tax mobilization, budget prioritization, reducing health budget underspending and efficiencies in delivering care.[18,19]

Health taxes are taxes on unhealthy products, such as tobacco, alcohol and sugar-sweetened beverages. A number of countries (e.g. Mexico, Panama, the Philippines, South Africa and Thailand) have raised significant revenue from these taxes. Governments sometimes take the opportunity to earmark some or all of these revenues for health or a particular area of health such as health promotion or NCDs.[20] Other innovative financial instruments to raise funds for the prevention and control of NCDs include solidarity levies, debt conversion, social impact bonds, risk or credit guarantees,[21] but these require considerable further assessment to understand better their potential in supporting action on NCDs.[22]

Development assistance funding for NCDs

External aid accounts for 29% of health spending in LICs and 12% in lower MICs.[23,24] As a proportion of official development assistance (ODA) in the health sector, that specified for NCDs was less than 1% in 2020 (Table 39.2), despite NCDs accounting for as much as 34% of DALYs lost in low-income

Table 39.2 Official development assistance (official donors, all channels, gross disbursements, for developing countries) in 2020[b]

	USD (million)
Total health	18,827
which includes …	
Infectious disease (other)	3,102
Malaria	2,187
Tuberculosis	921
NCDs	**174 (account for 0.92% of total health)**
Total population policies/programmes and reproductive health	10,287
which includes …	
Sexually transmitted disease control including HIV/AIDS	7,590
Reproductive health care	1,481
Total health and total population policies/programmes and reproductive health	29,114 **(NCDs account for 0.60%)**

(OECD. Stat. https://stats.oecd.org/Index.aspx?DataSetCode=crs1)

countries and 55% in lower-middle-income countries in 2019 (IHME, GBD Compare). The 2015 Addis Ababa Action Agenda on financing sustainable development emphasized that while NCDs should be financed primarily from domestic resources, development assistance for NCDs can play an important role in mobilizing domestic resources and investing in the prevention and control of NCDs to strengthen human capital, reduce poverty and inequity and improve workforce productivity.

In contrast to many other areas of health, the Organisation for Economic Co-operation and Development (OECD) Development Assistance Committee only recently (2019) started tracking annual official development assistance (ODA) spending on NCDs. ODA includes funds from bilaterals (e.g. government development agencies) and multilaterals (e.g. the World Bank). The focus of available development assistance is on providing technical and catalytic support, especially for LICs with a high NCD burden.

Arguments have been advanced that development assistance should primarily be targeted towards global public goods (GPGs) for health, such as improved surveillance, research and development (R&D), and the development of global tools.[25] This aligns well with a move away from verticalized funding although it is notable that many of the examples for GPGs remain disease-targeted (e.g. R&D for neglected tropical diseases, outbreak preparedness and antimicrobial resistance).

At the country level itself, examples where support can be helpful include:

- Strengthening public financial management (PFM), including the level and allocation of public funding (budget formulation), the effectiveness of spending (budget execution) and the flexibility in which funds can be used (pooling, sub-national PFM arrangements and purchasing).[26] For countries spending money on existing programmes but not attaining the health outcomes desired, this avenue can spotlight new opportunities for NCD investments.
- Identifying opportunities for increasing domestic financing for NCD prevention and control, for example, by increasing direct and indirect taxes to achieve a higher public contribution to health and enhancing social security systems. Political and economic analysis is a key element of such support. The extent to which direct and indirect taxes increase domestic financing for NCDs depends on the extent to which increased public revenues are allocated to health and the extent to which any increase for health is 'allocated to NCDs' (ideally through an integrated benefits package rather than vertical funding, except perhaps for dedicated population-based prevention programmes).
- Multilateral loans that support action on NCDs, either alone or as part of broader health and/or development programmes.
- Technical assistance to support the implementation of best buys and other interventions. This also requires strengthening governance in order to develop and implement such action, including, where appropriate, passing the necessary legislative and regulatory frameworks (e.g. for tobacco and alcohol control, and access to treatment).

In addressing some of these issues, WHO, UNICEF and the UNDP recently established Health4Life, a multi-partner trust fund, to provide catalytic support for low- and middle-income countries, including mobilization and effective use of domestic funds to scale up responses to NCDs.[27] However, a lack of investment in the prevention and control of NCDs is a major impediment to achieving domestic and international development goals.[28,29,30] Moreover, in many countries resources for NCD prevention and control have become even more limited because of COVID-19, even though people living with NCDs are often those most affected by the pandemic and will continue to be so in its aftermath.

The authors gratefully acknowledge the valuable inputs and critical review provided by Gabriela Flores, Matthew Jowett, Joe Kutzin, Andrew Siroka and Ke Xu, WHO, Geneva.

Notes

1. World Health Report. Health systems financing: the path to universal coverage. WHO, 2010.
2. Jowett M et al. Assessing country health financing systems: the health financing progress matrix (health financing guidance no. 8). WHO, 2020.
3. Yameogo P et al. *Strategic health purchasing policymakers' perspectives*. Nairobi, Kenya: Strategic Purchasing Africa Resource Centre (SPARC), 2022.
4. Cashin C, Gatome-Munyua A. The strategic health purchasing progress tracking framework: a practical approach to describing, assessing, and improving strategic purchasing for universal health coverage. *Health Syst Reform* 2022;8:e2051794.
5. Jowett M, Kutzin J. Raising revenues for health in support of UHC: strategic issues for policy makers. Health financing policy brief no. 1. WHO, 2015.
6. Bollyky TJ et al. Lower-income countries that face the most rapid shift in noncommunicable disease burden are also the least prepared. *Health Aff* 2017;36:1866–75.
7. Jakovljevic M et al. Comparative financing analysis and political economy of noncommunicable diseases. *J Med Econ* 2019;22:722–7.
8. Mihailovic N. Review of diagnosis-related group-based financing of hospital care. *Health Serv Res Manag Epidemiol* 2016;3:2333392816647892.
9. Moss JR et al. eHealth and mHealth. *Eur J Hosp Pharm* 2019;26:57–8.
10. Rantala R et al. Intersectoral action: local governments promoting health. *Health Promotion Int* 2014;29:i92–102.
11. Abuja declaration on HIV/AIDS, tuberculosis and other related infectious diseases. OAU/SPS/ABUJA/3, 2001.
12. Global spending on health 2020: weathering the storm. WHO, 2020.
13. A system of health accounts 2011: revised edition. Concise version. OECD/WHO, 2022.
14. Financial protection in the South-East Asia region: determinants and policy implications. Working paper prepared by WHO Regional Office for South-East Asia, 2017.
15. Global monitoring report on financial protection in health 2021. WHO and World Bank, 2021.
16. Jan S et al. Action to address the household economic burden of non-communicable diseases. *Lancet* 2018;391:2047–58.
17. Gill I, Nagle P. *Inflation could wreak vengeance on the world's poor*. Washington, DC: Brookings, 18 March 2022.

18 Barroy H et al. Can low-and middle-income countries increase domestic fiscal space for health: a mixed-methods approach to assess possible sources of expansion. *Health Syst Reform* 2018;4:214–26.
19 Allen LN. Financing non-communicable disease responses. *Global Health Action* 2017;10:1326687.
20 WHO and Imperial's Centre for Health Economics & Policy Innovation. In Lauer J et al. (eds.), *Health taxes: policy and practice*. Singapore: World Scientific, 2022.
21 Global Dialogue on Partnerships for Sustainable Financing of NCD Prevention and Control Meeting Report. WHO, 2019.
22 Hulse ESG et al. Use of social impact bonds in financing health systems responses to non-communicable diseases: scoping review. *BMJ Global Health* 2021;6:e004127.
23 OECD, *Multilateral development finance 2020*. Paris: OECD Publishing Paris, 2020.
24 Global expenditure on health: public spending on the rise? WHO, 2021.
25 Yamey G et al. Financing global common goods for health: when the world is a country. *Health Syst Reform* 2019;5:334–49.
26 Fiscal space, public financial management and health financing: sustaining progress towards universal health coverage. Health Financing Working Paper No 2, WHO, 2016.
27 UN Inter-Agency Task Force on NCDs. United Nations NCD and Mental Health Catalytic Trust Fund (Helth4Life). https://www.who.int/groups/un-inter-agency-task-force-on-NCDs/programmes/un-ncd-mental-health-catalytic-trust-fund
28 NCD Countdown 2030 Collaborators. NCD Countdown 2030: efficient pathways and strategic investments to accelerate progress towards the sustainable development goal target 3.4 in low-income and middle-income countries. *Lancet* 2022;399:1266–78.
29 Nugent R, Brouwer E. Economic benefit-cost analysis of select secondary prevention interventions in LMIC. *Global Heart* 2015;10:319–21.
30 Invest to protect. NCD financing as the foundation for healthy societies and economies. NCD Alliance, 2022.

40 Making the economic case for investing in NCD prevention and control

Anna Kontsevaya, Rachel Nugent, Alexey Kulikov, Nick Banatvala

Maximizing the impact of available resources is essential as part of a government's responsibility to ensure that its people enjoy the highest attainable standard of physical and mental health as a human right. The challenge is always to ensure these resources are allocated most effectively and efficiently for the greatest health gain across the population. In informing decisions on what should be funded, economics has an important role to play.

In 2001, the WHO Commission for Macroeconomics and Health concluded that investing in health is good for economic development.[1] More recently, a cross-country analysis has shown that reducing mortality and morbidity by 10% is associated with nearly 10 percentage points to GDP per capita growth over around 25 years.[2]

When it comes to NCDs, health economics has been used in high-income countries to measure their economic impact and to show which interventions are most cost-effective. The more recent increase in the NCD burden in low- and middle-income countries has turned attention to the economics of NCDs at the global level and also among countries that are now looking to increase their response to the increasing burden of epidemics of NCDs.

Those involved in developing and implementing policy and programming on health and specifically NCDs, benefit from the inputs of health economists in understanding the costs of NCDs to national economies, outlining the fiscal arguments for investing in NCDs as well as how best to use these resources for maximum impact. To make judgments about efficiency, economic evaluation has to compare health and social outcomes, however measured, with costs. Examples of approaches that can be used to measure outcomes include clinical endpoints, quality of life measures (e.g. quality of life years and disability-adjusted life years), and willingness to pay. Economic evaluation is a specific tool for comparing the costs and consequences of different interventions and has been key to developing the cost-effectiveness of the numerous interventions described in this book.

The economic argument for investing in NCD prevention and control

The economic arguments for investing in NCD prevention and control are quite straightforward:

DOI: 10.4324/9781003306689-45

- In most countries NCDs account for a large (and in many cases the largest) proportion of the disease burden.
- NCDs are responsible for substantial costs to the health system.
- NCDs result in a loss of income for families, communities, employers and countries.
- A large number of interventions for preventing and controlling NCDs are highly cost-effective and can provide a significant return on investment.

Healthier people are more productive, leading to greater economic productivity with improved quality of life. NCDs reduce the supply of labour and economic growth both through premature deaths and reduced performance of unwell workers who remain on the job. Those with NCDs are more likely to retire early, take time off from work (absenteeism) or work at reduced capacity while at work (presenteeism). The same applies to those caring for those with NCDs. Studies have shown that in European countries heart disease, cancer, and diabetes decrease employment rates and increase the likelihood of early retirement by at least 10%.[3] This adds to the large cost of health care for those with NCDs.

Healthy people are more likely to invest in the future, increasing savings rates and building financial capital. Children may be required to stop education prematurely because they are caring for unwell family members or because funds are no longer available for them to continue their studies.

The arguments above demonstrate that NCDs significantly affect not only the health of the population and the health sector but also a number of other sectors, highlighting the importance of tackling NCDs in order to meet the Sustainable Development Goal 8 (promote sustained, inclusive and sustainable economic growth, full and productive employment and decent work for all).

The direct and indirect costs of NCDs

Direct costs include tangible costs associated with diagnosis, treatment and care from the perspective of the provider, the payer and/or the user/patient. It usually includes the costs of medical care (inpatient, outpatient, and emergency) and medicines costs, non-medical costs such as the cost of transport to a health provider or disability payments can be included. *Indirect costs* are associated with lost productivity and income due to disability or premature death. Costs-of-illness studies are the sum of direct and indirect costs. Informal care, pain and quality of life reduction are also sometimes included in economic evaluations.

In most countries, especially low-income countries, direct costs are the smaller portion of the total economic burden.[4] This is because people living with NCDs in lower-income settings have less access to health services and therefore spend less on their care than people in higher-resource settings. Of course, when health care resources are available and affordable, costs to the health sector can be considerable, especially as treatment and care for NCDs are often required over many years.

The impact of NCDs on the economy

In 2011, a report from the World Economic Forum and the Harvard School of Public Health estimated the global economic burden of NCDs in 2010 and projected the size of the burden through 2030. The report concluded that while NCDs already pose a substantial economic burden, under a 'business as usual' scenario, this burden will evolve into a staggering one over the next two decades. Based on direct and indirect costs for the four main NCDs, the report suggested a cumulative output loss of US$ 30.4 trillion between 2011 and 2030 (Table 40.1).[5]

Despite the variations in the table above, in terms of GDP, NCDs are now having a significant impact on the economies of countries of all income groups. In addition, these data are now quite old and they almost certainly underestimate the future economic impact of NCDs, especially given the COVID-19 pandemic.

Cost-effectiveness of interventions to prevent and control NCDs

The 16 WHO best buys (effective interventions with cost-effectiveness analysis ≤ I$ 100 per DALY averted in low- and middle-income countries), 21 effective interventions (with cost-effectiveness analysis >I$ 100 per DALY averted in low- and middle-income countries) and 36 other recommended interventions (shown to be effective but the cost-effective analysis is not available) are described in Chapter 34 and a number of other chapters in the book. It is important to recognize that not having cost-effectiveness data does not mean that the intervention in question is not cost-effective; in some instances, it means the data are not available.

Health impact and economic returns that come from the prevention and control of NCDs at the global level

In 2021, WHO updated data first published in 2018 on the health and economic benefits of implementing the 16 most cost-effective and feasible

Table 40.1 Economic burden of NCDs, 2011–2030 (trillions of US$ 2010)*

Country income group	Diabetes	Cardiovascular diseases	Chronic respiratory Diseases	Cancer	Total
High	0.9	8.5	1.6	5.4	16.4
Upper-middle	0.6	4.8	2.2	2.3	9.9
Lower-middle	0.2	2.0	0.9	0.5	3.6
Low	0.0	0.3	0.1	0.1	0.5
Low- and middle-income	0.8	7.1	3.2	2.9	14
World	1.7	15.6	4.8	8.3	30.4

*Bloom DE et al. *The global economic burden of NCDs*. Geneva, Switzerland: World Economic Forum, 2011.

interventions to prevent and control NCDs (WHO best buys) in 76 low- and lower-middle-income countries – covering almost 4 billion people.[5] The analysis concluded that an additional US$ 0.84 per person per year between 2020 and 2030, would result in saving over seven million lives, including averting over 10 million cases of heart attacks and strokes, with US$ 230 billion in economic gains. The report concludes that every US dollar invested in the 16 WHO best buys would yield a return of at least US$ 7 by 2030. Despite this, there remains significant underuse of the best buys, especially in low- and middle-income countries.[6]

While the report above focused on implementing the most cost-effective interventions, it is well recognized that much health spending is on unproven and/or ineffective interventions and that around a fifth of total health spending in countries is ineffective.[7]

'Wasted buys' and 'contestable buys'

The concepts of 'wasted buys' and 'contestable buys' have recently been developed.[8] The principal criteria for best buys, 'contestable buys' and 'wasted buys' are cost and effectiveness. While the cost-effectiveness of various interventions is often considered universal, there will always be uncertainties at the margins with some dependence on local circumstances (context specificity) which may include political factors as well as acceptability to the community, feasibility and sustainability. While best buys are clearly those interventions that are more effective and less costly and 'wasted buys' the reverse, 'contestable buys' are those that are either more effective and more costly or less effective and less costly. The threshold to separate the cost-effective from the cost-ineffective therefore depends on how much a decision maker is willing to pay for additional health benefits and will therefore vary according to economic factors such as the budget for public expenditure.

Estimating the cost of NCDs and return on investment at the country level

In addition to global figures, those working in countries wish to have estimates for NCD prevention and control. In the last few years, a large number of country-specific case studies have been conducted. These assessments estimate that the average economic burden from NCDs is around 4% of GDP and, in some countries, exceeds 6%.[9,10] It is important that such analyses not only estimate direct and indirect costs of NCDs, the costs of interventions and the return on investment, but they also include a political analysis (or institutional and context analysis) to determine where opportunities exist (and don't exist) for implementing evidence-based policy and programming.[11] As with any research, it is important that the questions being answered have buy-in from relevant stakeholders and that are clear approaches for ensuring that the results are heard, understood and implemented. It is also important to recognize that these so-called 'NCD investment cases' depend on the assumptions being made in the model (including for example the impact of COVID-19) as well as the data available and their quality.

Table 40.2 provides examples of five-year returns on a set of intervention packages to prevent NCDs based on WHO-UNDP investment case methodology across a selection of countries.[11] The return on investment rises over time as the health benefits from prevention and disease management grow. Notwithstanding that there are cost-effective interventions for each NCD risk factor, the results show wide variations in the return on investment across countries. Reasons for this include differences in disease prevalence, intervention starting points and costs of implementing interventions. This underscores the importance of an economic analysis that takes into account the local context.

Investment cases based on similar methodology have been undertaken in the countries in the Gulf, with results indicating that returns on investment of the interventions include 290,000 averted premature deaths and US$ 4.9 for every US$ 1 invested over 15 years.[12]

While economic analyses are helpful in exploring how to use resources most effectively and advocating for investment in neglected areas, it is important that that they don't encourage vertical approaches to policymaking and programming, i.e. undermining a universal health coverage approach. Similarly, it is crucial not to pit economic analyses of different diseases against one another (for example, NCDs vs HIV/AIDS vs tuberculosis vs maternal and child health) as the methodology is often not comparable and a health system will need to ensure that it is providing care to the population across all areas. Even in the areas of NCDs, it is important not to take a simplistic and reductionist approach as many important interventions are unlikely to be included in the analysis and it would be inappropriate to focus attention too narrowly on a few interventions simply because they have a slightly higher economic return on investment.

Tax and other fiscal policies

Fiscal policies can generate substantial additional revenue for the government while improving public health. Price and tax measures are effective ways to encourage people to quit tobacco use, reduce consumption of alcohol as well as unhealthy foods and beverages. For example, almost all countries tax tobacco products to some extent. However, tobacco taxation is not sufficiently implemented in most countries: raising cigarette excise by US$ 0.75 per pack in all countries would generate an extra US$ 141 billion in revenue globally.[13] Health taxes are considered in more detail in other chapters. Conversely, fiscal measures can be used to encourage the consumption of healthy foods and healthy beverages (e.g. subsidizing fruit and vegetable sales and vendors, decreasing import duties on fresh fish).

Industry interference is a major challenge. Tobacco, alcohol and food companies often seek to influence governments with a number of misleading arguments

Table 40.2 Five-year returns on a set of intervention packages to prevent NCDs based on WHO-UNDP investment case methodology across a selection of countries[11]

	Armenia	Belarus	Turkey	Ethiopia	Philippines	Cambodia	Peru	Thailand	UAE	Kazakhstan	Russia	Uzbekistan
Five-year return of investment
Tobacco use	4.8	8.4	2.6	1.1	2.6	5.5	2.4	1.4	0.1	15.1	8.2	7.3
Harmful use of alcohol	1.0	3.2	0.2	0.5	1.5	3.1	0.7	2.6	N/A	4.9	3.2	0.4
Physical inactivity	1.6	1.9	1.1	0.6	3.0	7.7	N/A	1.7	0.2	10.7	7.2	3.9
Salt reduction	1.5	28.8	51.0	2.0	11.5	5.0	3.0	5.6	1.0	53.4	31.1	8.3

NA = Not available.

as to why they should not tax health-harming products. These include taxes being regressive and unfair to the poor. In reality, unregulated policy environments are unfair to the poor because such environments allow stark inequities in how NCDs and their risk factors are distributed. Further details are provided in other chapters.

The importance of non-financial considerations

While this chapter highlights the value of economic analyses in decision-making, it has limitations and should not be used as the sole basis for decision-making. Non-financial considerations are equally important when assessing the impact of NCDs and when determining interventions to be used for preventing and controlling NCDs. These are often determined by national circumstances, such as political opportunity, social justice and equal opportunities for all, implementation capacity, feasibility (including cultural acceptability, sustainability and scalability), the need to promote health equity, and the importance of combining a balance of prevention and treatment as well as population-wide and individual interventions.

Future health costs

The costs of NCDs on the economy highlight the need to increase spending on NCDs. Nevertheless, it is important to recognize that over time, health care costs for NCDs will rise because of an ageing population, the availability of new treatments, and consumer demand. Growth in economies from reducing premature death and ill health, along with the tax and fiscal policies described above, will provide resources to support the expansion of NCD prevention and control programmes. Countries need to plan for this: a number of countries with the highest projected increase in NCD burden are projected to have the smallest increase in per capita spending on NCDs. This suggests that many of the countries that face the most rapid shift in NCD burden are the least prepared.[14]

Monitoring and evaluation of economic and fiscal policies

Monitoring and evaluation of economic and fiscal policies are essential in order to assess their impact. This also includes assessing the capacity of NCD programmes to utilize funds. Monitoring and evaluation can also help assess, in an independent manner, the impact of those policies on the population's health and refute common industry arguments used to counter their implementation or expansion.

The authors gratefully acknowledge the valuable input and critical review provided by Edith Patouillard, WHO, Geneva.

Notes

1 WHO Commission on Macroeconomics and Health & World Health Organization. *Macroeconomics and health: investing in health for economic development.* WHO, 2021.

2. Rocco L et al. Mortality, morbidity and economic growth. *PLoS ONE* 2021;16:e0251424.
3. Feigl AB et al. The short-term effect of BMI, alcohol use, and related chronic conditions on labour market outcomes: a time-lag panel analysis utilizing European SHARE dataset. *PLoS ONE* 2019;14:e0211940.
4. WHO, UNDP. The WHO/UNDP global joint project on catalysing multisectoral action for non-communicable diseases. Report to the Ministry of health of the Russian Federation. 2021. WHO Geneva. https://cdn.who.int/media/docs/default-source/uni-taf/gjp-ncds-web-(003).pdf?sfvrsn=3843adb5_7.
5. Saving lives, spending less: the case for investing in NCDs. WHO, 2021.
6. Allen LN et al. Evaluation of research on interventions aligned to WHO best buys for NCDs in low-income and lower middle-income countries: a systematic review from 1990 to 2015. *BMJ Glob Health* 2018;3:e000535.
7. Tackling wasteful spending on health. OECD, 2017.
8. Isaranuwatchai W et al. Prevention of non-communicable disease: best buys, wasted buys, and contestable buys. *BMJ* 2020;368:m141.
9. Hutchinson B et al. The investment case as a mechanism for addressing the NCD burden: evaluating the NCD institutional context in Jamaica, and the return on investment of select interventions. *PLoS ONE* 2019;14:e0223412.
10. Bertram M et al. Using economic evidence to support policy decisions to fund interventions for non-communicable diseases. *BMJ* 2019;365:1648.
11. Non-communicable disease prevention and control: a guidance note for investment cases. WHO, UNDP. 2019.
12. Elmusharaf K. The case for investing in the prevention and control of noncommunicable diseases in the six countries of the Gulf Cooperation Council: an economic evaluation. *BMJ Global Health* 2022;7:e008670.
13. Goodchild M et al. Modelling the impact of raising tobacco taxes on public health and finance. *Bull World Health Organ* 2016;94:250–57.
14. Bollyky TJ et al. Lower-income countries that face the most rapid shift in NCD burden are also the least prepared. *Health Aff* 2017;36:1866–75.

41 Fiscal measures for NCD prevention and control

Franco Sassi, Ronald Cafrine, M Arantxa Colchero, Neena Prasad

Effective NCD prevention strategies require changes in the consumption and production of products that shape people's lives and health, from food to energy, from substances like tobacco and alcohol to leisure activities and transport. In a market economy, prices are key drivers of consumer and producer choices, and in many instances unhealthy products are cheaper than healthier alternatives.[1] Governments have powerful tools at their disposal to influence market prices, including consumption taxes, among others.

Taxes have been levied on alcoholic beverages and tobacco products for centuries. However, it took a long time before taxation became a tool for meeting public health objectives, gradually moving from the idea of 'sin taxes', targeting 'sins' to avoid interference with other consumption, to the idea of targeting consumption that has negative social impacts ('externalities', in the language of economics), and, finally, to the idea of 'health taxes' aiming to promote changes in consumption that may affect an individual's future health and social and economic outcomes (or 'internalities').[2] On the other hand, taxes on sugar-sweetened beverages (SSBs), which have become very common in the past decade, have been conceived first and foremost as a public health measure, thus representing a step change in the use of fiscal policies for health. Many countries are now considering building on the success of SSB taxes by applying similar taxes to foods high in fat, sugar and salt (HFSS).

Tobacco and alcohol taxes are among the WHO best buys, and SSB taxes are recommended as an effective means of reducing sugar intake, especially among children. The political declaration in 2018 of the Third High-level Meeting of the United Nations General Assembly on the Prevention and Control of NCDs presents fiscal measures as policies that can contribute to 'minimizing the impact of the main risk factors for NCDs, and promote healthy diets and lifestyles'.

> **BOX 41.1 TAXES – SOME BASIC DEFINITIONS**
>
> **Tax**: a compulsory contribution to state revenue, levied by the government on incomes, profits and assets, or added to the prices of some

DOI: 10.4324/9781003306689-46

goods, services and transactions. Taxes are classified as either direct or indirect.

Direct tax: a tax on the profit, income, property or wealth of persons or companies.

Indirect tax: a tax on goods and services.

Value-added tax (VAT): an indirect tax levied as a proportion of price through a cascading collection system throughout the supply chain, from raw materials to final products and services.

Sales tax: indirect tax typically levied as a proportion of price at the retail level.

Import duty: indirect tax on goods imported into a country for consumption in that country.

Excise tax: indirect tax applied to specific goods or services. Excises are commonly applied on tobacco, alcohol, fuel and sugar-sweetened beverages. There are two basic types of excise tax:

- Specific: levied as a monetary value per quantity of the product being taxed (e.g. per 1000 cigarettes, kilogram of tobacco); and,
- Ad valorem: levied as a percentage of the price of the product being taxed.

Hypothecation (also known as ring-fencing or earmarking): attribution of the revenue from a specific tax to a particular type of public expenditure purpose, e.g. health taxes being used for a health promotion fund.

How health taxes work

The most basic concept underlying health taxes is that people will reduce their consumption of products that may cause harm to their health if the prices of those products are raised. Taxation may produce stronger effects on consumption than price hikes due to other factors because it signals to consumers that certain products are unhealthy, and it therefore contributes to stigmatizing their consumption.[3] The expectation that higher prices will lead to reduced consumption is supported by strong empirical evidence for all the products that are potential targets for health taxes. However, the use of taxes for health promotion is not without challenges, and designing taxes that may achieve public health goals is complex. The main challenge is that health taxes are, and will always be, fiscal policies before anything else, despite them being viewed today as an integral part of the public health toolkit. This means that their design and use will have to follow fiscal rules, and they will always require close cooperation between health and finance ministries.

Targeted use of the revenues generated by health taxes (e.g. for health promotion and education programmes, whether through formal earmarking or not) can play an important role in the acceptability by the public and sustainability of health taxes. However, hard earmarking is often opposed by finance ministries because it can create unwarranted constraints in the public budgeting process.

If the expectation that raising prices will lead to lower consumption is sound, this is not necessarily sufficient for taxes to improve health, for which at least two conditions must be met:

- Levying taxes must raise the prices faced by consumers. This happens in most, but not all, cases, and when it does it may happen to varying degrees, depending on a range of characteristics of the market in which the taxed product is traded.[4] Only some of those characteristics are known to governments at the tax design stage.
- Increasing the price of the taxed product must not trigger wider changes in consumption patterns that may offset the benefits of reducing the consumption of the taxed product. The risk that consumers may end up with a less healthy overall consumption basket is higher when they have more opportunities to replace the taxed products with other potentially unhealthy products that are not taxed or are less expensive (e.g. foods, alcoholic beverages).

Taxes should be combined with synergistic measures such as product labelling, regulation of marketing and access to unhealthy products, as described in other chapters.

Tobacco products

Taxes are levied on tobacco products in most countries. On average, over 60% of the price of tobacco products is represented by taxes globally, based on the leading brand in each country. WHO provides detailed guidance on applying taxes to tobacco products[5] and recommends a minimum incidence of 75% of the market price, a recommendation that is met by 40 countries according to the latest estimates.

Taxation is an element of the WHO MPOWER package of effective policies to tackle tobacco use and it is a key component in the WHO Framework Convention on Tobacco Control. The evidence that taxes reduce the use of tobacco products is strong and the impact on smoking habits increases over time. Taxes are most effective on young people and people of low socio-economic status (who have a lower purchasing power and are more sensitive to product prices), both of whom are priority targets in the fight against smoking. However, concerns have been raised about the regressive effects of tobacco taxes, given that people of low income are significantly more likely to smoke than others and bear a larger financial tax burden. However, while low-income households undoubtedly spend a larger share of their income, on average, on tobacco taxes, they can also benefit disproportionately in terms of health improvement from reducing or quitting smoking, to the point that their productivity, income and risk of incurring catastrophic health care expenditures can be significantly improved, offsetting the regressive distribution of tax payments.

While the taxation of traditional tobacco products is now an established policy, governments are constantly catching up with a rapidly evolving market in which new products such as electronic nicotine delivery systems (ENDS) present new challenges for policymakers. While WHO recommends treating these new products just as traditional ones in terms of taxation, some countries are viewing them as an aid to smoking cessation and have applied more favourable tax regimes.

Alcohol beverages

The taxation of alcohol products is also very common and very effective in reducing beverage consumption and a wide range of alcohol-related harms, although taxes have not been as large as those levied on tobacco products and, in many countries, have not kept up with inflation, or even increased at all, over time. Alcohol markets, and alcohol consumption patterns, are complex and deeply rooted in the economic, social and cultural traditions of countries. Taxation systems applied to alcohol products tend to reflect this complexity and often involve different taxes and different rates for different types of beverages, sometimes also differentiated by place of consumption (e.g. alcohol consumed in bars and restaurants vs alcohol purchased in retail stores). As a result, taxes influence consumer choices on levels of consumption, types of beverages and places of consumption but are not always in line with public health objectives, which is a legacy of the use of alcohol taxes for the pursuit of more traditional fiscal policy goals, such as revenue generation and addressing externalities.

Strengthening the health rationale for alcohol taxes requires more uniform taxes, with relatively high tax rates based on the alcohol content of beverages, ideally aiming at a convergence of the prices per unit of alcohol from different types of beverages.

As with tobacco products, the population groups that are most responsive to prices are young people and those with low incomes, which allows for the targeting of taxation policies at some of the highest-risk drinkers. However, for taxation to be truly effective in deterring consumption in high-risk groups, substitutions towards cheaper beverages (also known as 'trading down') must be prevented through a careful tax design. Specific excise taxes tend to be better than ad valorem taxes in preventing consumers from trading down to cheaper products. Those who have the most harmful patterns of alcohol drinking tend to consume predominantly the cheapest alcohol, and taxation is not always effective in raising the prices of such products, partly because alcohol manufacturers are likely to shift taxes onto the prices of more expensive products, less responsive to price increases. For the reasons described, several governments have used, or considered using, price regulation measures alongside taxation, including bans of various forms of price promotions or minimum unit pricing policies, which set a floor price per unit of alcohol below which beverages cannot be sold. Additional measures may include the setting or raising of licence fees for retail outlets.

The equity impacts of alcohol taxes are more complex than those of other types of products, because of the characteristic distribution of alcohol drinking and harm in the population. Alcohol drinking is more prevalent in high-income than in low-income groups, at least for commercial (as opposed to home-made) beverages, consistently across countries, which means that high-income households, on average, tend to pay a larger share of their income in alcohol taxes. Most alcohol, however, is drunk by a minority of the population in most countries (partly because alcohol is addictive and those addicted tend to drink large amounts). Therefore, some heavy drinking low-income households may bear a substantial tax burden. Nevertheless, low-income households can benefit the most from alcohol taxes in terms of health improvement and the social and economic benefits that come with it.

Food and non-alcoholic beverages

In the case of food consumption, fiscal policies have traditionally focused on addressing food insecurity and the sustainability of national food systems, mainly through subsidies for production and consumption. Health improvement has become a prominent goal in recent years, with the adoption of taxes on SSBs and on some highly processed, energy-dense and nutrient-poor foods (e.g. salty or sugary snacks) in a rapidly increasing number of countries.

Several systematic reviews have shown that taxes on SSBs are effective and reduce purchases of taxed beverages in a similar or greater proportion to the price increase, with people of low income and heavy consumers often displaying a stronger response.[6,7]

However, existing health taxes on food and non-alcoholic beverages (FNABs) are typically small, and even in the few countries where they are applied to more than SSBs, the range of taxed FNABs is narrow; therefore the impact on overall dietary intakes is relatively small. In addition, while existing health taxes have been shown to be effective in reducing the consumption of taxed products, their impacts on consumers' overall diets are uncertain because little is known about the substitutions triggered by health taxes (e.g. people buying fewer SSBs because of a tax on SSBs may buy more sugary foods). This makes, for instance, the setting of an appropriate tax base a very challenging step in tax design, and the heterogeneity of tax bases used in different countries for certain taxes (e.g. inclusion or exclusion of artificially sweetened beverages or unsweetened fruit juices or milk-based products from the tax base of beverage taxes) is a demonstration of the difficulties involved in understanding the patterns and impacts of potential substitutions.

Taxes on SSBs are important, given the well-documented health harms of SSBs (see Chapter 22 on dietary sugars). They have provided a valuable proof of concept but should not be regarded as an endpoint in the use of health taxes in the domain of diet and nutrition.

There is wide scope for further innovation in these areas and a need to experiment with new models of taxation. New approaches that some countries are beginning to adopt include modulating value-added tax (VAT) rates to reflect the nutritional quality of food products or using subsidies to incentivize the consumption of healthy foods, although such subsidies can be difficult to design and implement. As a general solution to identifying what food products should be taxed, interest has been increasing around the use of nutrient profiling models (NPMs) as a basis for the design of fiscal policies aimed at improving the nutritional quality of people's diets. NPMs are increasingly used in several nutrition policies, e.g. in defining criteria for public procurement of foods, in the design of front-of-pack nutrition labelling systems (Chapter 24 on nutrition labelling) and in food advertising regulation, which makes them especially attractive for creating a convergence of incentives in food choices.

Monitoring

Monitoring and evaluation are key requirements for health taxes to make a useful contribution to public health action through NCD progress monitor indicators (5a) measures to reduce affordability by increasing excise taxes and prices on tobacco products and (6c) – increases of excise taxes on alcoholic beverages (Chapter 35).[8]

Notes

1. Colchero MA et al. Affordability of food and beverages in Mexico between 1994 and 2016. *Nutrients* 2019;11:78.
2. Lauer J et al. (Eds.). *Health taxes: policy and practice*. World Scientific with World Scientific Pub Co Inc. Singapore, 2022.
3. Leicester A et al. Tax and benefit policy: insights from behavioural economics. Institute for Fiscal Studies, 2012. https://ifs.org.uk/publications/6268.
4. Colchero MA et al. Changes in prices after an excise tax to sweetened sugar beverages was implemented in Mexico: evidence from urban areas. PLoS One 2015;10:e0144408.
5. WHO technical manual on tobacco tax policy and administration. https://apps.who.int/iris/rest/bitstreams/1341465/retrieve.
6. Ng SW et al. Did high sugar-sweetened beverage purchasers respond differently to the excise tax on sugar-sweetened beverages in Mexico? *Public Health Nutr* 2019;22:750–56.
7. Colchero MA et al. In Mexico, evidence of sustained consumer response two years after implementing a sugar-sweetened beverage tax. *Health Aff* 2017;36:564–71.
8. Noncommunicable diseases progress monitor. WHO, 2022.

42 Strengthening health systems and service delivery for NCD prevention and control

Cherian Varghese, Baridalyne Nongkynrih, Pascal Bovet, Nick Banatvala

NCDs are the major cause of ill health including premature mortality in almost all countries of the world and therefore place huge pressure on the health system and thereby causing them to be overwhelmed, with a significant impact on public health finances, and household expenditures for those paying out-of-pocket, in addition to the health and broader socioeconomic impact that result from NCDs. The demand for the health system is further exacerbated by the increasing availability of new and expensive diagnostics and treatments in a number of countries.

Many healthcare systems in low-resource settings are poorly oriented to meet the needs of those with NCDs, historically having been structured around treating infectious disease-related and maternal and child health conditions rather than NCDs, conditions which are mostly chronic and often asymptomatic to start with and require long-term care.

In addition, improvement in public health (e.g. smallpox, polio, HIV, tuberculosis and malaria) has often come from verticalized programmes which created a parallel delivery system. This is not a practical approach for NCDs with multimorbidity and acute complications requiring long-term care. NCDs therefore need to be managed through an integrated systems and care (horizontal) approach, recognizing that there remain times when disease-specific programmes are developed, often as a pragmatic entry point for adding new healthcare services before these specific programmes are fully integrated (e.g. hypertension, diabetes, cervical cancer control programmes) or for evaluating the quality of the services. NCD programmes should be undertaken in conjunction with interventions in multiple sectors to reduce exposure to the risk factors for NCDs across the whole population. Combining the vertical and horizontal is sometimes referred to as a diagonal approach.

Strengthening health systems is particularly important at the primary care level, where the most cost-effective interventions for the prevention and treatment of NCDs can be delivered. Most NCDs' conditions and advice on reducing their risk factors can be effectively managed at the primary care level, in addition to it being close to the patient's home, allowing for the development of long-term relationships to be developed with local health professionals. Primary care is the most cost-effective approach for delivering healthcare – and

DOI: 10.4324/9781003306689-47

conditions well managed at this level will reduce (but do not obviate) the need for more expensive secondary and tertiary care.

Challenges

WHO describes six building blocks for a health system in order to increase access, coverage as well as quality and safety: (i) service delivery; (ii) health workforce; (iii) health information systems; (iv) access to essential medicines, vaccines and technologies; (v) health financing; and (vi) leadership and governance. Challenges for improving NCD treatment and care apply across all the six elements of the building blocks but with a shift from acute conditions to long-term care, with partnerships required between health carers and patients, and the need to ensure integrated prevention and care across primary, secondary and tertiary health and social care services.

Lack of a structured approach, slow adaptation of fair allocation of limited resources to both acute and chronic care and long-term care plan with adequate financial support for patients lead to high, but potentially largely avoidable, premature morbidity, mortality, as well as financial losses. The challenges in emergency, humanitarian and complex emergency settings are even greater (Chapter 51). The need for integrated action across the continuum of care is illustrated for hypertension in Figure 42.1, using the example of how inadequate healthcare for hypertension can result in a preventive condition, such as cerebrovascular accident (stroke). It demonstrates the importance of the interaction of the different building blocks to ensure a continuum of care.

A WHO survey in 2019 revealed the inadequacy of NCD management. Of six essential technologies for early detection, diagnosis, and monitoring of NCDs, only half of 160 countries reported their availability in primary care facilities in the public health sector.[1] A recent study confirms inadequate guidelines, essential diagnostic tools, and treatment for hypertension and diabetes across primary healthcare facilities in the public sector in a number of African countries.[2] COVID-19 has made the management of NCDs an even greater challenge because (i) NCDs and their metabolic, behavioural and environmental risk factors have increased risks of severe disease and death from COVID-19;[3] (ii) the pandemic has severely disrupted diagnostic, treatment, rehabilitation and palliation services for people living with NCDs;[4,5] and (iii) pressure on health services is likely to increase in the long term because of possible increases in cardiovascular disease (CVD) and respiratory complications among COVID-19 survivors.

What needs to change

Health system building blocks

Action is required across all six health system building blocks if communities are to benefit from improvement in the management of NCDs.

310 Cherian Varghese et al.

Lack of:
- knowledge
- awareness of symptoms

Challenges:
- location, transport
- access to health facility
- financial

Lack of:
- unique ID and records
- protocol for diagnosis/management
- technology for clinical assessment
- medicines
- team-based care

Challenges:
- out-of-pocket expenses
- poor adherence to treatment
- inadequate follow up
- lack of care in the community

Stroke (with a delay in recognizing symptoms)

Lack of:
- established referral system
- prehospital care
- financial capacity to seek care from private facility

Limitations:
- system for triage
- diagnostic capacity
- capacity for intervention
- lack of rehabilitation services

Outcome:
- paralysis
- unable to work and participate fully in family activities
- requires care and support
- financial burden

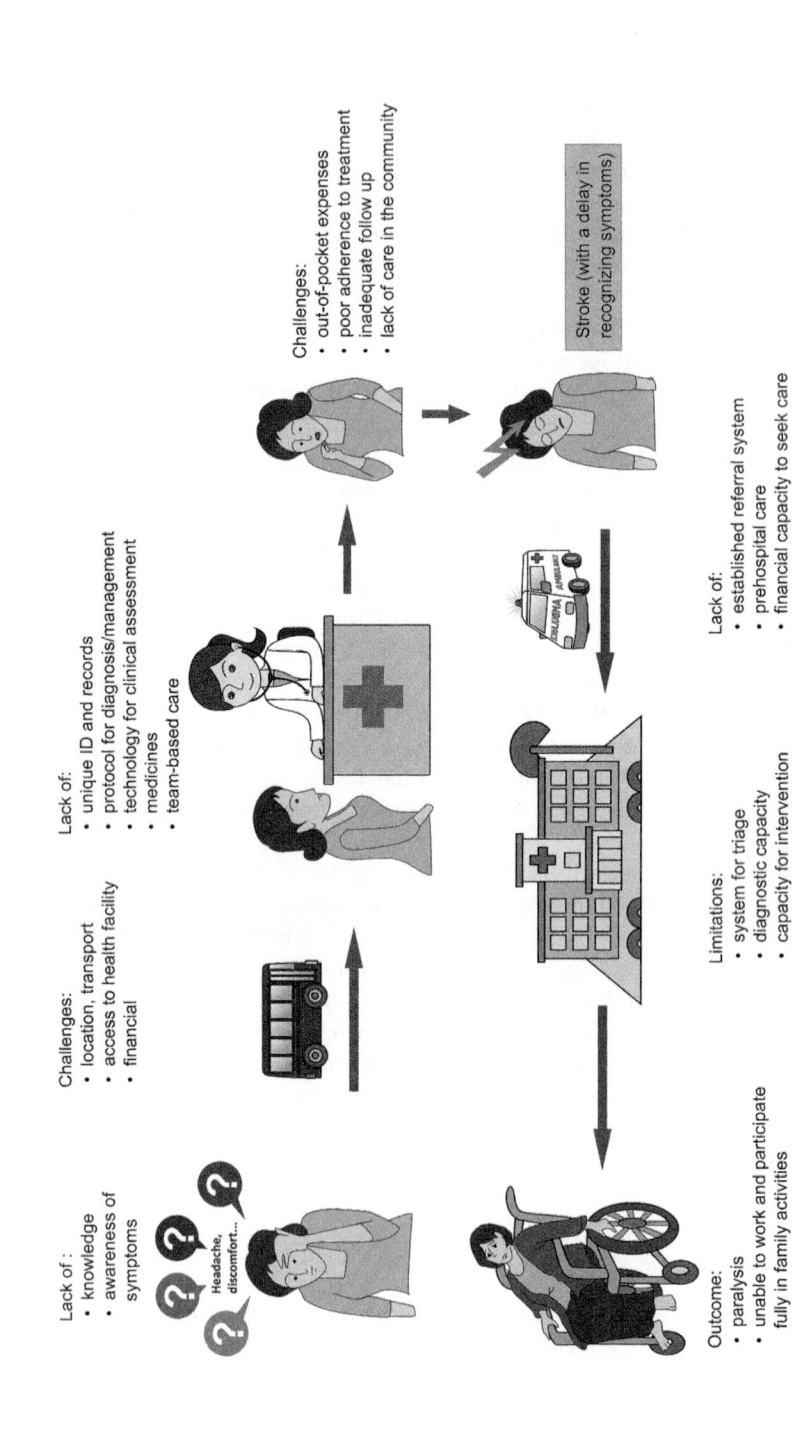

Figure 42.1 Challenges in providing optimal healthcare for NCDs.

Governance issues specific of particular importance for NCD prevention and control include:

- Development of health system policies and plans based on accurate situation analysis and priority setting, with specific and measurable outcome indicators.
- Strategies to translate these policies into actions and programmes for financing, human resources, pharmaceuticals, technology, infrastructure and service delivery, along with plans and monitoring and evaluation targets.
- Coalitions and alliances to be built across sectors with appropriate partners (across government, parliament and non-state actors) including people living with NCDs, to deliver effective health system policies, plans and strategies and hold all those involved accountable.

A robust *workforce* for NCDs requires:

- Strong leadership to ensure that NCDs are integrated into broader health workforce development and management, and health workforce policies in national health strategies.
- Pre-service educational curricula that include the necessary knowledge and skills required for essential NCD healthcare, and quality training and continuing education programmes for health workers.
- Multidisciplinary teams to provide integrated care for those with NCDs.
- Positive work environments, for example, ensuring availability of essential supplies, referral services and supportive management.

Health information systems are described in Chapters 4 and 5. Access to essential medicines, vaccines and technologies is considered in more detail in Chapters 44 and 45. Universal health coverage is described in Chapter 38, health financing in Chapter 39, and fiscal measures for tackling NCDs in Chapter 41.

Service delivery is critical for ensuring that people with NCDs and at risk of NCDs have access to good quality screening, diagnosis, management and palliative care in a way that is equitable and users do not incur financial hardships, whether this is delivered through the public or private sector or a mix of both. The rest of this chapter focuses on service delivery.

Service delivery for the management of individuals with or at risk of NCDs

A strategic shift is needed to ensure that health systems are 'NCD ready'. Indeed, the majority of preventive (including screening), diagnostic behavioural and pharmacological treatment, and long-term integrated and multidisciplinary care for NCDs (particularly hypertension and diabetes, which affect large proportions of the population), as well as palliative care, can be satisfactorily provided at the primary/community care level.[6]

Nevertheless, it is important to recognize that an acute event such as a heart attack or stroke, for which urgent re-vascularization treatment with thrombolytic drugs or invasive procedures within a few hours or complex cancer treatment requires care that can only be provided in secondary or tertiary care settings. It is therefore essential that robust referral systems are in place to allow rapid access to this level of care. Strategies that improve the continuity of primary healthcare can reduce the need and cost of secondary care (hospital admissions). This may also improve the experience of patients and those working in general practice.[7]

Examples of changes required across the primary healthcare system include:[8]

- Establishing multidisciplinary teams with diverse competencies (e.g. health education, dietary education, medication management and social care and support).
- Training mid-level non-physician care providers to prescribe treatment in certain situations.
- Ensuring that essential diagnostic tools, medicines and treatment are available and affordable for patients.
- Improving health information systems that use a unique patient identifier (particularly if electronic systems are available) to enable fast retrieval of clinical data (e.g. blood pressure, blood glucose, etc.).
- Develop family and community-based models of care (including collaboration with public health officials to tackle local determinants of health) that enable the provision of high-quality patient-centred long-term care of chronic conditions).

Technical packages and tools to support integrated approaches to NCDs in primary care

The WHO package of essential noncommunicable (PEN) disease interventions provides a set of cost-effective interventions for a large range of NCD conditions that can be delivered in primary healthcare.[9] The package also provides guidance on the use of essential medicines and technology to deliver interventions for hypertension, diabetes, total cardiovascular risk, asthma, chronic obstructive pulmonary diseases and cancer early detection and management. Palliative care is also added as an entity to be provided in primary care. The package is now available as an App and can be adapted to all settings, including low-resource ones.[10]

The HEARTS technical package provides a strategic approach to improving cardiovascular health in countries. It comprises six modules and an implementation guide. The practical, step-by-step modules are supported by an overarching technical document that provides a rationale and framework for this integrated approach to the management of NCDs.[11] The six modules are shown in Table 42.1, which, when supported by the necessary financing and governance, provide the key elements for a health system that is well-placed to respond to NCDs.

Table 42.1 The six HEARTS modules to strengthen the management of NCDs in primary care

Module	Measures for strengthening NCD management	Financing	Service delivery & governance
Healthy-lifestyle counselling.	• Health facilities should be designed to promote a 'whole person' approach that promotes health along integrated services (e.g. that persons with HIV have their blood pressure (BP) checked and managed). • Regularly train health professionals in relation to NCDs and their risk factors, including awareness of relevant guidelines and protocols locally used.		
Evidence-based protocols.	• Evidence-based protocols help in standardizing treatment. Global protocols can be adapted to the local context and made part of the in-service training and standard clinical guidance. • It is important that protocols specify which tasks can be handled by different health professionals for more efficient provision (task shifting/sharing). • Ensure that health services can provide appropriate medicines recommended by protocols, in sufficient amounts and sustained manner, with the available funds. • Regularly evaluate healthcare outcomes (e.g. proportions of patients who have BP or blood glucose to target) and adjust protocols and their implementation accordingly.	Affordable, if possible free of charge, provision of long-term treatment (e.g. hypertension, diabetes) to patients is essential for long-term adherence to treatment. This can be addressed through national health systems (healthcare paid by tax), mandatory assurance systems (with fees waived for the poor), or other systems (e.g. health maintenance organizations) or a mix of these measures.	Regularly assess and revise which services and therapies can be offered to people living with NCDs based on the available or predicted resources (nationally, but also at the level of any health centre, based on their situation). This requires that a number of indicators are collected e.g. proportions of patients attending heath care have risk factors controlled, etc., health service surveys of service availability and readiness assessments (SARA).
Access to essential medicines and technology.	• Promote the availability and use, as much as possible, of once-daily combinations of medications for long-term treatment (e.g. hypertension, diabetes, cholesterol) to reduce the number of pills to be taken by patients and improve adherence as well as simplify their provision by healthcare professionals. • Regularly check instruments for accuracy (e.g. weighing scales, stadiometers, sphygmomanometers, glucose monitors, etc.). • Regularly assess the list of essential medications for possible additions or changes for more cost-effective and/or affordable options (including fixed-dose combinations).		
Risk-based management.	• Total cardiovascular risk assessment is a means of cost-effectively managing multiple risk factors (and lab-based and non-lab-based risk assessment can be used, e.g. WHO CVD risk charts or other nationally used risk prediction charts).		

(*Continued*)

Table 42.1 (Continued)

Module	Measures for strengthening NCD management	Financing	Service delivery & governance
Team-based care and human resources.	• Promote task shifting/sharing with/by non-physician health workers (e.g. to assess BP/diabetes control and, possibly, allowing them to make minimal adjustments to therapy). • Involve a variety of healthcare (e.g. pharmacists) and non-healthcare providers in different settings to promote screening of risk factors (e.g. hypertension, diabetes), e.g. at work wellness programmes, workplaces, hairdressers. • Ensure that health professionals can assign sufficient time to patients with NCDs, including payment for these services in fee-for-service systems, in order to allow them to adequately advise and follow their patients with regard to smoking cessation, healthy diet and lifestyle.		
Systems for monitoring.	• Monitor patients' risk factor control (tobacco use, BP, diabetes, body mass index (BMI), etc.) at healthcare level (to identify trends over time) preferably using electronic medical files (which help assess trends over time). • When using electronic medical file systems, develop mechanisms that automatically highlight patients with poorly controlled risk factors levels and/or patients who do not attend follow-up visits and options that can automatically send to patients results, related advice and reminders of follow-up visits (e.g. through SMS, etc.). • E-health interventions (SMS, smartphone apps, phone calls) can improve patients' self-management of chronic NCDs, including improving adherence to treatment and reducing risk factors (e.g. BP, diabetes).		

Monitoring

A number of global NCD targets require action across the health system. They include:

A 25% relative reduction in the overall mortality from CVD, cancer, diabetes or chronic respiratory diseases.

The unconditional probability of dying between the ages of 30 and 70 from CVD, cancer, diabetes or chronic respiratory disease.
Cancer incidence, by type of cancer, per 100,000 population.

A 25% relative reduction in the prevalence of raised BP or contain the prevalence of raised BP, according to national circumstances.	Age-standardized prevalence of BP among persons aged 18+ years (defined as BP ≥140/90 mmHg).
At least 50% of eligible people receive drug therapy and counselling (including glycaemic control) to prevent heart attacks and strokes.	Proportion of eligible persons (e.g. aged ≥40 years with a ten-year CVD risk ≥20%, including those with existing CVD) receiving drug therapy and counselling (including glycaemic control) to prevent heart attacks and strokes.
An 80% availability of affordable basic technologies and essential medicines, including generics, is required to treat major NCDs in both public and private facilities.	Availability and affordability of quality, safe and efficacious essential NCD medicines, including generics, and basic technologies in both public and private facilities.

Table 42.2 Fifteen health system challenges and opportunities to improve NCD outcomes

Political commitment to NCDs.	Explicit priority-setting approaches.	Interagency cooperation.	Population empowerment.
Effective model of service delivery.	Coordination across providers.	Regionalization.	Incentive systems.
Integration of evidence into practice.	Distribution and mix of human resources.	Access to quality medicines.	Effective management.
Adequate information solutions.	Managing change.	Ensuring access and financial protection.	

A number of tools have been developed to assess the effectiveness of health systems in their ability to respond effectively to NCDs. One example is that developed by the WHO Regional Office for Europe, which provides guidance on questions to ask to explore 15 areas of the health system in order to make recommendations on improving NCD outcomes across each of the 15 areas as well as highlight examples of good practice (Table 42.2).[12] Examples of country assessments in the WHO European Region based on this tool are also available.[13]

Notes

1 Assessing national capacity for the prevention and control of noncommunicable diseases: report of the 2019 global survey. WHO, 2020.
2 Bovet P et al. Availability of protocols, equipment and medicines for cardiovascular disease risk management in primary care health facilities in nine African countries. *Ann Cardiol Vasc Med* 2021;4:1043.

3 Williamson EJ et al. Factors associated with COVID-19-related death using OpenSAFELY. *Nature* 2020;584:430–36.
4 The impact of the COVID-19 pandemic on NCD resources and services: results of a rapid assessment. WHO, 2020.
5 Splinter MJ et al. Prevalence and determinants of healthcare avoidance during the COVID-19 pandemic: a population-based cross-sectional study. *PLoS Med* 2021;18:e1003854.
6 Frenk J. Reinventing primary health care: the need for systems integration. *Lancet* 2009;374:170–3.
7 Barker I et al. Association between continuity of care in general practice and hospital admissions for ambulatory care sensitive conditions: cross sectional study of routinely collected, person level data. *BMJ* 2017;356:j84.
8 Varghese C et al. Better health and wellbeing for billion more people: integrating non-communicable diseases in primary care. *BMJ* 2019;364:l327.
9 *WHO package of essential noncommunicable (PEN) disease interventions for primary health care.* WHO, 2020.
10 WHOPEN. https://apps.apple.com/gb/app/whopen/id1566338877.
11 WHO package of essential noncommunicable (PEN) disease interventions for primary health care. WHO, 2020.
12 *Better NCD outcomes: challenges and opportunities for health systems. Assessment guide.* Copenhagen: WHO Regional Office for Europe, 2014.
13 Farrington J et al. Better noncommunicable disease outcomes: challenges and opportunities for health systems. Kazakhstan country assessment. WHO Regional Office for Europe, 2018.

43 Screening and health checks for NCD prevention and control

Kevin Selby, Nick Banatvala, Pascal Bovet, Jacques Cornuz

The purpose of screening is to identify people in an apparently healthy population who are at higher risk of a health problem or related condition so that an early treatment or intervention can be offered, in order to lead to better health outcomes in those screened.[1] Criteria for identifying a disease suitable for screening have been in existence for over 50 years (Box 43.1).[2]

BOX 43.1   CRITERIA FOR IDENTIFYING A DISEASE SUITABLE FOR SCREENING

- The condition sought is an important health problem.
- The natural history of the condition, including development from latent to declared disease and sequels is well understood.
- There is a recognizable latent/early symptomatic stage.
- There is a suitable and acceptable test or examination.
- There is an accepted, cost-effective and affordable treatment.
- Facilities and resources for diagnosis and treatment are available.
- There should be an agreed policy on whom to treat as patients (protocols for diagnosis and treatment).
- The cost of case-finding (including diagnosis and treatment) is economically balanced in relation to expenditure on medical care as a whole.
- Case-finding is a continuing process and not a 'once and for all' project.

More recently, policy-orientated criteria have been proposed (Box 43.2).[3]

BOX 43.2   POLICY CRITERIA FOR SCREENING

- The screening programme should respond to a recognized need.
- The objectives of screening are defined at the outset.
- There is a clearly defined target population.

DOI: 10.4324/9781003306689-48

- There is scientific evidence of screening programme effectiveness (the benefits of the screening programme should outweigh the harm).
- There are mechanisms to maximize quality assurance and minimize potential risks of screening.
- The programme ensures informed choice, confidentiality and respect for autonomy.
- The programme promotes equity and access to screening for the entire target population.
- Programme evaluation is planned from the outset.
- The overall benefits of screening should outweigh the harm.

Population-level screening programmes

Mass screening is particularly important for NCDs as many cancers and other NCDs fulfil the criteria set out above, particularly high frequency in the population, a long symptomless period before clinical events develop and effective treatments. The impact of screening is best assessed on the number of deaths avoided or years of life gained per 1000 individuals screened compared with these outcomes in the same population if was not being screened – and the evidence for screening programmes for a number of NCDs has grown substantially over the years.

In addition to the outcomes described above, it is important to take into account the cost-effectiveness of screening programmes. Costs need to include the financial, human, technical and other resources (including for quality assurance and accountability) that are required to establish and maintain a programme – which is usually very significant. But in addition, there are costs to individuals and the health system and wider society for those that fall into false-positive and false-negative categories (e.g. the former requiring unnecessary further investigation and possibly unnecessary treatment, and the latter being falsely reassured) (Figure 43.1). For example, in the United Kingdom, for every 1000 women 50–70 years old invited to screening for breast cancer every three years, it is estimated that four women will have their life saved from breast cancer but 13 women will be incorrectly diagnosed, and possibly treated, for cancer that would not have harmed them.[4] In Belgium, a similar approach estimates that for every 1000 women 50–59 years screened every two years, three women will have their life saved from breast cancer and three women will be overdiagnosed and possibly harmed by unnecessary treatment.[5]

It is also important to appreciate that screening programmes can sometimes be established because of pressure from lobby groups. Overall, these groups as well as the public tend to overestimate the benefits and underestimate the harm that comes from screening. Importantly, once established, screening

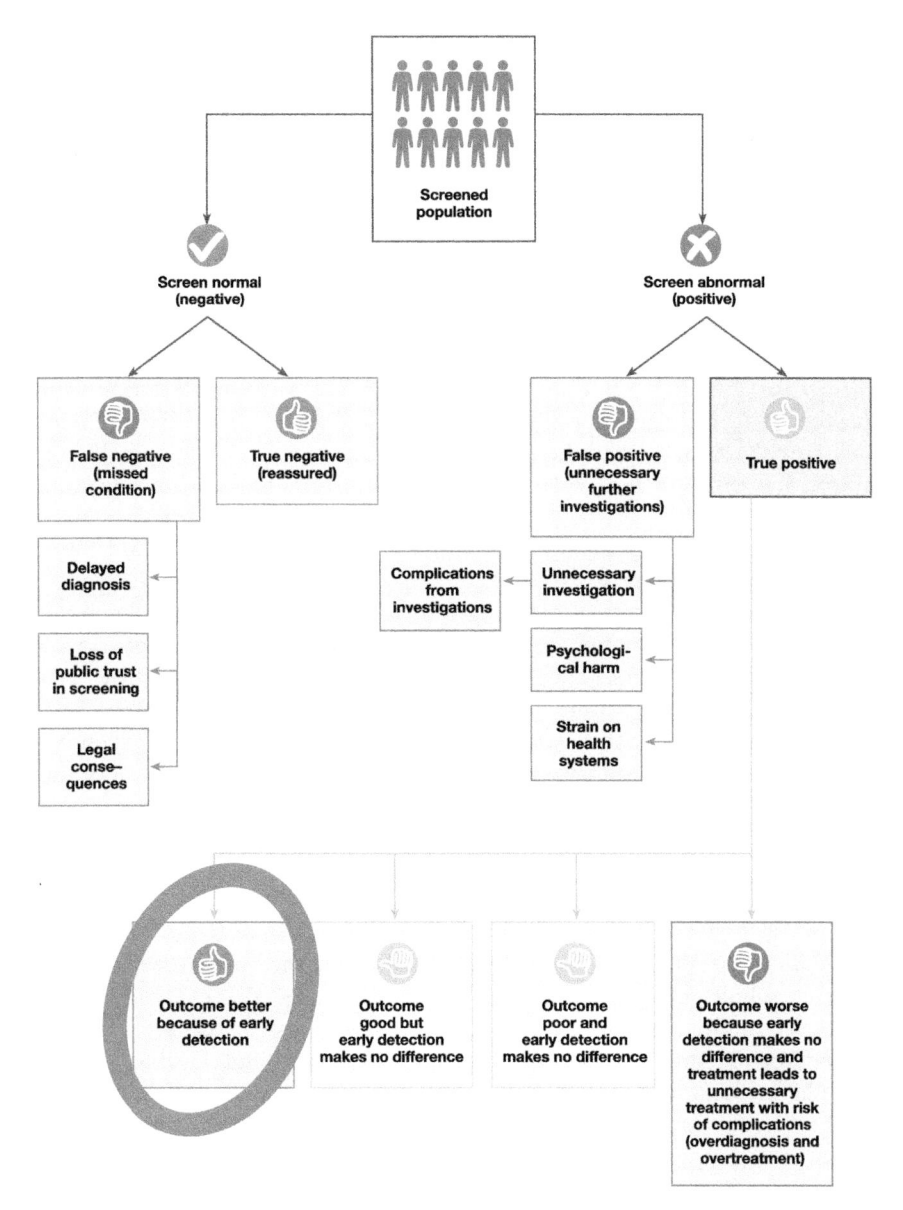

Figure 43.1 The benefits and harms associated with a screening programme. (Screening programmes: a short guide. Increase effectiveness, maximize benefits and minimize harm. WHO Regional Office for Europe; Copenhagen, 2020).

programmes can be very difficult to disband. Piloting a screening programme in a small area before scaling it up to the regional or national level is therefore a prudent approach. It goes without saying that a screening programme should be established only if there is access for all those screened as positive to the necessary diagnostic tests, treatment and follow-up required – and this needs to be factored into the decision (including budget) on setting up a screening programme.

In addition, care needs to be taken when extrapolating the results of an evaluation of a screening programme for the same condition from one country to another. Differences in disease burden, population structure and health systems mean that conclusions in one country may not apply to another country. Again, this highlights the importance of undertaking pilots. Nevertheless, national and international guidance (for example from WHO, the International Agency for Research on Cancer (IARC), the UK's National Institute for Health and Care Excellence (NICE), the United States Preventive Services Task Force (USPSTF), and the European Commission) is available (including information on how and when to establish, and how to evaluate screening programmes).

Traditionally, the evaluation of screening programmes has focused more on the risks and benefits for individuals than on the overall cost-effectiveness (e.g. $ per DALY averted) and long-term affordability of the programme. More recently, greater emphasis is being placed on the economics of screening programmes. Economic arguments need to take into account that even programmes that may require an expensive screening tool and/or treatment can be cost-effective if they reduce mortality and future need for expensive treatment and follow-up that would arise from treatment at later stages of the diseases (e.g. colonoscopy for colorectal cancer screening).

Organized systematic screening programmes for NCDs targeting the entire population

These are designed and managed by national or regional health services and target the whole population (or groups of them) to ensure that everyone has an equal opportunity to participate and benefit. Everyone who takes part is therefore offered the same services, information and support. High levels of quality control, external monitoring and evaluation and accountability are in place.

They usually involve a large engagement of primary health care but also require strong support from secondary levels (e.g. colonoscopy for colon cancer, complex imagery or biological techniques for breast cancer, complex and/or long-term treatment and/or surgery). These programmes must be carefully considered because of the large resources involved and the difficulty to stop them once started. Decisions will depend on resources in a country. As in Figure 43.1, the benefits and harm need to be weighed up carefully.

Screening programmes for cervical, colon, prostate and breast cancers are described in chapters on these diseases. Those for other NCD conditions such as aortic artery aneurysm are not covered in this compendium.

Opportunistic screening for NCDs

Opportunistic screening is when individuals are screened outside an organized programme. Although this is not screening in the formal sense, such activities are often referred to as 'screening' in popular parlance. Opportunistic screening may not be subject to the same checks, balances and quality control as for an organized screening programme. Opportunistic screening may be used when organized screening is not available, for example for lack of resources (e.g. in countries where cervical cancer programmes have yet to be established) or for an individual who does not meet the criteria for participating in an organized screening programme (e.g. screening for breast cancer in a young woman where there is a strong family history). The benefits, risks and harms of opportunistic screening (for example PSA testing for prostate cancer) need to be discussed with the individual before a shared decision is made on whether to undergo screening.

Opportunities should be taken by health professionals to use consultations to 'screen' for NCD risk factors (e.g. tobacco use, harmful use of alcohol, unhealthy diet and sedentary habits) in order to provide appropriate counselling. It is devoid of harmful effects and can be cost-effective, e.g. simple advice to smokers to quit.[6] Such 'screening' is perhaps better considered as a routine component of quality whole-person care.

Health checks for NCDs

Periodic health examinations, commonly called 'check-ups' can take place along organized or opportunistic circumstances, and are undertaken in the community, for example in primary care, the workplace or schools. The main aim of check-ups (in relation to NCDs) is to identify behavioural, physical and metabolic risk factors (e.g. smoking, high blood pressure, elevated blood lipid or sugar levels) among apparently healthy persons.

As NCDs increase with age, the usefulness of check-ups also increases with age, particularly after age 40–50 years. Check-ups may also be extended to those with a strong familial history of a particular condition or those with potential comorbidities (e.g. screening for hypertension among the obese or those with diabetes of any age), although this latter example may be better considered the provision of ongoing health care for unhealthy persons. Importantly, health checks also allow for a discussion around ways to reduce exposure to risk factors (and where required, the need for medications). Health checks are likely to be more effective when they are done with a health worker who knows the individual well and a trusted relationship is more likely to result in more personalized counselling.[7]

While there appears to be a growing trend towards more health checks of NCDs and risk factors, fuelled by the growing availability of tests for many conditions including point-of-care ones and demand from patients, clear evidence of their effectiveness is often lacking. For example, general health checks provided in primary care in Denmark did not result in improved mortality,[8,9] perhaps in part because routine health care is already of high quality. A number of issues that pertain to screening apply equally to health checks, e.g. selecting the most appropriate age group, ensuring that those with the greatest need attend (rather than just the 'worried well' or those who can easily access or afford health care), maximizing efficiency by dealing with multiple issues at one time, and establishing the right intervals between repeat health checks.

Decisions on what is made available to a particular population through organized screening, opportunistic screening, or well-health checks depend on a number of factors, including resources, access, availability and affordability of health care.

A framework for the prevention of NCDs at the primary care level

Primary care needs to ensure that screening (both organized and where appropriate opportunistic), counselling and other preventive interventions, such as vaccination, are available for their population. Figure 43.2 is adapted from a more comprehensive illustrative framework recommended for those managing and delivering primary care in Switzerland. The schedule was developed using GRADE (Grading of Recommendations Assessment, Development and Evaluation), which is a systematic approach based on available evidence for making recommendations for clinical practice.[10] Those developing frameworks in a particular country will need to take into account a number of factors, including the available resources, the strength of the evidence base and related recommendations (e.g. what to do when evidence is weak, such as screening for lung cancer with low dose CT among smokers[11] or for prostate cancer using PSA in some individuals[12]), the way health care is organized (e.g. where and how screening and check-ups are provided and financed), and the expectations of the public and the response of primary care to that demand.

Health checks to 'screen' for NCDs at the workplace

Health checks ('screening') may also be offered as part of services granted to employees (similar to subsidized and/or healthy meals or provision of facilities to practice physical activity at a work), and can promote the health and work productivity of the employees. However, this may raise ethical concerns about people's autonomy when people are under pressure to undergo screening either to obtain or retain a certain job.

Health checks to 'screen' for NCDs in schools

Screening at school for some NCD conditions (e.g. body weight) is common in some countries. This can provide good opportunities to assess and address

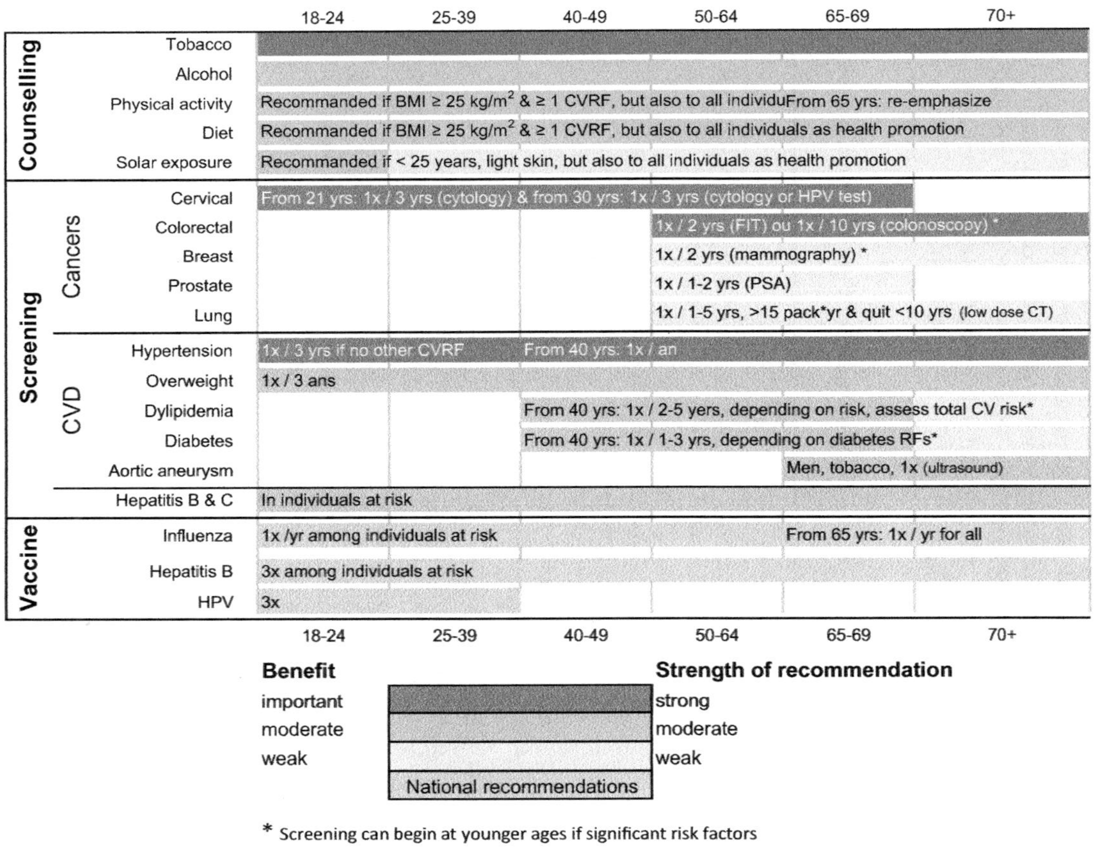

Figure 43.2 Example of a framework for screening, counselling and vaccination for the prevention of NCDs and their risk factors at the primary care level in Switzerland. (adapted from Jacot Sadowski I et al. Recommandations suisses pour le bilan de santé au cabinet médical. *Forum Médical Suisse* 2021;21:888–94).

unhealthy behaviours if relevant services are available to provide quality support (e.g. tobacco use, healthy diet, etc.) on site (e.g. by school nurses) and/or through referral to health services. Respect for dignity and autonomy should be a priority and include, as often as possible, informed consent by schoolchildren.

WHO best buys and other interventions for NCDs that can benefit from screening

The WHO best buys and other recommended interventions include several NCD conditions that can benefit from early detection and treatment (Table 43.1). While some are clearly best undertaken through organized systematic screening, others may be delivered through opportunistic screening programmes or health checks, including when organized screening programmes are not available. It is important to re-emphasize that for any condition screened, treatment must be available and delivered affordably. The interventions in Table 43.1 are described in more detail in other chapters.

Table 43.1 Screening and health checks consistent with the WHO best buys and other interventions for NCD conditions

Screening approach	WHO recommended interventions
Organized screening, opportunistic in some settings.	• Cervical cancer for women aged 30–49 years. • Breast cancer for women aged 50–69 years. • Colorectal cancer at age >50 years. • Oral cancer screening in high-risk groups (e.g. tobacco users, betel-nut chewers). • Assessment of cardiovascular disease (CVD) risk to enable drug therapy and counselling to be provided to those at high risk of a CVD event.
Health checks, including 'screening' questions on healthy behaviours in order to advise about…	• Advise smokers to quit and seek support from tobacco cessation services (including telephone based). • Provide brief psychosocial intervention for persons with hazardous and harmful alcohol use. • Provide counselling on healthy lifestyles (including physical activity and diet) as part of routine patient-centred primary health care services, particularly to those at increased CVD risk (e.g. persons with overweight, diabetes and hypertension).
Ongoing care, but referred to as screening in WHO's recommended interventions.	• Screening of people with diabetes for proteinuria and treatment with angiotensin-converting enzyme inhibitor for the prevention and delay of renal disease. • Drug therapy (including antiplatelet therapy) and counselling for individuals who have had a heart attack or stroke.

Notes

1. Raffles A, Mackie A, Muir Gray JA. *Screening: evidence and practice*, 2nd ed. Oxford: Oxford University Press, 2019.
2. Wilson JMG, Jungner G. *Principles and practice of screening for disease*. WHO, Public Health Papers 34, 1968.
3. Andermann A et al. Revisiting Wilson and Jungner in the genomic age: a review of screening criteria over the past 40 years. *Bull WHO* 2008;86:317–9.
4. Marmot MG et al. The benefits and harms of breast cancer screening: an independent review. *Br J Cancer* 2013;108:2205–40.
5. Kohn L et al. *Informed choice on breast cancer screening: messages to support informed decision*. Brussels: Belgian Health Care Knowledge Center, 2014.
6. Stead LF et al. Physician advice for smoking cessation. *Cochrane Database Syst Rev* 2008;16:CD000165.
7. Brett AS. The routine general medical checkup: valuable practice or unnecessary ritual? *JAMA* 2021;325:2259–61.
8. Krogsbøll LT et al. General health checks in adults for reducing morbidity and mortality from disease. *Cochrane Database of Syst Rev* 2019;1:CD009009.
9. Bjerregaard AL et al. Effectiveness of the population-based 'check your health preventive programme' conducted in a primary care setting: a pragmatic randomised controlled trial. *J Epidemiol Community Health* 2022;76:24–31.
10. What is GRADE? BMJ best practice. https://bestpractice.bmj.com/info/toolkit/learn-ebm/what-is-grade/.
11. Krist AH et al. In high-risk adults aged 50 to 80 y, USPSTF recommends annual lung cancer screening with LDCT (moderate certainty). *Ann Intern Med* 2021;174:JC86.
12. Dickinson JA. Guideline: USPSTF recommends against PSA screening except in men 55 to 69 years who express a preference for it. *Ann Intern Med* 2018;169:JC28.

44 Access to medicines for NCD prevention and control

Cécile Macé, David Beran, Raffaella Ravinetto, Christophe Perrin

Ensuring access to safe, effective, quality and affordable essential medicines is a key part of the 2030 Sustainable Development Agenda and critical for meeting global and country targets for NCDs. Target 3.8 of the Sustainable Development Goals is to 'achieve universal health coverage (UHC), including financial risk protection, access to quality essential health care services, and access to safe, effective, quality, and affordable essential medicines and vaccines for all'. Access to medicines is included in the WHO Global NCD Action Plan and supported by the WHO road map for access to medicines, vaccines and other health products 2019–2023.[1,2]

To address barriers that prevent access to quality-assured affordable medicines, strong political commitment and action is needed internationally, to help shape the global market, as well as at a national level to build and maintain well-functioning regulatory, procurement and supply systems.[3] Although a number of these issues have been partially addressed over the last few decades for HIV/AIDS, tuberculosis, malaria, and other communicable diseases, the response for NCD medicines has been much weaker.[4] The COVID-19 pandemic has further impacted the ability of those with NCDs and those at risk of NCDs to access treatment. A rapid assessment done by WHO in the first half of 2020 showed that one in five countries (20%) reported disruptions or discontinuation of NCD services due to the shortage of medicines, diagnostics, and other technologies.[5] Disruptions to global supply systems as well as national lockdown measures and (more recently) health systems shifting their focus to the COVID-19 response were some of the reasons for this.

WHO framework on essential medicines

In 2004, WHO adopted a framework to guide and coordinate collective action on access to essential medicines. This chapter is structured around the four themes of the framework (rational selection and use, availability and affordability, sustainable financing, and functioning health and supply systems for NCD management and care) and includes global and national commitments to achieving UHC.

DOI: 10.4324/9781003306689-49

Rational selection and use

Rational selection aims to ensure that the most effective, safe, and cost-effective medicines are chosen and provided to people needing them to ensure optimal health benefits and appropriate adherence to their treatment. Unfortunately, irrational choices are made in both high-income countries (HICs) and low- and middle-income countries, for instance by favouring newer, only marginally better, and more expensive medicines.

This may be the result of the inclusion of newer but non-essential medicines in national essential medicines lists (EML) or clinical guidelines, where evidence-based data, technology assessments and/or the context do not justify their use, as well as the influence of the pharmaceutical industry on policy-makers, doctors and patients. These medicines, when included in national reimbursement lists or partly/fully subsidized, can have a large impact on health care budgets. Where costs are paid out-of-the-pocket, this can have a significant impact on household expenditure. For example, in Kyrgyzstan, in 2009 71% of insulin purchased met WHO recommendations (human insulin in vials) and accounted for 43% of total expenditure. The remaining 29% of insulin comprising analogue insulin and insulin in pen devices consumed 57% of the insulin budget. Therefore, by following WHO recommendations Kyrgyzstan would have been able to reduce its annual insulin expenditure by around 40%.[6]

Ministries of health should regularly update their EML, national treatment guidelines, reimbursement guidelines, and procurement catalogues for the public sector, and guidance for private sector providers, ensuring that these are aligned. The WHO Model EML provides useful guidance to national policy-makers in helping define a list of essential medicines that should be prioritized. However, achieving international consensus on algorithms for the treatment of NCDs applicable to all contexts, and that can then be adopted at national or more local levels, is difficult given the variation in the way different health systems operate, including levels of financing. For the development of WHO and the country's EMLs and treatment guidelines, as well as for the training of health professionals on guidelines and protocols, it is crucial that this is done in a transparent way and is not influenced by those with vested interests.

Availability and affordability

How medicines are purchased by the health system, their availability and affordability and how costs are passed on to patients vary from country to country and even within countries, as well as by type of product. In 2016 for example, the availability of medicines to treat asthma in low- and middle-income countries was 30.1% and 43.1% in the public and private sectors, respectively.[7] Studies done in nine African countries have found that several classes of the main medicines for hypertension treatment (thiazide diuretics, calcium channel blockers, ACE inhibitors/angiotensin receptor blockers and beta blockers) were only consistently available in the 3–4 countries with the highest GDP per capita.[8]

In line with the WHO 2020 Country Pharmaceutical Pricing Policy, prices of medicines should be affordable for the health system and individuals, without compromising on quality, equitable access, and rational use. Many medicines for treating NCDs, such as amlodipine, furosemide, metformin or statins, can be affordable for health systems when several generic versions and competition exist. These often have a cost as low as US$ 0.05 per treatment per day, although for long-term treatment of conditions such as cardiovascular disease and their risk factors, there may be significant issues around availability and affordability for individuals who are poor.[9]

The price and affordability of medicines can be influenced by a variety of factors. For instance, prices of newer medicines, such as cancer treatments,[10] are high mainly because the patent holder has a monopoly. For other medicines, such as insulin, despite being developed over 100 years ago, the concentration of the market with three manufacturers and the fact that insulin is a biological product, more complex to manufacture, means that its availability and affordability are reduced in many settings.[11] Fixed-dose combinations for hypertension, which have been included in the WHO Model EML since 2019, can be more expensive than the sum of their standalone formulations.[12] Finally, in some countries mark-ups, including tariffs and taxes within the supply chain, can further increase the price to the end-user to a greater or lesser extent.

Robust procurement and supply chain systems are required to ensure the continued availability of quality-assured products in an efficient way, even for migrant populations, refugees and those in disaster and humanitarian settings. NCD-specific kits have been developed to support humanitarian responses (Chapter 51).

Lack of standardized international criteria for regulatory assessment and registration can act as a significant barrier, for example in the case of some biosimilars (biotherapeutic products which are similar in terms of quality, safety and efficacy to an already licensed reference product), including insulin, monoclonal antibodies that may be used in treating cancer, and in many inhaled medicines for asthma and chronic obstructive pulmonary disease. Issues also arise from reliance on donations and on preferential pricing policies that fall under pharmaceutical company access programmes. Even if these programmes result in savings in the short term, reliance on single suppliers may lead to higher prices than those from alternative manufacturers, and in the long term can disrupt national supply chains and encourage dependence.

Responding to the challenges above require actions at the global level, for example those related to global innovation and intellectual property rights. At the national level, actions should include an improvement in the efficiency of expenditure and strengthening pricing policies. The latter requires transparency on price-setting and enforcement of price control by a competent body, which could be achieved by: (i) adoption of external reference pricing; (ii) robust mark-up regulation along supply chains; (iii) promoting price transparency; (iv) using quality-assured generic and biosimilars; and (v) adopting pooled procurement. Governments should also require transparency on the modalities and timelines of donations and preferential pricing programs and ensure there are adequate exit strategies from the onset.

UHC and sustainable financing

As part of UHC, essential medicines including those for NCDs should be included in national benefit packages and ideally provided for free or at least at a very low cost to patients either at the point of delivery or through reimbursement mechanisms.[13] To do this, adequate mechanisms for the sustainable financing of NCD medicines need to be in place that take into account the increasing burden of NCDs and the effectiveness of treatment.

High-, middle- and low-income countries struggle, in different ways, to ensure sustainable financing for long-term care for NCDs including for medicines. In HICs, the procurement costs of new and expensive medicines are a significant threat to publicly funded health care budgets and/or out-of-pocket expenditures, for those not covered through national health services or health insurance. In low- and middle-income countries the combination of the lack of health insurance schemes and lack of availability and affordability of medicines in the public sector, with the often-higher prices in the private sector, can result in catastrophic health expenditure for many people with NCDs.[14] These patterns are inflated when the selection of procured medicines is based on efficacy alone (as is often the case in HICs) as opposed to cost-effectiveness.

Irrespective of the country's economic level, it is critical that funds are used most efficiently and for the biggest public health gain (i.e., considering both cost-effectiveness and affordability). Governments should also explore opportunities to raise sustainable funding for medicines through health taxes (e.g. tobacco, alcohol and sugar-sweetened beverages). Countries receiving development assistance should consider using this support to strengthen procurement and supply chains for medicines, including NCD medicines. The above measures will however only be successful in making an effective contribution to UHC if essential medicines for treating those with NCDs are systematically included in health insurance and reimbursement systems.

Functioning health and supply systems for NCD management and care

Access to quality assured affordable NCD medicines is an essential component of a functioning health system. Procurement mechanisms need to be in place to guarantee that only quality-assured *and* affordable medicines are purchased. This includes purchasing generic/biosimilar quality-assured medicines whenever possible. Multi-country and global pooled procurement mechanisms are options to consider when national volumes alone are insufficient.

NCD medicines procured in both public and private sectors should be effective and safe, and systems should ensure no substandard or falsified medicines are provided which will not only harm individuals but reduce trust in the services being provided. Assuring the quality of medicines and sharing accurate and understandable information on approved products with the population and health workers is the responsibility of national regulatory authorities. In many countries, these authorities are not well-functioning and integrated into the health system, and they should be strengthened. An expansion of the scope of the WHO Prequalification Programme for specific categories of products, as has been done for insulin and some cancer medicines and could be done for other medicines, for example inhalers and other cancer medicines, may also be helpful in supporting the work of national authorities with limited capacities.

Those working to improve access to medicines need to be aware of other relevant barriers to effective care for patients with NCDs. These include broader challenges to accessing health services, disproportionate investment in expensive tertiary level facilities that only reach a small proportion of the population, lack of trained staff and diagnostic tools that prevent confidence in providing optimal treatment, as well as inadequate data around service provision and utilization, and low awareness on the importance and opportunities to prevent and treat NCDs and their risk factors in the population.

A particular challenge is that treatment for many NCDs, such as diabetes, hypertension, dyslipidaemia, coronary heart disease and chronic respiratory diseases is required daily for many years which implies sustained availability of large volumes of medicines. This necessitates logistic management information systems supported by IT systems to be in place and trained staff to generate and monitor data and accurately forecast needs. Medicines for the treatment of the most common NCD conditions should be available in primary care so that they are easily accessible for patients, with patients being empowered to be fully involved in the management of their conditions, with a detailed understanding of their treatment. Consideration should also be given to the possibility for populations to access medicines directly from community pharmacists without having to revisit medical centres, which can improve adherence to the long-term treatment that is required for NCDs by reducing costs, as well as travel and waiting times. Ensuring continuity of care should be the foundation of NCD management and care and continuous access to affordable medicines is a critical element of this and needs to be included in the global and national response to NCDs.

Global targets and indicators

The WHO NCD Monitoring Framework includes two indicators specific to access to medicines:

- At least 80% of essential health products required for major NCDs should be available, quality-assured and affordable in public and private facilities.
- At least 50% of NCD patients should receive therapy and counselling to prevent outcomes such as heart attacks and strokes.

In 2022 the WHA endorsed the following indicators:

- 60% of people with diabetes of 40 years or older receive statins.
- 100% of people with type-1 diabetes have access to affordable insulin treatment (including devices for insulin delivery, such as syringes and needles) and blood glucose self-monitoring.

Notes

1. Hogerzeil HV et al. Promotion of access to essential medicines for noncommunicable diseases: practical implication of the UN political declaration. *Lancet* 2013;381:680–89.
2. Road map for access to medicines, vaccines, and other health products 2019–2023: comprehensive support for access to medicines, vaccines, and other health products. WHO, 2019.
3. NCD Alliance Briefing Paper. Access to essential medicines and technologies for NCDs. NCD Alliance, 2011.
4. Minghui R et al. Gaps in access to essential medicines and health products for noncommunicable diseases and mental health conditions. *WHO Bulletin* 2020;98:582–582A.
5. The impact of the COVID-19 pandemic on noncommunicable disease resources and services: results of a rapid assessment. WHO, 2020.
6. Beran D et al. Diabetes in Kyrgyzstan: changes between 2002 and 2009. *Int J Health Plann Manage* 2013;28(2):e121–37.
7. Bissel K et al. Access to essential medicines to treat chronic respiratory disease in low-income countries. *Int J Tubercul Lung Dis* 2016;20:717–28.
8. Bovet P et al. Availability of protocols, equipment, and medicines for cardiovascular disease risk management in primary care health facilities in nine African countries. *Ann Cardiol Vasc Med* 2021;4:1043.
9. Husain MJ et al. Access to cardiovascular disease and hypertension medicines in developing countries: an analysis of essential medicine lists, price, availability, and affordability. *JAMA* 2020;9:e015302.
10. Leighl NB et al. An arm and a leg: the rising cost of cancer drugs and impact on access. *Am Soc Clin Oncol Educ Book* 2021;41:1–12.
11. Beran D et al. A global perspective on the issue of access to insulin. *Diabetologia* 2021;64:954–62.
12. Negi S et al. Prices of combination medicines and single-molecule anti-hypertensive medicines in India's private health care sector. *J Clin Hypertens* 2021;23:738–43.
13. Beran D et al. Noncommunicable diseases, access to essential medicines and universal health coverage. *Glob Health Action* 2019;12:1670014.
14. Wirtz VJ et al. Essential medicines for universal health coverage. *Lancet* 2017;389:403–76.

45 Access to medical technologies for NCD prevention and control

Adriana Velazquez Berumen, Nicolò Binello, Sasikala Thangavelu, Gabriela Jiménez Moyao

Medical technologies or devices are essential for preventing, diagnosing, monitoring and treating NCDs and are essential to deliver quality health care and universal health coverage. Medical technologies include instruments, apparatus, machines, implants, reagents and software, and range from relatively basic equipment such as stethoscopes or glucometers to highly advanced technology used for radiotherapy, implantable devices such as coronary stents, genetic testing, genetic manipulation of living tissue, robotic surgery and remote patient management. The rapid advancement of technologies and medical devices means that there are now over two million different kinds of medical devices.

Challenges exist for the effective use of medical technologies and devices in all countries and health systems have demand that surpasses resources. Decisions on the introduction of new technologies and devices therefore require an appreciation of costs and benefits.

Ensuring access to the appropriate medical technology requires collaboration between scientists, biomedical engineers, health care professionals, health economists and policymakers and end users.[1] Regulatory oversight should ensure the medical technology is safe and compliant with quality standards before it reaches the market.

Health technology assessment should consider a range of social, organizational and ethical issues to ensure that medical devices are effective and that there is a cost–benefit. Health technology management should address the availability, accessibility and affordability of medical devices given the resources available in a given setting. It includes planning, needs assessment and procurement, as well as installation, maintenance and disposal/decommissioning to ensure safe and effective use of medical devices.

A number of the WHO best buys and recommended interventions (Chapter 34) require access to medical technologies and the importance of ensuring access to affordable basic technologies for primary health care is included in one of the nine targets of the WHO Global NCD Action Plan, and is described at the end of the chapter. To complement this, WHO's Priority Medical Device Project, provides a continuously updated list of priority

DOI: 10.4324/9781003306689-50

medical devices needed for the management of high-burden diseases, including cardiovascular disease and cancer and for specific populations.[2]

Public health, intellectual property and trade

Access and availability to medical technologies and devices require collaboration across health policy, intellectual property and trade, with action from policymakers as well as lawmakers, government officials, researchers, international organizations and NGOs.[3] Medical devices are usually protected by different patents. For example, blood glucose monitors used by people living with diabetes can have multiple patents relating to user interface, transducers, software, battery, memory, power management system, integrated circuits and wireless or internet connectivity. Intellectual property (IP) and their management are important for various stages of the product life cycle. The research & development and marketing stages often rely on non-disclosure agreements, patent, design, trademark and copyright protection. For example, molecular diagnostics have been protected by patents on foundational technologies, such as nucleic acid amplification testing technologies, which underpin the ever-increasing number of newer technologies.

Governance and economic issues for developing policies on medical devices

Countries need to have effective policies and strategies for medical technologies (which should include those used for the diagnosis or treatment of NCDs and their risk factors). An overarching health technologies policy is an important first step and needs to be aligned with broader health policies and plans.[4] However, around one-half of countries do not have this in place.[5] Issues that can hamper the availability of quality and safe medical devices include the lack of regulatory mechanisms, particularly, in some low- and middle-income countries. The manufacturer needs to register the technology in the country where it will be commercialized and has to report any problems or recalls in case the product malfunctions or is unsafe or can cause an adverse event (in a similar way to the automobile industry). Post-marketing surveillance may be extremely difficult to implement, especially in low- and middle-income countries, which may have limited access to registries and therefore analysis of clinical data.[6] The WHO global model regulatory framework for medical devices provides guidance around legal requirements, implementation and monitoring and regulatory authorities, conflicts of interest and impartiality, along with a step-by-step approach for regulating medical devices.[7]

Procurement

Good procurement practice is important to ensure the provision and performance of quality health technologies at an appropriate market cost. Technical specifications need to be developed in order to procure the medical technology, and these should be adapted to the health care facility setting where it will be used. Before making a decision to purchase a medical technology (or receiving a donation), the technical and procurement should provide in-depth guidance to fully capture the financial, infrastructural, and human resource implications.[8] Different brands often require different consumables (e.g. strips for glucometers, consumables for clinical chemistry and immunoassays equipment), and this needs to be taken into account. Overall, a lack of consideration of maintenance services and user training and incomplete budgeting during procurement planning are primary drivers of suboptimal device uptake and utilization in the frontline.[9]

Affordability

Access to medical technologies requires that they are affordable. Imaging, nuclear medicine and radiotherapy technologies are examples where many considerations should be met in order to promote a financially sustainable solution because of the high capital cost implied (infrastructure, utilities, associated devices and the technology itself) and the ongoing operational costs (reagents, specialized maintenance, regular calibration/quality assurance), which are often not planned sufficiently early. These issues are particularly relevant for NCDs as medical devices for diagnosis and treatment for NCDs (e.g. cardiovascular disease, cancer) beyond the most basic ones, are often expensive to install and maintain. In low- and middle-income countries, where there is often no or limited local production, limited services for testing, commissioning and maintenance, and challenging supply chain systems, the costs of medical technologies, both essential and more complex medical equipment are often substantially higher.

Pooled procurement

While there has been widespread use of pooled procurement for medicines, this is much less advanced for a medical device. Reasons for this include equipment changing rapidly over time, the large range of models and brands, devices often procured less frequently and in smaller volumes and the different accessories required for different settings (i.e. compliance with local standards, such as plugs, electric voltage and frequency or software interface languages).

Training and technology acceptability

While large numbers of medical devices and technologies require trained medical staff, engineers, technologists, technicians and/or health care workers, an increasing number of devices are being developed for home use by the patient and have significant potential to improve access to diagnostic testing, treatment and monitoring of long term conditions such as NCDs. This is especially helpful for increasing access to health care among rural or isolated communities,[10] but requires the individual to develop basic knowledge about the technology and follow manufacturer's conditions and instructions in order to ensure safety and performance.[11]

Maintenance and decommissioning

A number of medical devices require complex installation, testing and commissioning by technical experts and once installed stable temperature and humidity, electrical power supply, supply of clean water, maintenance management programme and spare parts, including the provision of consumables (e.g. radiological film, ECG graph paper, primers for PCR assays, filters and solutions for haemodialysis, software updates). A full assessment of the requirements is critical before purchasing or receiving any medical devices. A reasonable assumption is that at least 10% of the initial cost of the device will be required each year for ongoing maintenance,[12] in addition to day-to-day operational costs. It is also critical to have systems in place for the safe disposal of waste, decontamination and/or decommissioning.[13]

Innovation

Medical devices possess an incremental (often very rapid) nature of innovation. Innovation is important to improve the detection and treatment of NCDs (e.g. ability to measure new markers for cancer, imagery with higher definition, etc.) but upgrading to newer generations should be carefully weighed against available resources. It is important that those considering new acquisitions or upgrades are well informed on the added value in specific terms of newer models and if the added cost can translate to cost-effective NCD reduction).

Selection of priority medical devices

With the ever-increasing number of new medical technologies, it is imperative to prioritize those that have been subjected to a full technology assessment, which takes into account the issues described above, with a focus on those that ensure that best buys (e.g. retinopathy screening for all diabetes patients and laser photocoagulation for prevention of blindness and standard home glucose monitoring for people treated with insulin to reduce diabetes complications) or main WHO Global NCD Action Plan targets (e.g. ensure basic equipment is available to assess a person's cardiovascular risk) are fully implemented before more complex technologies are considered. Medical technologies and devices should be explicitly linked and identified as part of an intervention for prevention, diagnosis, screening, treatment, follow-up and palliative care. In many countries this is undertaken formally by a health technology assessment agency,[14] in order to understand the cost-effectiveness, efficacy, safety and evidence underpinning the medical device, and its role in improving the health of the individual and the local population.[15]

For these purposes, medical device assessment should rely on real-world data sources, including evidence-based clinical trials, the cost of equipment and consumables in a particular country. However, this process is often hindered by limited access to available data, a lack of standardized health and economic outcome parameters and the use of inappropriate comparators.

There is often considerable pressure on policymakers and practitioners from manufacturers, lobbyists or the public to invest in the latest technology without a full and rigorous assessment. Examples of new technologies that may be used without sufficient evidence of their efficacy or cost-effectiveness compared with the existing technology include devices for screening and/or diagnosis (e.g. genetic or immunohistology markers for certain cancers), and treatment (e.g. stents for coronary revascularization, robotic surgery). It is important, therefore, that market entry and diffusion of medical devices are both well-managed and transparent.[16] Countries looking to identify the most cost-effective medical technologies for the prevention, diagnostic, investigation, treatment and monitoring of NCDs, including for national insurance or benefits packages, can refer to a number of WHO priority medical device lists,[17,18,19] which are available for cancer, CVD and diabetes as well as MeDevIS (Priority Medical Devices Information System open access electronic platform).[20] In countries where the health care system can afford it, it is the efficacy of the technology more than cost-effectiveness that often drives the use of new technologies (e.g. effective but extremely expensive cancer therapy, or haemodialysis to manage kidney failure resulting from diabetes).

Major gaps in the availability of essential medical technologies exist, particularly in primary care in low- and middle-income countries settings.[21,22] WHO has published a core set of NCD diagnostic and monitoring tools for primary care (Box 45.1).[23]

BOX 45.1 CORE SET OF NCD DIAGNOSTIC AND MONITORING TOOLS IN SETTINGS WITH LOW RESOURCES

Technologies

Thermometer, stethoscope, validated electronic blood pressure measurement device,[a] measurement tape, weighing machine, peak flow meter,[a] spacers for inhalers, glucometer, blood glucose test strips, Semmes-Weinstein 10 g monofilament, urine protein test strips, urine ketones test strips.

When resources permit the following should be included: nebulizer, pulse oximeter, blood cholesterol assay, lipid profile, serum creatinine assay, troponin test strips, urine microalbuminuria test strips, tuning fork, electrocardiograph,[b] defibrillator.

Tools

WHO CVD risk prediction charts, evidence-based clinical protocols, flow charts with referral criteria, patient clinical records, medical information register, audit tools.

a Disposable mouthpieces are required. Peak flow meters with one-way flow are preferable.
b Where training to read and interpret electrocardiograms is available.

The REASSURED criteria are a set of characteristics developed for assessing diagnostic and monitoring tools for communicable diseases.[24] They have recently been adapted for NCDs.[25]

BOX 45.2 'REASSURED' CRITERIA FOR ASSESSING DIAGNOSTIC AND MONITORING TOOLS FOR NCDs IN PRIMARY CARE

R*eal-time connectivity*: tests are connected and/or a reader or mobile phone is used to power the reaction and/or read test results to provide required data to clinicians and users.

E*ase of specimen collection*: tests should be designed for use with non-invasive specimens.

A*ffordable*: tests are affordable to end-users and the health system.

S*ensitive*: avoid false negatives.

S*pecific*: avoid false positives.

U*ser-friendly*: procedure of testing is simple — can be performed in a few steps, requiring minimum training.

R*apid and Robust*: results are available to ensure treatment of patient at first visit (typically, 15min to 2h) and the tests can survive the supply chain without requiring additional transport and storage conditions such as refrigeration.

E*quipment free and environmentally friendly*: ideally the test does not require any special equipment or can be operated in very simple devices that use solar or battery power. Completed tests are easy to dispose of and manufactured from recyclable materials.

D*eliverable to end-users*: accessible to those who need the tests the most.

Guidance is available to enable countries to expand on this core set of primary care technologies and tools according to their needs and resources available, through the WHO list of priority medical devices[2,17,18,19] and the online database MeDevIS.[20]

WHO Global NCD Action Plan targets and indicators

Target: An 80% availability of affordable basic technologies and essential medicines, including generics required to treat major NCDs in both public and private facilities. For technologies, this refers to the percentages of public and private primary health care facilities which have all of the following available: blood pressure measurement device, a weighing scale, height measuring equipment, blood sugar and blood cholesterol measurement devices with strips and urine strips for albumin assay.

Indicator: Availability and affordability of quality, safe and efficacious essential NCD medicines, including generics and basic technologies in both public and private facilities.

Notes

1. Human resources for medical devices, the role of biomedical engineers. WHO, 2017. https://www.who.int/publications/i/item/9789241565479.
2. Prioritizing medical devices. WHO. https://www.who.int/activities/prioritizing-medical-devices.
3. Promoting access to medical technologies and innovation - second edition, WHO, WIPO, WTO, 2020.
4. Development of medical device policies. WHO, 2011.
5. Global atlas of medical devices. WHO, 2017.
6. Guidance for post-market surveillance and market surveillance of medical devices, including in vitro diagnostics. WHO, 2020.
7. WHO global model regulatory framework for medical devices including in vitro diagnostic medical devices. WHO, 2017.
8. Procurement process resource guide. WHO, 2011.
9. Diaconu K et al. Methods for medical device and equipment procurement and prioritization within low- and middle-income countries: findings of a systematic literature review. *Global Health* 201718;13:59.
10. Fleming KA et al. The Lancet Commission on diagnostics: transforming access to diagnostics. *Lancet* 2021;398:1997–2050.
11. Trainings for medical devices. Webpage, WHO.
12. Medical equipment maintenance programme overview. WHO, 2011.
13. Decommissioning medical devices. WHO, 2019.
14. 2015 global survey on health technology assessment by national authorities. WHO, 2015.
15. Pongiglione B et al. Do existing real-world data sources generate suitable evidence for the HTA of medical devices in Europe? Mapping and critical appraisal. *Int J Technol Assess Health Care* 2021;37:e62.
16. Drummond M et al. Economic evaluation of medical devices. Oxford Research Encyclopedias, Economics and Finance, 2018.
17. WHO list of priority medical devices for cancer management. WHO, 2017.
18. WHO list of priority medical devices for management of cardiovascular diseases and diabetes. WHO, 2017.
19. Velazquez Berumen A et al. Defining priority medical devices for cancer management: a WHO initiative. *Lancet Oncol* 2018:e709–19.
20. MeDevIS (Priority Medical Devices Information System) webpage. WHO.
21. Yadav H et al. Availability of essential diagnostics in ten low-income and middle-income countries: results from national health facility surveys. *Lancet Glob Health* 2021;9:e1553–60.

22 Sabet Sarvestani A, Sienko KH. Medical device landscape for communicable and noncommunicable diseases in low-income countries. *Global Health* 2018;14:65.
23 WHO package of essential noncommunicable (PEN) disease interventions for primary health care. WHO, 2020.
24 Land KJ et al. REASSURED diagnostics to inform disease control strategies, strengthen health systems and improve patient outcomes. *Nat Microbiol* 2019;4:46–54.
25 Bernabé-Ortiz A et al. Diagnostics and monitoring tools for noncommunicable diseases: a missing component in the global response. *Global Health* 2021;17:26.

46 Law and NCD prevention and control

Benn McGrady, Kritika Khanijo, Suzanne Zhou

Laws are important in preventing and controlling NCDs. This chapter provides a brief introduction to the roles played by law in the context of NCDs. More detail is available elsewhere.[1,2,3,4]

For the purposes of this chapter, the concept of law includes a variety of legally enforceable instruments, including, but not limited to: (i) national constitutions; (ii) legislation passed by bodies with legislative powers; (iii) regulations, decrees, ordinances, administrative orders and other instruments promulgated by the executive branch of government and using powers created by legislation; and (iv) case law, as decided by courts.

Law determines the duties, rights and obligations of government – simultaneously creating the powers under which different branches of government can act and placing limits on those powers.[5] Law functions as an instrument of public policy, linked to political declarations, policies, strategies, action plans and other instruments that are not ordinarily legally enforceable. But in practice, both policy and law are shaped by public and private interests, and thereby influence commercial determinants of health.

The functions served by law and regulation

Laws serve a number of different functions for altering exposure to NCD risk factors in the population and enabling access to health care (described at the very end of this chapter). First, they are used to implement public policy. Many WHO best buys and other recommended interventions are implemented through law – and are often the purview of ministries beyond health, such as finance, trade, the economy or education.[6] These include:

- Taxes and other fiscal measures relating to tobacco, alcohol and foods and beverages.
- Restrictions on the marketing of tobacco, alcohol, foods and beverages, and breast-milk substitutes.
- Labelling, such as health warnings on tobacco products and alcoholic beverages, and nutrition labelling.
- Laws on smoke-free areas and the availability of alcohol.

DOI: 10.4324/9781003306689-51

Other examples of legal interventions include urban planning, occupational health and safety, and regulating the services provided by community organizations such as those responsible for delivering sports and leisure activities[7] as well as environmental laws on transport and factory emissions that impact air pollution.[8] Health is also shaped by laws with a less direct impact, such as those relating to housing, social protections, competition law or general taxation.

Second, legal considerations influence the development, implementation and enforcement of policy. Although domestic interventions to address NCD risk factors may be evidence-based; political, economic and social factors also shape those interventions. For example, the design of an intervention may depend substantially on how powers are divided within governments, on any applicable international norms, or relevant political commitments or national priorities.

Third, economic operators such as manufacturers, importers and distributors can bring legal claims challenging interventions to address risk factors for NCDs. Most obviously, producers of harmful commodities, such as tobacco companies, often use litigation to stymie attempts to regulate their activities.[9] In recent years, a number of high-profile international and domestic legal disputes have arisen to challenge measures that governments have taken to address risk factors for NCDs, for example on tobacco plain packaging,[10] minimum unit pricing on alcoholic beverages[11] and restrictions on the marketing of foods and beverages to children.[12]

Litigation highlights the central reason of why laws and regulations are so important in addressing NCD risk factors: it compels economic and other operators to reduce risks to public health where doing so is not aligned with their private interests (Chapter 56 on the private sector).

International instruments

International instruments take the form of legally binding treaties as well as instruments that do not directly bind States. National laws and norms influence the development of international instruments. These, in turn, influence national laws and norms, although the extent of national implementation varies.

The WHO Framework Convention on Tobacco Control (WHO FCTC) is the only legally binding treaty under the auspices of WHO focused on an NCD-specific issue, with obligations for the Parties (i.e. the countries that have joined the treaty). Nevertheless, Parties still have to 'domesticate' the treaty by passing the relevant national tobacco control laws and regulations.

In contrast to the WHO FCTC, States are not legally bound to implement other international instruments specific to NCDs that are under the auspices of WHO (Box 46.1). These instruments are frequently implemented by WHO Member States, often through domestic laws and regulations, and can also be relevant when international or domestic legal disputes arise regarding specific interventions.

> **BOX 46.1 EXAMPLES OF INTERNATIONAL INSTRUMENTS FOR THE PREVENTION AND CONTROL OF NCDs**
>
> - Codex Alimentarius (FAO & WHO, 1981).
> - Global Strategy for the Prevention and Control of NCDs (WHO, 2000).
> - Global Strategy on Diet, Physical Activity and Health (WHO, 2004).
> - Recommendations on the Marketing of Foods and Non-Alcoholic Beverages to Children (WHO, 2010).
> - Global Strategy to Reduce Harmful Use of Alcohol (WHO, 2010).
> - UN Political Declaration on NCDs (UN, 2011 and 2018) and outcome document (UN, 2014).
> - WHO Global NCD Action Plan 2013-2030 (WHO, 2013).
> - 2030 Sustainable Development Agenda (UN, 2015).

International instruments of all types influence domestic laws on NCDs. For example, Codex standards are frequently domesticated through mandatory food laws or voluntary national standards, (e.g. nutrition labelling) despite Codex not creating a legal obligation to implement domestically.

A variety of international instruments also affect the relationship between law and NCDs at the national level. For example, in the UK, tobacco companies challenged domestic legislation for tobacco plain (standardized) packaging[13] implementing obligations under the WHO FCTC[14] and the 2014 EU Tobacco Products Directive[15] on the grounds that it infringed international trade agreements and breached UK law protecting property rights, EU law and the European Convention on Human Rights. Related legal challenges also called on the UK and other courts (e.g. Australia, Uruguay and Thailand) to interpret WTO agreements on similar grounds. Contentions that plain packaging violated standards of treatment under bilateral investment treaties (BITs) were also assessed by an ad-hoc investment tribunal.[16] Similarly, Swedish Match, a snus manufacturer, challenged the application of plain packaging to snus before the courts in Norway on the ground that it was not proportional to the comparatively lesser risk posed by snus. The Courts dismissed the case and held that the measure was appropriate and proportional, in fact, the State enjoyed a wide margin of appreciation in the area of health.[17] In these examples, international law provides both an impetus for implementing the intervention (through the WHO FCTC) and defines limits on the powers of what the government can implement (EU law, WTO law and European human rights law) or creates a chilling effect through the dispute settlement provisions (BITs, Treaties with Investment Provisions [TIPs]).

Non-binding international instruments can also play an important role. For example, when Chile sought to enforce laws prohibiting the marketing of unhealthy foods and beverages to children by preventing the depiction of cartoon characters on unhealthy foods, the Government was challenged on the grounds that removing trademarked characters from packaging interfered with a company's right to property. Chile was in part implementing WHO guidance on regulating marketing to children, the right to the highest attainable standard of health, and the rights of the child, in the face of rising levels of obesity. But WTO rules on trademark protection and international human rights laws concerning the protection of property rights were also an issue in domestic litigation that was ultimately resolved in favour of the government.[18]

Domestic implementation of laws and regulations with respect to risk factors

Domestic implementation of international laws and norms depends significantly on governance arrangements, legal traditions, the burden of disease associated with specific risk factors, the importance attached to health, as well as the political economy. But there are some typical approaches that can be identified. Examples of domestic laws and regulations for implementing the best buys and other recommended interventions include:

- *Health taxes* (e.g. excise taxes on tobacco, alcohol, sugar-sweetened beverages). These are typically implemented through national finance legislation, which is amended periodically through national budgetary processes (e.g. updates of regulations and/or schedules on different taxes for various products). Other fiscal laws, such as those addressing tax administration, are relevant for purposes of enforcement, and other laws establishing governance arrangements, such as in the case of earmarked taxes, are sometimes present. Health taxes are not frequently challenged before domestic courts, but litigation does sometimes arise with respect to whether subnational governments are acting within the scope of their limited powers,[19] as well as whether tax has been correctly assessed on a given product. Chapter 41 describes health taxes in more detail.
- *Restrictions or bans on marketing.* These are most common in the context of tobacco products, where they are often found in national tobacco control legislation and implemented in combination with laws governing broadcasting (including over the internet), advertising, consumer protection and the retail environment. Frequently, the enforcement mechanisms available under these and other laws will be used for the purposes of implementing tobacco-specific restrictions. Restrictions on alcohol marketing and marketing of foods and non-alcoholic beverages to children are less widely implemented, but where in place are typically implemented in a similar manner. Restrictions on marketing have been challenged before the courts in many countries, particularly on grounds that they interfere with freedom of expression and occasionally on grounds that restrictions on the use of trademarks interfere with the right to property.

- *Packaging and labelling.* Interventions are typically implemented through a combination of national standards, regulations (possibly in a food safety Act or public health Act) and laws specific to a given risk factor (e.g. tobacco control Act). Laws and regulations are often developed by ministries of health or other bodies, such as food and drug regulatory agencies, whereas standards typically sit with national standard-setting bodies. For the reasons described above, tobacco control labelling measures have been challenged frequently (and usually unsuccessfully) before domestic courts, sometimes on grounds relating to freedom of expression,[20] but often on grounds relating to the protection of property rights in the form of trademarks and associated goodwill.[21]
- *Regulations on sale, use and exposure.* These may include measures to restrict smoking areas, set minimum ages for purchase, regulate access and placement of products, regulate hours and places of sale, or implement licencing schemes with conditions on the sale of products such as tobacco and alcohol.

Laws such as smoke-free area laws and laws governing the sale and service of alcohol, including licensing laws, tend to be implemented through a variety of legal mechanisms that depend more on the country context, including the allocation of authority between national and sub-national governments. This can also be true for other interventions. For example, in some countries authority to make laws governing the retail environment may sit with sub-national governments, as may limited powers to levy taxes and charges. Laws governing smoke-free areas have been challenged on grounds relating to the right to conduct a business,[22] and it is reasonably common for decisions administering licensing laws to be challenged before the courts.

In the context of tobacco control, these provisions are often part of a Tobacco Control Act or similar, that typically falls under the ministry of health (Chapters 18 on tobacco use and Chapter 33 on the WHO FCTC).

The role of laws in controlling NCDs

In addition to the roles played by laws in addressing NCD risk factors, laws play a foundational role in the provision of health services to treat and control NCDs. For example, laws govern who is authorized to provide health services and what quality standards they must meet (licensing and qualifications), on what financial terms services are provided (financing and financial protection), who may access services (equity and non-discrimination), how personal data collected in the context of health services may be stored and used (privacy and data protection), accountability for the provision of services (liability and statutory obligations), regulation of medicines and medical devices, and broader governance arrangements, including allocation of authority to government agencies. The mix of these and other laws collectively influences the availability, accessibility and quality of care for NCDs.

The potential for law to influence treatment in substantial ways was illustrated early in the acute phase of the COVID-19 pandemic, with some governments limiting under emergency orders the provision of what they deemed non-essential health services in order to prioritize COVID-19 response, or dedicating specific health facilities to COVID-19 response. In some countries, these arrangements were challenged before the courts, with patients invoking the right to the highest attainable standard of health to ensure access to care.[23]

Notes

1 Magnusson RS, Patterson D. The role of law and governance reform in the global response to non-communicable diseases. *Global Health* 2014;10:44.
2 Voon T et al. (Eds.). *Regulating tobacco, alcohol and unhealthy foods: the legal issues*. London and New York: Routledge, 2015.
3 Magnusson RS et al. Legal capacities required for prevention and control of noncommunicable diseases. *Bull WHO* 2019;97:108–17.
4 Key considerations for the use of law to prevent noncommunicable diseases in the WHO European Region. Report of an intensive legal training and capacity-building workshop on law and noncommunicable diseases. WHO Regional Office for Europe, 2016.
5 Gostin L, Wiley L. *Public health law: Duty, power restraint*, 3rd ed. Oakland, CA: University of California Press, 2016.
6 What legislators need to know. WHO, UNDP, 2018.
7 Nau T et al. Legal strategies to improve physical activity in populations. *Bull WHO* 2021;99:593–602.
8 Regulating air quality: the first global assessment of air pollution legislation. UN Environment Programme, 2021.
9 Tobacco Control Laws. Tobacco litigation database. Washington DC: Campaign for Tobacco-Free Kids.
10 Report of the appellate body, *Australia — certain measures concerning trademarks, geographical indications and other plain packaging requirements applicable to tobacco products and packaging*, WT/DS435/AB/R, WT/DS441/AB/R (9 June 2020).
11 *Scotch Whisky Association and Others v The Lord Advocate and another (Scotland)* [2017] UKSC 76.
12 Causa n° 46253/2017 (Proteccion). Resolución n° 58 de Corte de Apelaciones de Santiago, 2017.
13 British American Tobacco vs Secretary of State for Health. England and Wales Court of Appeal Civ 1182, 2016.
14 WHO framework convention on tobacco control. WHO, 2003 (updated 2005).
15 Approximation of the laws, regulations and administrative provisions of the member states concerning the manufacture, presentation and sale of tobacco and related products. European Union Directive 2014/40/EU.
16 *Philip Morris Brands Sàrl & Others v Oriental Republic of Uruguay*, ICSID Case No. ARB/10/7; *Philip Morris Asia Limited v The Commonwealth of Australia*, UNCITRAL, PCA Case No. 2012-12; See also Thow AM et al., Protecting noncommunicable disease prevention policy in trade and investment agreements. *Bull WHO* 2022;100:268–75.
17 *Swedish Match v The Ministry of Health & Care Services,* [2017] Case No. 17-110415TVI-OBYF.
18 Causa n° 46253/2017 (Proteccion). Resolución n° 58 de Corte de Apelaciones de Santiago, 2017.

19 For example *Lora Jean Williams et al. v. City of Philadelphia et al.* NOS. 2077, 2078 CD 2016.
20 United States Court of Appeals, District of Columbia Circuit. *R.J. Reynolds Tobacco Company, et al., Appellees v. Food and Drug Administration*, et al., Appellants. Nos. 11–5332, 12–5063.
21 See examples above relating to tobacco plain packaging.
22 See https://www.tobaccocontrollaws.org/.
23 See for example Sentencia T-195/21, available at https://www.corteconstitucional.gov.co/Relatoria/2021/T-195-21.htm and summarized at https://www.covid19litigation.org/case-index/colombia-constitutional-court-sentencia-t-19521-2021-06-18.

47 Changing behaviour at scale to prevent NCDs

Theresa M Marteau, Gareth J Hollands, Devaki Nambiar, Marcus R Munafò

Changing the behaviour of entire populations. This chapter describes behaviour change at scale using interventions that can impact the behaviour of individuals at the level of *entire populations*, or specific groups within populations, by altering aspects of the contexts or environments in which the behaviour occurs. This contrasts with approaches to changing behaviour through individuals engaging with healthcare professionals (Chapter 48). Implementing interventions that change behaviour at this scale most often requires legislative, regulatory and fiscal policies.

Changing environments to change behaviour. By creating environments that encourage healthy behaviour, interventions that target the whole population have the potential additional benefit of increasing the effectiveness of interventions targeting individuals. For example, one-to-one stop-smoking counselling can be more successful in areas where there are fewer tobacco retail outlets or where a smoking ban in public places is well enforced.

Interventions to change behaviour at scale

Broadening the range of interventions. Behaviour change interventions at scale can be categorized by the *outcome* of the intervention (i.e. the change in behaviour sought). For example, tobacco tax and health warning labels on tobacco packaging both reduce tobacco use at scale, even though the interventions use different approaches (e.g. fiscal measures reduce purchasing; health warning labels provide information and associate negative feelings with tobacco use).

Categorizing interventions by systems or environments changed. Interventions can also be categorized by the *system* or *environment* in which the change occurs. This includes interventions that change some aspect of the physical environment – for example increasing the availability of lower energy foods and drinks in cafeterias or increasing the availability of attractive green public open spaces – and interventions that change some aspect of the economic environment to increase the affordability of healthier options and/or decrease the affordability of unhealthier ones, e.g. taxes on tobacco, alcohol and sugar-sweetened beverages.[1,2,3] Interventions that change some

DOI: 10.4324/9781003306689-52

aspect of the physical environment to alter behaviour in a predictable way are sometimes known as nudges.[4]

Structural changes make healthy behaviour easier. Interventions designed to create environments that make healthy behaviour easier and/or unhealthy behaviour more difficult are often referred to as 'structural'. Such interventions generally place lower demands on the cognitive, social and material resources of individuals than those based on advice, e.g. advice to eat more fruit and vegetables or to increase levels of physical activity. The mechanisms by which interventions that alter some aspect of physical environments – sometimes known as nudges – have their effects are little studied, but generally involve greater regulation of behaviour by systems that are sometimes described as automatic or non-conscious.[5] These effects are therefore based less upon reflection and more upon feelings, relative to interventions based on information provision and requiring planning and goal setting. Price-based interventions may also have some of their effects through these less conscious mechanisms, e.g. by signalling danger in the case of taxes on harmful products, an effect that explains why taxes on sugary drinks can reduce sales by more than the reduction expected from price alone.

Structural changes to reduce health inequalities. Structural measures can have a greater overall impact than individual measures as they target the whole population. Importantly, structural interventions are often more equitable in producing behaviour change. This contrasts with mass media campaigns to change behaviour at scale, which can require individuals to have many resources – including time, understanding and money – to respond. This can serve to widen health and other inequalities. Interventions based on awareness and information can be 'regressive' – i.e. less effective among the less educated and wealthy (and often unhealthier) individuals who may be less able to understand the key messages and have fewer resources including the time and money needed to adopt them. In many cases, populations already facing disadvantage see their exclusion becoming further pronounced through such interventions. In some cases, such populations are essentially invisible to authorities responsible for decision-making, as in the case of the urban poor in many parts of the world, including the poorest billion.[5,6]

Examples of structural changes to physical and economic environments. Examples of population-level interventions that are designed to change behaviour at scale are shown in Table 47.1. These include both WHO best buys and other interventions. They can be distinguished from individual-level (high-risk) interventions (Chapter 36). These are divided into those that change the physical environment, those that are centred around health information and those that change the economic environment. It should be noted that some of the WHO best buys are not behaviour change interventions per se – such as reformulating foods or beverages to eliminate trans fats or reduce levels of salt or sugar.

Changing behaviour at scale to prevent NCDs 349

Table 47.1 Population-level interventions to change behaviour at scale to prevent NCDs: WHO best buys (in bold) and other related interventions

	Tobacco use	Harmful alcohol use	Unhealthy diets	Physical inactivity
Physical environments **Availability** *of products or opportunities for behaviour:*				
by product range in stores/cafes.		• Reduce the proportion of drinks that are alcoholic.[7]	• **Reformulate to low salt.** • **Increase low salt options.** • Reduce the proportion of foods that are less healthy (vs healthier) in retail settings.[8]	
by age.	• Minimum age and raise legal age for sales and smoking.[9]	• **Minimum age and raise age for sales and drinking.**		
by time (e.g. store hours).		• **Reduce hours of sales (particularly at nights and weekends).**		
by area level (local).	• Reduce density of outlets.[10]	• **Reduce density of outlets.**	• Reduce density of fast-food outlets.	• **Urban design to connect neighbourhoods with walkable street networks and public transport.**

(*Continued*)

Table 47.1 (Continued)

	Tobacco use	Harmful alcohol use	Unhealthy diets	Physical inactivity
by area level (national).	• Minimize illicit trade • Ban smoking in indoor public spaces, workplaces and on public transport.		• Ban industrial trans-fats.	• Convenient and safe access to quality public open space with infrastructure to support walking and cycling.
Size reduce portion and pack sizes.	• Regulate minimum and maximum pack sizes.[11]	• Reduce sizes of portions (servings), packs (bottles and cans) and glasses.[12]	• Reduce portion and pack size to lower size and volume of unhealthier food and beverages.	
Information-based. Labelling. Packaging. Advertising & promotions. Mass media campaigns.	• Graphic health warning labels. • Plain packaging. • Comprehensive ban on advertising, promotion & sponsorship. • Educate on the harms of smoking.	• Health warning labels. • Comprehensive restrictions on advertising. • Restrict or ban promotions related to sponsorship and activities targeting young people. • Educate on the harms of alcohol including a link to different cancers.[14]	• Front-of-pack labelling including food content and interpretative information (e.g. traffic light system). • Restrictions on advertising, promotion and sponsorship.[13] • Educate on the harms of salt. • Educate on a healthy diet.	• Educate on the benefits of physical activity.

| Economic environments. Taxes and other price-based interventions (e.g. minimum unit price on alcohol), to reduce demand. Subsidies to increase demand. | • Increase tax and prices. | • Increase tax and prices. | • **Tax on sugar-sweetened drinks.**
• Tax on sugary and salty foods.[15]

• Subsidize selected healthier foods.[19]
• Subsidize locally produced, indigenous healthier food options (to promote food security and sovereignty).[20] | • Increase taxes on fuel.[16]
• Road user charging for private vehicles.[17]
• Remove subsidies on fossil fuels.[18]

• Subsidize public transport.[21]
• Increase affordability of bikes, including e-bikes and rental schemes for bikes.[22] |

Instead, they are interventions that, if applied at scale and made widely available at affordable prices, would lead to reduced exposure to risk factors (in this case intake of trans fats) at the population level sufficient to contribute to preventing NCDs.

Key issues for implementing interventions to change behaviour at scale

The following are important considerations when it comes to implementing NCD programmes and policies aimed at changing behaviour at scale.[23]

1. *Strengthening political leadership and governance*

Transparent and accountable whole-of-government, whole-of-society governance structures at local, national and international levels are needed to minimize conflicts of interest and to be responsive to the needs and values of citizens. Collective action from healthcare professionals, civil society organizations, invoking relevant rights-based frameworks (see Chapter 52 on human rights) can be instrumental. NCD plans at all levels should include structural and social interventions that encourage behaviour change in a way that promotes fairness and equity. Robust, equity-oriented evaluations should be incorporated into all programmes and interventions.

2. *Engaging with industry and the private sector while safeguarding against corporate interference in policy*

Changing behaviour at scale will sometimes require engagement with industry, with the exception of the tobacco industry (Article 5.3 of the WHO Framework Convention on Tobacco Control – the protection of public health policies with respect to tobacco control from commercial and other vested interests of the tobacco industry). Any such engagement, however, needs to protect against conflicts of interest and corporate interference in policymaking. The latter includes preventing and delaying the implementation of evidence-based policies to reduce NCDs. These activities are well-documented in the food, alcohol and fossil fuel industries (and of course the tobacco industry). Of particular concern is the influence of vested corporate interests in UN bodies and activities including WHO[24] (see Chapter 56 on the private sector).

Systems for preventing and managing conflicts of interest in public health-oriented government policy include setting up independent panels to advise on corporate actor engagement in policy.[25] The effectiveness of these systems requires evaluation. Governments need to fully implement relevant legal frameworks as well as systems that enable corporations to engage with policymakers without interference in effective policymaking.

3. Increasing public demand

Public support (including civil society organizations) is vital for policies that encourage the successful establishment and enforcement of interventions that change behaviour at scale. Unfortunately, public support is often inversely related to the size of the intervention effect – i.e. it is highest for information-based interventions (which often have a small overall impact) and lowest for price-based interventions (which generally have a larger overall impact). Public support of interventions is increased by communicating their effectiveness,[26] and ensuring they are fair – e.g. not disproportionately impacting the poorest, applying equally to the wealthy.

The three considerations listed above are strongly interlinked. For example, inadequate governance allows effective policies with low levels of public demand to be stopped or delayed by commercial opposition. The corollary is that interventions to address one of the above issues can enhance others, for example increasing public demand for effective policies can result in more effective governance systems that prevent interference from commercial actors.

In conclusion, realizing the WHO Global NCD Action Plan requires policymakers and practitioners to prioritize best buys and other interventions in Table 47.1 that can change behaviour at scale. Regular monitoring of the outcomes of these interventions as part of evaluations will ensure that they can be refined to optimize their impact. Critically, the WHO Global NCD Action Plan needs to be urgently updated to include more explicitly specific structural and social interventions that can enable healthier behaviour to address the burden of NCDs in all populations, including the poorest.

Notes

1. Hollands GJ et al. The TIPPME intervention typology for changing environments to change behaviour. *Nature Hum Behaviour* 2017;1:0140.
2. Marteau TM et al. Increasing healthy life expectancy equitably in England by 5 years by 2035: could it be achieved? *Lancet* 2019;393:2571–3.
3. Bloomberg MR et al. *Health taxes to save lives: employing effective excise taxes on tobacco, alcohol, and sugary beverages: the task force on fiscal policy for health.* New York: Bloomberg Philanthropies, 2019.
4. Thaler RH, Sunstein CR. *Nudge: improving decision about health, wealth and happiness.* New Haven, CT: Yale University Press, 2009. (note: Thaler is the 2017 Nobel Prize winner in Economic Sciences and the book was a New York Times bestseller).
5. Hollands GJ et al. Non-conscious processes in changing health-related behaviour: a conceptual analysis and framework. *Health Psychol Rev* 2016;10:381–94.
6. Nambiar D, Mander H. Inverse care and the role of the state: the health of the urban poor. *Bull WHO* 2017;95:152.
7. Blackwell AK et al. The impact on selection of non-alcoholic vs alcoholic drink availability: an online experiment. *BMC Public Health* 2020;20:526.
8. Reynolds JP et al. Impact of decreasing the proportion of higher energy foods and reducing portion sizes on energy purchased in worksite cafeterias: a stepped-wedge randomised controlled trial. *PLOS Medicine* 2021;18:e1003743.

9. Bonnie RJ et al. (Eds.). *Public health implications of raising the minimum age of legal access to tobacco products*. Washington, DC: National Academies Press, 2015.
10. Valiente R et al. Tobacco retail environment and smoking: a systematic review of geographic exposure measures and implications for future studies. *Nicotine Tob Res* 2021;23:1263–73.
11. Lee I et al. Cigarette pack size and consumption: an adaptive randomised controlled trial. *BMC Public Health* 2021;21:1420.
12. Pilling M et al. The effect of wine glass size on volume of wine sold: a mega-analysis of studies in bars and restaurants. *Addiction* 2020;115:1660–7.
13. Mytton OT et al. The potential health impact of restricting less-healthy food and beverage advertising on UK television between 05.30 and 21.00 hours: a modelling study. *PLoS Med* 2020;17:e1003212.
14. Weerasinghe A et al. Improving knowledge that alcohol can cause cancer is associated with consumer support for alcohol policies: findings from a real-world alcohol labelling study. *Int J Environ Res Public Health* 2020;17:398.
15. Scheelbeek PF et al. Potential impact on prevalence of obesity in the UK of a 20% price increase in high sugar snacks: modelling study. *BMJ* 2019;366:l4786.
16. Brown V et al. Obesity-related health impacts of fuel excise taxation- an evidence review and cost-effectiveness study. *BMC Public Health* 2017;17:359.
17. Hosford K et al. The effects of road pricing on transportation and health equity: a scoping review. *Transp Rev* 2021;4:766–87.
18. Erickson P et al. Why fossil fuel producer subsidies matter. *Nature* 2020;578:E1–4.
19. Blakely T et al. The effect of food taxes and subsidies on population health and health costs: a modelling study. *Lancet Public Health* 2020;5:e404–13.
20. Weiler AM et al. Food sovereignty, food security and health equity: a meta-narrative mapping exercise. *Health Policy Plan* 2015;30:1078–92.
21. Martin A et al. Financial incentives to promote active travel: an evidence review and economic framework. *Am J Prev Med* 2012;43:e45–57.
22. Scheepers CE et al. Shifting from car to active transport: a systematic review of the effectiveness of interventions. *Transp Res Part A Policy Pract* 2014;70:264–80.
23. Swinburn BA et al. The global syndemic of obesity, undernutrition, and climate change: the Lancet Commission report. *Lancet* 2019;393:791–846.
24. Lauber K et al. Big food and the World Health Organization: a qualitative study of industry attempts to influence global-level non-communicable disease policy. *BMJ Glob Health* 2021;6:e005216.
25. Buse K et al. Thinking politically about UN political declarations: a recipe for healthier commitments—free of commercial interests (comment). *Int J Health Policy Manag* 2021 (August 9).
26. Reynolds JP et al. Communicating the effectiveness and ineffectiveness of government policies and their impact on public support: a systematic review with meta-analysis. *R Soc Open Sci* 2020;7:190522.

48 Promoting health behaviours at the individual level for NCD prevention and control

Paul Aveyard, Wendy Hardeman, Robert Horne

Tobacco use, harmful use of alcohol, unhealthy diet and lack of physical activity are strong, shared, and modifiable behavioural risk factors for NCDs. While many of the chapters in this book (including Chapter 47 on changing behaviour at scale) describe actions at the population level to reduce these risk factors, the focus of this chapter is on behaviour change and improving adherence to treatment at the individual level to reduce NCD risk.

Governments rarely include explicit action and specific resources to support individuals to change their behaviour as a priority in basic health service packages. Underlying this is a common misconception that individuals can change health behaviours with ease (e.g. that information imparted in the clinic through a poster, a factsheet or minimal advice from a health care worker will rapidly result in a change in behaviour). This is in large part because the actual impact of free choice on behaviour is considerably less than most people imagine.

Understanding behaviour change

Sociology, genetics and neuroscience all make a significant contribution to shaping an individual's behaviour and their role needs to be considered and then addressed when aiming at changing a particular individual's behaviour:

- Sociology can help explain how personal decisions are largely governed by broad social structures such as socioeconomic category, gender and ethnicity.
- Genetics explains how behaviour choices (e.g. dietary intake, alcohol consumption and exercise) are in part determined biologically.
- Neuroscience explains how behaviours are often subconsciously influenced by the environment, with internal impulses and need for immediate rewards (e.g. through the dopamine brain system) underlying, for example, why individuals may engage in pleasurable but possibly unhealthy behaviours (e.g. the 'reward centre' of the brain valuing foods high in both fat and carbohydrates).

DOI: 10.4324/9781003306689-53

Understanding that behaviour is the result of both impulses and conscious reflection is important for triggering and supporting behaviour change. The PRIME theory of motivation (Box 48.1), for example recognizes the importance of a number of interlinked conscious and subconscious forces when it comes to smoking, alcohol use, exercising and dietary behaviours.

BOX 48.1   PRIME THEORY OF MOTIVATION[1]

PRIME theory proposes that **R**esponses are determined by a set of interlinked drivers:

- **P**lans – self-conscious intentions to behave in a particular way.
- **I**mpulses and inhibitions – both instinctive and learned.
- **M**otives – wants (imagined future states of the world with associated feelings of anticipated pleasure or satisfaction), and/or needs (imagined future states of the world with associated feelings of anticipated relief from distress or discomfort).
- **E**valuations – beliefs about what is good or bad, right or wrong, harmful or beneficial.

PRIME theory posits that individuals act in any single moment in the way that they most need or want or act. The primary drivers of behaviour, the impulse to act or inhibitions of impulse, are driven by competing wants and needs. Want represents desire, while a need is a negative emotion that is relieved by acting. In this context, the want to smoke competes with the need for relief of anxiety that is generated because higher cognitive functions, including evaluations of what is right or wrong, tell one that smoking is harmful.

Individual behavioural programmes for NCD prevention therefore need to recognize and martial forces to help people use their conscious reflective motivation and psychosocial resources to counteract those other drivers that they do not perceive to affect them, but which can derail attempts to change behaviour. The principle of behavioural programmes is thus to boost motivation and enhance the individual's capacity to change behaviour. Behaviour change often requires both a trigger and follow up supportive action.

Triggering behaviour change

Population-level interventions can trigger individual behaviour change by, for example, creating a strong sense that smoking is harmful and, in that sense, bad, and the need for relief from anxiety can trigger smoking cessation attempts.

Events such as New Year, or national no-smoking days, act to crystallize the need to act into an impulse to do so, capitalizing on this latent motivation. By concentrating on the value of the momentary impulse, dual process theory prompts public health agencies to provide programmes, often light-touch interventions, that crystallize latent motivation to change behaviour by providing prompts.

Very brief (<2 minutes) opportunistic counselling[2,3] for smoking, unhealthy diet and obesity and harmful alcohol consumption are effective,[4,5,6,7] and can be cost-effective in triggering change,[8,9] while longer (up to 30-minute) counselling is required to increase physical activity.[10]

The behaviours of clinicians are similarly determined by competing for conscious and less conscious forces so that context-specific policies and incentives are needed to motivate them to trigger patients to change their behaviours.[11] In addition, clinicians may lack the knowledge and skills and resources (time and financial) to deliver the required interventions.

Supporting behaviour change

While brief counselling is useful to trigger behaviour change, broader behaviour support programmes are important to provide sustained support to individuals for maintaining their willpower and motivation and enable long-term behaviour change.

The momentary balance between wants and needs helps explains relapse and possible responses to reduce relapse. Take the example of smoking, at every moment where smoking is possible, the 'need not to smoke' has to be strong enough to overcome the 'want to smoke'. This means that inhibition must overcome the impulse to smoke at all times. This is particularly important given that if smoking occurs, this will immediately interfere with the neuroadaptation to non-smoking with a rapid return to needing to smoke. Secondary cognitive factors, such as catastrophizing in response to a lapse, will also kick in and undermine motivation by lowering a person's perception of their capability to maintain abstinence and, again, it is important to discuss those aspects with the individual concerned to help them find adequate responses.

This 'quit attempt' model applies to alcohol, but less so to losing weight. Unlike smoking and alcohol, weight loss does not easily lead to neuroadaptation to the lower body weight state because obesity is less of a learnt addiction. Biological forces that regulate appetite (e.g. the adipocyte-gut-brain neuro-hormonal loops) and energy balance (e.g. resting metabolic rate, which decreases in response to body weight loss) tend to lead to long-term weight regain (i.e. a 'reset' to status quo ante) when the attempt ceases. This explains why most people who lose weight in the short term regain it (often within months). Therefore the aim is to strengthen motivation in maintaining the new behaviour and sticking to behavioural rules that can help with robust habit formation and thereby protect against relapse.

Behavioural support programmes aim to identify and equip individuals with resources to combat the forces of compulsions, urge or craving, which are often cue-provoked or habitual, and can be highly distressing (e.g. smoking). Behavioural support programmes also help patients identify and address the challenges associated with broader social and physical environments. Such barriers are also important in understanding why those from lower educational and socioeconomic groups find it more difficult to change their behaviour.

A successful behavioural support programme includes:

- *Setting a goal*, both the end goal and intermediary behavioural goals.
- *Creating an action plan*. This is sometimes referred to as 'implementation intentions', which helps people make specific plans for how, when and where key behaviours should be enacted, and plan for what to do if those initial plans are interrupted or deviated.[12]
- *Monitoring and feedback*. While this can increase effectiveness (e.g. measuring body weight every day), it can also undermine motivation because it reinforces notions of guilt and shame when the expected change does not occur. Programmes should therefore frame behaviour change as a learning opportunity that will include successes and failures, with self-experimentation at its heart.[13]

Behavioural support programmes are often provided by specialists, either face-to-face or remotely via telephone or digital devices. Behavioural support programmes have been shown to be effective in reducing intake of alcohol, quitting smoking and treating obesity, but there is less evidence that such programmes improve long-term physical activity.[14,15,16] Clinicians are increasingly looking to prescribe behavioural interventions[17] (e.g. face-to-face or digital tobacco quit support services, gym subscriptions, pedometer-based programmes or a written prescription for regular walking every week).[18]

A number of medications can improve the success of behaviour change attempts. Medications for smoking cessation reduce the intensity of the urge to smoke and are of modest cost, with nicotine replacement treatment being included in the WHO essential medications list. Medications to support alcohol abstinence (e.g. disulfiram) are usually prescribed in specialist settings, such as addiction services, as these drugs can cause unpleasant effects if alcohol is consumed in any amount. Medications for obesity are effective (particularly GLP-1 agonists that act on appetite regulation and can reduce body weight by up to 15% (Chapter 10 on obesity), but are costly, which currently limits their use.

Individual interventions to improve medication adherence

Behavioural interventions to improve medication adherence require action from/by: (i) health policy and practice (e.g. whether training in delivering behavioural interventions is available (ii) patient-health care provider interactions and social support (e.g. where a trusted long-term patient-doctor relationship is available); and (iii) the patient themselves (e.g. science literacy and education).

Adherence rates vary, not just between individuals, but also within individuals, over time and for different treatments. For this reason, interventions to improve a patient's adherence should focus on understanding the interactions between the individual, the individual's life context and the particular disease/treatment. Non-adherence often results from patient's beliefs (possibly echoing those that are socially or culturally prevalent in a particular setting), e.g. how individuals judge their personal need for the treatment (necessity beliefs, e.g. 'Do I really need this treatment?') relative to their concerns about potential negative consequences (e.g. side effects, stigma, interference in daily life, financial cost). From a patient's perspective, non-adherence is often 'logical', given their understanding of the condition(s), experiences and expectations of symptoms (e.g. absence of symptoms associated with hypertension and dyslipidaemia) and background beliefs (e.g. suspicions of medicines in general and/or the pharmaceutical industry more broadly, or concerns about dependence), even if these are not substantiated by evidence.

One approach shown to be cost-effective in increasing adherence to treatment is the Perceptions and Practicalities Approach[19,20,21] (Box 48.2), which can also be delivered digitally.[22]

BOX 48.2 THE PERCEPTIONS AND PRACTICALITIES APPROACH (PAPA)

- A patient-centred, 'no-blame' approach that encourages patients to reveal and discuss treatment doubts and concerns and that patients' beliefs and preferences influence the way treatment is prescribed.
- Three essential components:
    - Providing a 'common-sense' rationale for treatment necessity that takes account of patients' perceptions of the illness (including current and long-term consequences), their experiences, expectations, and answers to the two fundamental questions that constitute a necessary belief: *'Why do I need to do this to achieve a goal that is important to me?'* and *'Can I get away without doing it?'*.
    - Eliciting and addressing concerns.
    - Making it as easy and convenient as possible to adhere by attending to practicalities influencing the ability to adhere.
- A range of behaviour change techniques can be applied to elicit and address perceptions and practicalities (e.g. misconceptions and concerns) and practical barriers (e.g. limitations in capability and resources).
- Interventions can be integrated into more comprehensive approaches that also address environmental and societal causes of non-adherence.

The importance of policy frameworks to support individual behaviour change programmes

Policies are required to create and implement behavioural interventions in routine health care services (e.g. protocols, training, and structures that support brief interventions), which imply that these interventions are explicitly and adequately costed and funded and routinely provided within health care services.[23] More broadly, behaviour change programmes at health care level are more likely to be successful where population-level policies and programmes are in place to encourage the individual to embark on healthy behaviour (e.g. cities that encourage cycling, walking and public transport; bans on indoor smoking; and taxes on tobacco, alcohol and sugar-sweetened beverages).

Similarly, policy needs to support monitoring of service delivery to assess the provision of behaviour change interventions, and related training for health care providers about these interventions.[24] Such monitoring can drive up quality standards of service delivery. The provision of behavioural interventions, particularly among individuals with NCD risk factors, should be assessed in population-based surveys (e.g. STEPS) and surveys of health services (e.g. SARA, including the protocols used).

Notes

1 West R, Michie S. UBC briefing 9: a brief description of the PRIME theory of human motivation, London: Unlocking Behaviour Change, 2019.
2 Krist AH et al. Interventions for tobacco smoking cessation in adults, including pregnant persons: US Preventive Services Task Force Recommendation Statement. *JAMA* 2021;325:265–79.
3 Alcohol-use disorders: prevention. Public health guideline [PH24]. NICE, 2010.
4 Kaner EFS et al. Effectiveness of brief alcohol interventions in primary care populations. *Cochrane Database Syst Rev* 2018;2:CD004148.
5 Stead LF et al. Physician advice for smoking cessation. *Cochrane Database Syst Rev* 2008;2:Cd000165.
6 Aveyard P et al. Screening and brief intervention for obesity in primary care: a parallel, two-arm, randomised trial. *Lancet* 2016;388:2492–500.
7 Hardeman W et al. Evaluation of a very brief pedometer-based physical activity intervention delivered in NHS health checks in England: The VBI randomised controlled trial. *PLOS Med* 2020;17:e1003046.
8 Retat L et al. Screening and brief intervention for obesity in primary care: cost-effectiveness analysis in the BWeL trial. *Int J Obes* 2019;43:2066–75.
9 Solberg LI et al. Repeated tobacco-use screening and intervention in clinical practice: health impact and cost effectiveness. *Am J Prev Med* 2006;31:62–71.
10 Lamming L et al. What do we know about brief interventions for physical activity that could be delivered in primary care consultations? A systematic review of reviews. *Prev Med* 2017;99:152–63.
11 Williams SJ, Calnan M. Perspectives on prevention: the views of general practitioners. *Sociology Health & Illness* 1994;16:372–93.
12 Sheeran P. Intention—behavior relations: a conceptual and empirical review. *Eur Rev Soc Psychol* 2002;12:1–36.
13 Kangovi S, Asch DA. Behavioral phenotyping in health promotion: embracing or avoiding failure. *JAMA* 2018;319:2075–76.

14 Curry SJ et al. Behavioral weight loss interventions to prevent obesity-related morbidity and mortality in adults: US Preventive Services Task Force Recommendation Statement. *JAMA* 2018;320:1163–71.
15 Curry SJ et al. Screening and behavioral counseling interventions to reduce unhealthy alcohol use in adolescents and adults: US Preventive Services Task Force Recommendation Statement. *JAMA* 2018;320:1899–909.
16 Mangione CM et al. Behavioral counseling to promote a healthful diet and physical activity for cardiovascular disease prevention in adults without cardiovascular risk factors: US Preventive Services Task Force Recommendation Statement. *JAMA* 2017;318:167–74.
17 Thornton JS et al. Physical activity prescription: a critical opportunity to address a modifiable risk factor for the prevention and management of chronic disease: a position statement by the Canadian Academy of Sport and Exercise Medicine. *Clin J Sport Med* 2016;26:259–65.
18 Gc VS et al. Cost-effectiveness and value of information analysis of brief interventions to promote physical activity in primary care. *Value Health* 2018;21:18–26.
19 Horne R et al. Supporting adherence to medicines for long-term conditions: a perceptions and practicalities approach based on an extended common-sense model. *Eur Psychol* 2019;24:82–96.
20 Clifford S et al. Patient-centred advice is effective in improving adherence to medicines. *Pharm World Sci* 2006;28:165–70.
21 Elliott RA et al. The cost effectiveness of a telephone-based pharmacy advisory service to improve adherence to newly prescribed medicines. *Pharm World Sci* 2008;30:17–23.
22 Chapman S et al. Personalised adherence support for maintenance treatment of inflammatory bowel disease: a tailored digital intervention to change adherence-related beliefs and barriers. *J Crohns Colitis* 2020;14:1394–404.
23 van den Brand FA et al. Healthcare financing systems for increasing the use of tobacco dependence treatment. *Cochrane Database Syst Rev* 2017;9:CD004305.
24 Brose LS et al. Changes in success rates of smoking cessation treatment associated with take up of a national evidencebased training programme. *Prev Med* 2014;69:1–4.

49 Digital technologies for NCD prevention and control

*Surabhi Joshi, Cheick Oumar Bagayoko,
Awa Babington-Ashaye, Antoine Geissbuhler*

Digital health technologies are solutions that use technology to improve health and healthcare delivery, including the prevention and control of NCDs. Although digital technologies have been used in healthcare for decades, recent advances in network connectivity, cloud computing, the Internet of Things (IoT) and artificial intelligence (AI) have dramatically increased the potential efficacy and ability to scale up and their adoption. Definitions used in this chapter are provided in Box 49.1.

BOX 49.1 DEFINITION OF SELECTED TERMS

- *Digital health:* technology-aided and -enabled solutions for care delivery, disease management and promoting wellness.
- *Digital health technologies:* technology solutions used for digital health.
- *Artificial intelligence (AI):* the ability of a computer to do tasks that are usually done by humans because they require human intelligence and discernment, such as providing counselling and treatment recommendations based on specific patient conditions.
- *Blockchain:* an example of distributed ledger technology (DLT). DLT refers to technological infrastructure and protocols that allow the simultaneous access, validation and updating of records that use a computer network spread over multiple entities or locations. Unlike traditional databases, DLT has no central data store or administration functionality, which allows for information exchange without intermediaries and thus provides high levels of security and confidentiality.
- *Chatbot(s):* computer programme(s) designed to simulate conversation with human users, especially over the internet.
- *Data mining:* a process of extracting usable data from a larger set of raw data.
- *Internet of Things (IoT):* a system of interrelated computing devices, machines, objects or people that are provided with unique identifiers (UIDs), which have the ability to share data over a network

---

DOI: 10.4324/9781003306689-54

without requiring human-to-human or human-to-computer/device interactions.[1]
- *Interoperability:* refers to the capability of digital technologies to exchange and make use of data amongst each other based on common standards and norms.
- *mHealth:* a subset of digital health aimed at utilizing mobile technology to improve health outcomes.

Digital health and digital health technologies are an increasingly important part of the health system because if used effectively they can: (i) improve access to healthcare; (ii) reduce inefficiencies in the healthcare system; (iii) improve the quality of care; (iv) lower the cost of healthcare; (v) enable patient empowerment and education, and (vi) provide more personalized healthcare for patients.[2] Examples include:

- Strengthening coordination and continuity of care (e.g. electronic patient records, tools for improving clinical decisions, communication tools, telemedicine). This is particularly important for NCDs in order to enable healthcare providers to easily and quickly assess health behaviours, risk factors and clinical parameters (e.g. tobacco use, hypertension, diabetes, body mass index) of patients over time in order to calibrate counselling and treatment. In addition, centralized electronic systems are also very useful to get hold of data (e.g. blood pressure, medications, etc.) from patients when they attend healthcare at different providers.
- Enabling patient empowerment and education, in particular through the information that patients can seek on the internet (e.g. web sites advised by health providers, WHO, Wikipedia and other trusted websites), electronic games with strong educational potential (also known as 'serious games'), symptom checkers, chatbots, interactive social robots[3] and other behaviour change tools.
- Improving patient-reported outcome measurements (e.g. blood pressure [BP] or blood sugar self-measured by patients at home and which can be shared electronically and automatically with health providers to help adjust management).
- Training healthcare workers through electronic media (teleconferences, online tutorials, etc.)
- Strengthening the capacity of health professionals on the way they obtain and use data, e.g. for planning or real-time forecasting.

Strengthening the delivery of healthcare for NCD prevention and control

Digital technologies are primarily used by caregivers for patient data collection, care delivery and coordination through various levels of care delivery, as emphasized above. With regard to NCDs, which evolve over many years, electronic medical records (EMR) are particularly useful for maintaining and accessing patient data. In addition, EMR can record and track behavioural and physiological risk factors of individuals (e.g. tobacco or alcohol use, blood cholesterol and glucose levels, BP, body weight) that would not have been done and/or recorded if the caregiver had not been prompted to enter the data into the system. Software for EMR can also offer support in the clinical decision by making use of algorithms based on data and information on a patient (e.g. suggestions about differential diagnosis, reminders for preventive measures, further investigations required, treatment and potential adverse consequences to treatment). Teleconsultation (e.g. face to face consultations or access to radiological or cardiac investigation results) enables audio and/or video remote communication between patients and caregivers, either in real time or at a later date. Teleconsultation improves access to expert care for those in remote locations.

Example: The collaboration between Babyl (a healthcare services mobile app developed by a Rwandan private company) and the government of Rwanda led to the launch of video teleconsultation and SMS alert services in the country through government health centres.[4] To encourage the adoption and use of these electronic services, the government has extended insurance coverage for teleconsultations and worked with Babyl to establish protocols and standards (including safety procedures when sharing personal data with third parties) for the use of digital health services.

Example: The use of tele-expertise in Senegal in the fight against diabetic retinopathy. This activity, which was initiated by the Senegalese Ministry of Health with the support of WHO and the International Telecommunication Union (ITU), links diabetes clinics in remote areas to ophthalmologists of the Fann University Hospital in Dakar. The eye exams (e.g. eye fundus) are carried out by general practitioners, nurses or community health workers and results and/or images are sent to specialists for advice using the tele-expertise platform developed by the Francophone Africa Network of Telemedicine. The images and diagnoses are, in parallel, used to train an AI platform, with the goal of automatizing and improving the screening process.

Improving health promotion, health literacy and patient empowerment

In addition to information on health that individuals can find themselves on the internet, some advanced digital technologies are customer-facing and can support education, access to health records (e.g. when a patient can retrieve his/her medical data from the healthcare provider's website) and quality of life management. This includes promoting 'digital inclusion', which refers to the activities necessary to ensure that all individuals and communities, including the most disadvantaged, have access to and use of digital tools.[5] Examples of newer and potentially powerful technologies include medical chatbots, which use natural language processing to understand patient queries and AI to provide the responses to the queries. Chatbots vary in their level of sophistication and can range from informational, which only provides prerecorded responses to a limited number of patient queries, to prescriptive which used data mining and AI. Chatbots can also be used to support health literacy and encourage behavioural change.

Example: WHO Be He@lthy Be Mobile SMS programme in collaboration with the government of India for tobacco cessation. This was the world's largest mobile SMS-based initiative aimed at smoking cessation and had a documented quit rate of 7.2% after six months.[6] Another example is the use of remote patient monitoring devices (e.g. electronic devices that record patient vital signs, blood glucose or BP measurements), which can connect to other devices and mobile phones using IoT protocols (i.e. modes of communication that protect and ensure optimum security to the data being exchanged between connected devices). The data fed through these devices can then be used in advanced analytics and AI algorithms to identify patients at risk and suggest early interventions. Obviously, such systems that involve data exchanges with third parties require high levels of safety in terms of confidentially and use of data; this may be regulated at the national level by specific laws.

Strengthening health systems

Digital technologies are important tools to strengthen the infrastructure that covers network connectivity, cloud computing (i.e. the use of remote servers hosted on the internet to store, manage, and process data, rather than a local server or a personal computer), interactions with suppliers, regulators and insurance providers. Large government healthcare IT strategies and projects to collect and use vast quantities of patient data have not always been successful or cost-effective.[7,8]

Example: The World Bank is using blockchain to track shipments of prescription medication in order to increase the level of security and confidentiality when sharing data of patients with third parties. In this example, the aim is to reduce counterfeit drugs, theft and improve accountability in the prescription medication supply chains. While the issue of security is relevant for all diseases, it has particular importance for NCDs given the huge volumes of medication trade (e.g. hundreds of millions of patients worldwide need BP lowering medication for many years). An additional example is the use of multiple geospatial data sources and computerized models to improve the evaluation of the accessibility of healthcare facilities, and better inform strategies to scale-up healthcare services.[9]

Implementation challenges and mitigation strategies

Although digital technologies hold a huge potential for improving the quality of healthcare delivery and alleviating capacity constraints (e.g. to improve access and minimize long-term costs), there are a number of challenges associated with their adoption.

Costs and benefits

Digital technologies require a significant upfront investment in procurement, customization, training and management before benefits are realized. For example, implementing an EMR system could cost US$ 600 million for a large US hospital network.[10] In view of many challenges related to the deployment of reliable EMRs, the benefits of using digital technologies may not be straightforward, with some studies showing an overall benefit,[11,12] while others show a negative impact of digital technologies on quality of care outcomes.[13,14,15]

Implementation of digital technologies (including EMRs) is followed by a period of lower performance due to adaptation where organizational processes and the technology itself go through a series of updates before stable technology-mediated processes are streamlined. Additionally, some studies have also documented that the benefits of digital technologies may only be realized when they are fully integrated throughout the healthcare services instead of operating independently in silos. Hence, organizations adopting digital technologies should be aware of these challenges and be advised and guided by independent experts (i.e. not only by the manufacturers of the envisaged electronic systems) who have a large experience in implementing such systems.

Interoperability

Interoperability is the capability of digital technologies to exchange and make use of data amongst each other, based on common standards and norms. As discussed earlier, it is essential that multiple digital technologies can work in an integrated manner in order to maximize their full benefits. Interoperability is key to achieving this objective.

Technical interoperability ensures that multiple electronic systems can connect and exchange data fluently, reliably and safely. This is the main challenge as different health providers (e.g. public and private hospitals, government or private practitioners, pharmacies, etc.) often use different electronic systems and software that have been implemented at different times and can therefore not connect easily with each other.

Semantic interoperability ensures that the meaning of the data exchanged is understood properly by all systems. Interoperability can enable real-time alerts based on patient information, faster access to comprehensive EMRs, advanced data analytics, and better patient engagement, all of which can result in improved care delivery outcomes.

Achieving interoperability is challenging due to different data storage structures and terminologies used by different vendors, and customizations made by individual organizations. Standardized communication protocols, terminologies and formal descriptions of knowledge domains (ontologies) are necessary to achieve interoperability. When designing systems related to health, it is important to ensure that their developers are well aware of the existing main electronic systems and plans in a particular country used by the government and other main health care and allied providers.

Communication infrastructure

The cost and quality of the communication infrastructure (e.g. mobile broadband, internet connectivity) is also an impediment to the adoption and use of digital health technologies. This problem can be particularly pronounced in low- and middle-income countries, and in rural areas in other countries, where internet connectivity is very poor or inexistent. This provides opportunities for 'leap-frogging' using the latest technology. Digital health technologies often transmit high volumes of encrypted information amongst each other and across multiple connected devices. Often the information transmitted is comprised of high-resolution scans and images – requiring good internet connectivity and large bandwidth. Hence, government support in developing communication infrastructure can be critical to the successful adoption and use of digital technologies.

Regulatory challenges

Transformation to a technology-enabled or mediated healthcare delivery environment, which implies sharing individual data with third parties, needs to be supported by an adequate regulatory frame. There are a number of aspects that need supportive regulatory actions. For example, policymakers can incentivize organizations to adopt digital technologies by cost sharing with further monetary incentives based on milestones for technology usage. Such legislation (or legal agreements) may help organizations overcome challenges associated with the high cost of transformation, adoption, and integration of multiple digital technologies. An example of a legislative action along these lines is the HITECH Act – which was passed by the US Congress in 2009 and was aimed at incentivizing hospitals for the adoption and use of EMR technologies.

Further, legislation around patient safety, data privacy and interoperability standards are necessary conditions that can help enhance the adoption, use, safety, confidentiality and benefits of digital technologies. In some countries, these laws can be very restrictive and limit the use of personal data and/or require that patients provide informed consent on which use is done and for which specific data before data can be shared.

Resilience and safety of health systems

Data stored on servers and all interconnected devices (including IoT) may be cyber-attacked with consequences such as ransoms being asked by cybercriminals, data being wiped out or made public on the Darknet, and/or devices being made non-functional or destroyed. This has happened to many hospitals. This emphasizes that electronic platforms must be adequately secured, have the risk of cyber-attacks regularly assessed and analysed by specialized IT companies, whose work is to detect security weaknesses and address them including certification (security intelligence).[16] Healthcare professionals must specifically be trained on these issues.

Notes

1. Malhotra P et al. Internet of things: evolution, concerns and security challenges. *Sensors* 2021;21:1809.
2. Global strategy on digital health 2020–2025. WHO, 2021.
3. Bouchard K et al. The social robots are coming: preparing for a new wave of virtual care in cardiovascular medicine. *Circulation* 2022;145:1291–93.
4. LaRock Z. Telehealth unicorn Babylon signed a decade-long deal with the Rwandan government to give consumers free access to its services, 2020. Insider Inc. (Axel Springer). https://www.businessinsider.com/babylon-lands-10-year-deal-with-rwandan-government-2020-3.
5. Rodriguez JA et al. Digital inclusion as health care – supporting health care equity with digital-infrastructure initiatives. *NJEM* 2022;386;1101–03.
6. Gopinathan et al. Self-reported quit rates and quit attempts among subscribers of a mobile text messaging-based tobacco cessation programme in India. *BMJ Innov* 2018;4:147–54.
7. Godlee F. What can we salvage from care data? *BMJ* 2016;354:i3907.
8. Greenhalgh T, Bowden T. There is goes again. *BMJ* 2011;343:d5317.
9. Lyer HS et al. Geospatial evaluation of trade-offs between equity in physical access to healthcare and health systems efficiency. *BMJ Glob Health* 2020;5:e003493.
10. Barlas S. Hospitals scramble to meet deadlines for adopting electronic health records: pharmacy systems will be updated slowly but surely. *Pharmacy & Therapeutics* 2011;36:37.
11. Jha AK et al. Use of electronic health records in US hospitals. *NEJM* 2019;360:1628–38.
12. McCullough JS et al. The effect of health information technology on quality In U.S. hospitals. *Health Affairs* 2010;29:647–54.
13. Koppel R et al. Role of computerized physician order entry systems in facilitating medication errors. *JAMA* 2005;293:1197–203.
14. Linder JA et al. Electronic health record use and the quality of ambulatory care in the United States. *Arch Intern Med* 2007;167:1400–05.
15. DesRoches CM et al. Electronic health records' limited successes suggest more targeted uses. *Health Affairs* 2010;29:639–46.
16. Kim Y et al. Analysis of cyber attacks and security intelligence. In Park J et al. (eds.), *Mobile, ubiquitous, and intelligent computing -lecture notes 274, in electrical engineering* (pp. 489–94). Berlin, Heidelberg: Springer-Verlag, 2014.

50 Effective communication for NCD prevention and control

Jaimie Guerra, Elorm Ametepe, Pascal Bovet, Nick Banatvala

Public health communication has been described as 'the scientific development, strategic dissemination, and critical evaluation of relevant, accurate, accessible, and understandable health information communicated to and from intended audiences to advance the health of the public'.[1] Disciplines that contribute to public health communication include communication, health education, commercial and social marketing,[2] journalism, public relations, psychology and behavioural science, informatics and epidemiology.

When well-conceived, carefully implemented and sustained over time, public health communication programmes have the capacity to elicit change among individuals and populations by raising awareness, increasing knowledge, shaping attitudes, promoting motivation and ultimately changing behaviours. Without public health communication campaigns that effectively explain why and how people should adopt healthy behaviours, many of the interventions described throughout this compendium are less likely to be translated into significant health gain, even in environments that are supportive for promoting public health. In addition to promoting healthy behaviours among those targeted, public health communication initiatives can also help change social norms and promote policy changes that promote a more conducive environment for people to adopt healthy behaviours.

Public health communication can be factual (e.g. 'salt increases your blood pressure'), elicit fear (e.g. 'smoking kills', 'bigger snacks, bigger slacks'), encourage action (e.g. providing a telephone number for tobacco cessation services, or urging people to get their blood pressure tested) or highlighting benefit (e.g. 'kiss a non-smoker, enjoy the difference', or 'with a healthy heart, the beat goes on'). The impact can be greatest by using a mix of these. Communication needs to use channels appropriate for the audience; in the 2020s, this increasingly means the use of social media rather than print, which for many belongs to a bygone era.

Too often, health communication campaigns are paternalistic, with one-way communication from 'beneficent' experts to passive audiences.[3] To be effective, communication programmes need to be consistent with the audience's ideas, needs and values.[4] This requires an understanding of the audience's health literacy, culture and diversity. Communication campaigns are

DOI: 10.4324/9781003306689-55

more likely to be effective when there is two-way communication between promoters and receivers to ensure that messages are accessed, understood and acceptable, and that communities are involved and invested in the aims of the programmes, and that messages are modified as needed.

This chapter describes: (i) the challenge of communicating about NCDs and their risk factors; (ii) the principles of effective communication and targeting the audience; (iii) the role and impact of mass media campaigns; and (iv) the opportunities and challenges of social media.

The challenge of communicating on NCDs

The term 'noncommunicable diseases' is a barrier to communication in the first place. Although widely used by public health and policy professions, especially at global, regional and national levels, most people do not easily understand what is meant by the term NCDs.[5,6] The term unfortunately suggests what the diseases are not (i.e. 'noncommunicable') rather than what they are (disease of the heart and blood vessels, cancer, chronic lung disease or diabetes). This makes NCDs a difficult and unexciting concept to grasp, resonate with and raise attention and resources for. People do not talk about having an NCD, they talk about having a heart attack, a stroke or diabetes. Or breast, cervical or prostate cancer. Or chronic bronchitis or asthma. Similarly, people do not think in terms of NCD risk factors, but rather of having high blood pressure or raised blood cholesterol, or being overweight, or smoking or drinking too much alcohol.

Even focusing on specific diseases or risk factors can be a challenge. Those with risk factors or engaging in unhealthy behaviour may be asymptomatic. Furthermore, the impact of behaviour change (or adherence to treatment for NCDs) at a population level may not be guaranteed for the individual concerned (e.g. some people with a healthy diet or taking antihypertensive treatment may still have a heart attack and there will be some smokers that live to old age).

Nevertheless, behaviour change can result in rapid benefits for many (e.g. quitting smoking leading to improved respiratory function, a reduction in flare-ups of bronchitis, financial savings; reducing intake of alcohol leading to better physical and mental health; losing weight and increasing physical activity leading to a reduction in blood pressure and looking and feeling better, with enhanced self-esteem). Such 'quick wins' are important to emphasize in health education campaigns.

Explaining to patients, policymakers and funders that long-term treatment for hypertension will reduce the risk of stroke by a given percentage over the next ten years is a considerably greater challenge than explaining that antimicrobial or antiviral therapy will be effective in treating infection over a short period.

Attempts have been made to frame NCDs as a health security issue,[7,8] but this has not had the same level of resonance as has been the case for infectious diseases.

Principles of effective communication

To communicate effectively, language and terminology must resonate with the audience and be as simple, concise and concrete as possible. There is also only a finite capacity to take on board new information: today, individuals are subjected to more information in one day than people were in their entire life a few generations ago, hence the need to provide clear and easily digestible information in a convincing and attractive way. Humour can also play an important role. Many people will pay attention to an issue for just a few seconds, especially when the message was not solicited by the individual. To date, the NCD agenda has largely been led by professionals, where complexity is recognized and even celebrated. However effective public health communication requires that this model is inverted: messages must be simple, clear and unambiguous. Messages must be able to resonate immediately given the myriad of competing information individuals receive every day. Key principles for effective communication are accessibility, actionability, credibility, relevance, timeliness and understandability.[9]

Finger-wagging, paternalistic approaches that are negative or judgemental are unlikely to result in behaviour change (and may be counterproductive, particularly among youth), particularly when the environment is not conducive to changing behaviour. Consistent, positive, empowering messaging at the right time and in a sustained way is more likely to succeed in a supportive environment (e.g. a '5 a day' campaign encouraging people to eat five portions of fruit and vegetables a day is more likely to succeed where they are accessible and affordable, and local social media and influencers are promoting appealing ways of eating them). Educational campaigns to alert individuals to the risks of an unhealthy diet (which may be seen by the public as boring and negative) are unlikely to have a large impact if other media are providing (exciting and positive) messages on the undoubted instant pleasure that can be derived from the same unhealthy behaviour (e.g. consuming a sugar-sweetened beverage, or a cream cake). Messages should therefore emphasize opportunities for 'healthy' pleasure (e.g. 'more herbs, less salt') or encourage positive action (e.g. 'eat wise, drop a size', 'commit to be fit', 'walk the talk'). Again, these will be more effective where regulatory and other interventions are in place to reduce marketing on unhealthy alternatives.

Targeting the right audiences in the right way

There are a number of audiences when it comes to NCDs. The first group include: (i) people living with cardiovascular disease, diabetes, cancer and/or chronic respiratory disease; (ii) those with risk factors (or at high risk) of one or more of these conditions; and (iii) the rest of the (healthy) population. The second group includes community leaders, including social and other influencers. The third groups are health professionals. The fourth group includes policymakers across government and society, including development partners.

Identifying the key message for the targeted audience is critical as this determines the tools that will be used (e.g. social media, television, radio, newspapers, flyers, letters, petitions), the approaches (advertising and marketing, mail shots, detailed reports) and the content and tone of the message.

Many communication experts highlight the importance of having a single overarching communication outcome/objective (SOCO). Developing this requires an understanding of: (i) what the issue is; (iii) why focus on this issue – and why now; (iii) who needs to change behaviour (that is the target audience); (iv) what change is required, and (v) the benefits that will ensue. There is little point in trying to communicate public health messages if it is unclear why the issue is important to the audience, and why the audience should care, i.e. how the change will benefit them and/or those around them (e.g. the benefit of quitting tobacco for their unborn child, or quitting will make them more attractive; or implementing a policy change will enable a government official to meet his or her annual objectives and result in career progression).

It is also important to be aware of (and have plans for managing) different groups that can impact the outcomes being targeted (Table 50.1).

A communication strategy should aim to actively engage with champions and influencers, shift blockers to avoiders, shift avoiders to silent boosters and shift silent boosters to champions.

Mass media campaigns

These are widely used to expose high proportions of large populations to messages repeatedly, over time, at a low cost per head, through adequate media including television, radio, social media and print media. Exposure is generally passive, particularly with traditional media (newspapers, billboards, television). In contrast, social media allow more active participation of the targeted audience, and evaluation of the campaign can include levels of user engagement.

Educating the public about the harms of smoking/tobacco use and second-hand smoke, reducing salt intake across the population and increased physical activity, alongside other community-based education, motivational and environmental programmes aimed at supporting behavioural change, are all WHO best buys. Mass media campaigns on healthy diets, including social marketing to reduce the intake of total fat, saturated fats, sugars and salt, and

Table 50.1 Stakeholder or audience analysis for a single overarching communication outcome/objective (SOCO)

Blockers (active resisters): those with high energy levels and disagree with the SOCO.	**Champions** (active supporters): those with high energy levels that agree with the SOCO.
Avoiders (passive resisters): those with low energy levels and disagree with the SOCO.	**Silent boosters** (passive supporters): those with low energy levels that agree with the SOCO.

promoting the intake of vegetables and fruits is a recommended intervention. Further details on the impact of behaviour change from mass media campaigns targeting the prevention and treatment of NCDs are available elsewhere.[10]

Mass media campaigns can work by targeting the individual directly (e.g. to quit smoking or do more physical activity) or indirectly (e.g. individuals that have not seen the campaign can be influenced to change behaviour by those that have been exposed to the campaign).[10] Mass media campaigns (particularly those through social media) can also prompt public discussion of health issues that can collectively lead to changes in public policy (e.g. a campaign discouraging smoking because of its second-hand effects on non-smokers may increase public support for a new policy that restricts smoking in specific places).

The resources that the private sector has for large-scale, highly researched, intensive and sustained commercial marketing campaigns, largely exceed those available for public sector health campaigns. Where there is alignment between public health messages across private sector entities (e.g. sports goods industry and businesses specializing in healthy foods and drinks) and public health authorities, there may be opportunities to work together (Chapter 57).

The role of social media in the prevention and control of NCDs

Social media, mobile technologies and access to the internet have revolutionized communication, providing low-cost, powerful tools for communicating issues around NCD prevention and management.[11] Social media include social networking platforms, e.g. Facebook/Meta,[12] YouTube, Instagram, Twitter, LinkedIn, TikTok, which all have enormous global reach (each having over one billion users). Message and chat applications (including some of the above as well as WhatsApp, Snapchat, Telegram, Signal, WeChat, Skype, Viber) are viewed and used by billions of people daily. Together, these media are often seen/used by individuals for several hours each day. Social media therefore provides significant opportunities for health education and information sharing, and can provide social, peer or psychological support, encourage self-care and self-management, support public health campaigns, promote health professionals' capacity building, and endorse and support policymaking.[13,14]

Despite the opportunities described above, there remains limited evidence, so far, in terms of the impact of social media on NCD prevention and management. Furthermore, social media have a number of risks and challenges, including: (i) mix of high- and low-quality information (with users often unable to distinguish unreferenced, inadequate or misleading information, often focusing on and amplifying individual, sensational, overly emotional or controversial stories or indeed 'fake news', bad stories or misinformation, which can quickly become widely circulated and 'viral'); (ii) patient confidentiality and privacy; (iii) risks to professional reputation;[15] (iv) commercial interests (e.g. food and beverage marketing on social media and some 'influencers' or users who promote unhealthy behaviours); (v) lack of monitoring and regulation; and (vi) equity of access, magnifying the digital divide.[13]

Monitoring and evaluation

Regular assessments of communication campaigns are important to determine how and to what extent strategies and activities are reaching the targeted audiences and what impact they are making. Examples of frameworks and guides are available, that assess the relationship between inputs, activities, outputs, outcomes and impact.[16,17] A challenge is that the impact of awareness on healthy behaviour campaigns targeting the population as the benefit of NCDs (or risk factors) is often distant in time and influenced by many other factors and process indicators are therefore often used, e.g. rapid telephone surveys to assess how many people have heard about the campaign and any action taken as a result.[18] A protocol for the systematic review of reviews evaluating the effectiveness of mass media interventions for the prevention and control of NCDs has recently been developed.[19]

Notes

1 Bernhardt JM. Communication at the core of effective public health. *Am J Public Health* 2004;94:2051–3.
2 Hunt L. How social marketing differs from commercial marketing. San Diego: Civilian (web site).
3 Guttman N. *Public Health Communication Interventions: Values and Ethical Dilemmas.* Thousand Oaks, CA: Sage Publications, 2000.
4 Institute of Medicine. *Speaking of Health: Assessing Health Communication Strategies for Diverse Populations.* Washington, DC: National Academy Press, 2002.
5 Adjaye-Gbewonyo K, Vaughan M. Reframing NCDs? An analysis of current debates. *Glob Health Action* 2019;12:1641043.
6 Dugan A. Global study: harm from noncommunicable diseases underrated. Gallup Blog. 21 September 2022. https://news.gallup.com/opinion/gallup/401279/global-study-harm-from-noncommunicable-diseases-underrated.aspx
7 Three Ways NCDs Impact Global Health Security. US Centres for Disease Control and Prevention, 2018.
8 Saha A, Alleyne G. Recognizing noncommunicable diseases as a global health security threat. *Bull WHO* 2018;96:792–3.
9 Principles for effective communications. WHO, https://www.who.int/about/communications/principles.
10 Wakefield MA et al. Use of mass media campaigns to change health behaviour. *Lancet* 2010;376:1261–71.
11 Hawn C. Take two aspirin and tweet me in the morning: how Twitter, Facebook, and other social media are reshaping health care. *Health Aff* 2009;28:361–8.
12 Menefee HK et al. Mechanisms of communicating health information through Facebook: implications for consumer health information technology design. *J Med Internet Res* 2016;18:e5949.
13 Islam SMS et al. The role of social media in preventing and managing non-communicable diseases in low-and-middle income countries: hope or hype? *Health Policy and Technol* 2019;8:96–101.
14 Freeman B et al. Social media campaigns that make a difference: what can public health learn from the corporate sector and other social change marketers? *Public Health Res Pract* 2015;25:e2521517.

15 Bernhardt JM. A social media primer for professionals: digital dos and don'ts. *Health Promot Pract* 2014;15:168–72.
16 Evaluate complex campaigns. WHO, https://www.who.int/about/communications/evaluation/campaigns-evaluation.
17 Asibey E et al. Are we there yet? A Communications Evaluation Guide. Naperville, IL: The Communications Network, 2008.
18 Bovet P et al. Impact and cost of a 2-week community-based screening and awareness program for diabetes and cardiovascular risk factors in a Swiss canton. *Diabetes Metab Syndr Obes* 2011;4:213–23.
19 Jeet G et al. Protocol for a systematic review of reviews evaluating effectiveness of mass media interventions for prevention and control of non-communicable diseases. *BMJ Open* 2020;10:e032611.

51 NCD prevention and control in emergencies and humanitarian settings

*Éimhín Ansbro, Nick Banatvala,
Sylvia Kehlenbrink, Kiran Jobanputra*

Over 80 million people across the world are displaced from their homes as a result of conflict or natural disasters.[1] Displacement may be due to an acute event or a chronic situation, which can last many years or even decades. As with any population, a significant proportion of those displaced are living with NCDs or are at risk of developing NCDs. Displaced populations may be particularly vulnerable during crises due to poor health and limited access to healthcare prior to their displacement. Furthermore, displacement itself increases the risk of poor health outcomes for people with NCDs and creates specific challenges for health systems and for those providing emergency or long-term medical humanitarian assistance (Box 51.1).[2] In addition, refugees and internally displaced people (IDPs) are likely to have reduced social capital and limited access to community resources, such as labour markets, education, healthcare and social welfare systems, further undermining their health and wellbeing.[3]

BOX 51.1 CHALLENGES AND STRESSES FOR NCD PREVENTION AND CONTROL AMONG DISPLACED POPULATIONS

- Populations experiencing humanitarian emergencies are likely to have a greater incidence of NCD complications (e.g. cardiovascular mortality may be up to 2–3 times greater during a humanitarian emergency).[4,5]
- Access and continuity of healthcare may be poor, with limited available diagnostic facilities and treatment, resulting in increased mortality due to acute complications (e.g. diabetic ketoacidosis in type-1 diabetes or myocardial infarction in cardiovascular disease) or increased morbidity and poorer long-term health due to interruptions in long-term treatment (e.g. development of irreversible disability in type-2 diabetes).
- NCDs may lead to disability (for example, impaired vision due to diabetes or mobility problems due to cardiovascular disease), limiting

---

DOI: 10.4324/9781003306689-56

an individual's resilience to cope with displacement or another type of emergency.
- Displaced populations are also more likely to be exposed to NCD risk factors because of the psychosocial stresses of displacement as well as exposure to violence, disrupted social support and marginalization. This may lead to increased tobacco use, harmful use of alcohol, unhealthy diet, lack of opportunity for physical activity, and degradation of environmental conditions, with the inhalation of smoke and other toxic chemicals.

Legal frameworks and mandates

Whilst, in principle, refugees (those crossing international boundaries) can access a number of services as a result of internationally binding legal frameworks and treaties, including the provision of healthcare, these frameworks do not apply to IDPs (those that do not cross a country boundary) who, therefore, are not assured of the same protections. Nevertheless, the political declarations from the high-level meetings on NCDs, the UN Economic and Social Council (ECOSOC) and World Health Assembly resolutions[6] and the WHO Global NCD Action Plan highlight the impact of NCDs on refugees and IDPs, and the need to ensure that they can access appropriate prevention, treatment and care.

Agencies with mandates to support the health of those caught up in emergencies include governments (both those hosting displaced populations and those that channel support through their development assistance programmes), UN agencies, such as the UN Refugee Agency (UNHCR), UN Relief and Works Agency for Palestinian Refugees (UNRWA) and WHO. A number of (non-mandated) international organizations such as the International Committee of the Red Cross (ICRC), the International Federation of Red Cross and Red Crescent Societies (IFRC), Médecins sans Frontières (MSF), International Rescue Committee and Save the Children, as well as local civil society organizations are also key providers of healthcare in humanitarian crises. The WHO Cluster System has been developed to enhance collaboration and coordination between these various agencies on the ground.[7]

Key actions to ensure that populations in humanitarian settings have access to NCD prevention and care

Over the last two decades, humanitarian actors have adapted their models of healthcare for emergencies, which traditionally focused on acute episodic care for malnutrition, reproductive health and communicable diseases, to better address the chronic care requirements of NCDs. The Sphere handbook sets out actions to ensure that populations in humanitarian settings have access to preventive programmes, diagnostics and essential therapies for acute complications and long-term management of NCDs (Box 51.2).[8]

BOX 51.2 KEY ACTIONS TO ENSURE THAT POPULATIONS IN HUMANITARIAN SETTINGS HAVE ACCESS TO NCD PREVENTIVE AND TREATMENT SERVICES

1. Identify the NCD health needs and analyse the availability of services pre-crisis.
   - Identify groups with priority needs, including those at risk of life-threatening complications, such as insulin-dependent diabetes or severe asthma.

2. Implement phased-approach programmes based on life-saving priorities and relief of suffering.
   - Ensure patients diagnosed with life-threatening complications (for example, severe asthma attack, diabetic ketoacidosis) receive appropriate care, including palliative and supportive care.
   - Avoid sudden treatment disruption for patients diagnosed before the crisis.

3. Integrate NCD care into the health system at all levels.
   - Establish a referral system to manage acute complications and complex cases in secondary or tertiary care, and to palliative and supportive care.
   - Refer patients for nutrition or food security responses where required.

4. Establish national preparedness programmes for NCDs.
   - Include essential medicines and supplies in pre-positioned or contingency emergency medical supplies.
   - Prepare individual patients with a backup supply of medications and instructions on where to access emergency care should a crisis occur.

Despite this, NCD care remains inadequate in humanitarian settings. The remainder of this chapter describes key actions for strengthening NCD care in humanitarian emergencies.

Strengthening NCD care across the Humanitarian Programming Cycle

The humanitarian programming cycle (HPC) was developed by the Inter-Agency Standing Committee and is used widely by humanitarian agencies. It divides the emergency humanitarian response into phases consisting of preparedness and readiness, needs assessment and analysis, strategic planning, resource mobilization, implementation and monitoring, and evaluation and early recovery.[9] WHO and other agencies have highlighted the gaps and priorities for integrating NCD care into the HPC.[10] We highlight priorities for strengthening the operational response across the HPC phases.

Preparedness and readiness

Disaster and Emergency Response Plans should include ensuring: national NCD profile and capacity assessment completeness; health facility readiness; and availability of essential medicines/equipment, including those for NCDs.[11] Individualized NCD patient strategies for emergencies should be in place, including the availability of backup medicine supplies and the identification of alternative sources of clinical care. Attention should be given to the provision of emergency care for NCDs, including forming pre-established partnerships (e.g. the Renal Disaster Relief Task Force and Insulin for Life). Importantly, NCDs should be included in national disaster risk analysis initiatives.

Needs assessment and analysis

Up-to-date information is required on population demographics and baseline epidemiology, existing health services and infrastructure, access and barriers to NCD-specific services (human resources, medicines, equipment) at different healthcare levels, referral pathways and transport, procurement and supply chains, and existing NCD-related health information systems (patient files, registers, health information systems). Preliminary information on NCDs in countries that have humanitarian crises can be obtained through a desk review of WHO NCD country profiles, STEPS surveys (Chapter 5) and interagency data. In addition, the Multi-Sector Initial Rapid Assessment (MIRA)[12] can be used to provide real-time information on immediate needs. Health Resources and Services Availability Monitoring System (HeRAMS) and the Health Cluster 3/4W (who, what, where, when) tool can provide a rapid overview of response capacity.[13]

Strategic response planning

This involves defining priority NCD programme elements for inclusion in the global response, defining the service delivery model, and planning the transition to the protracted (or recovery) phase of the emergency. In contrast to some health domains (such as reproductive health), there is no agreed set of priority activities or Minimum Initial Service Package (MISP)[14] for NCDs in the emergency response phase. However, WHO South-East Asia Regional Office guidance on the integration of NCD care in emergency response and preparedness[15] and WHO operational guidance on maintaining essential services during the COVID-19 pandemic provides a list of priorities for NCD care that could apply to many humanitarian contexts.[16] The informal interagency NCD working group has developed operational guidance for NCD care in emergencies that can support the definition of the service delivery model. This includes: (i) triage, lifesaving and follow-up care – including referral pathways; (ii) prevention, including health promotion and patient education, including reducing the risk of COVID-19 (as people living with NCDs are at increased risk of developing the disease and complications); (iii) community engagement; (iv) training; and (v) surveillance and record keeping, including the importance of data protection.[17]

Minimizing mortality is the immediate priority. People living with NCDs (who are often neglected in crises) may be triaged as follows: first, those with life-threatening conditions (e.g. severe asthma crisis, heart attack, diabetic ketoacidosis, as well as those requiring pain relief, including for palliative care); second, those at immediate risk of complications if care is not given or is interrupted (e.g. insulin-dependent diabetes, unstable angina); third, those that are stable but at risk from treatment interruption (e.g. antihypertensive or anticoagulant therapy); and, finally, those that are undiagnosed and symptomatic.

Resource mobilization

An NCD Emergency Health Kit has been developed and included in the Inter-Agency Emergency Health Kit. Each NCD kit includes primary care treatment for hypertension, cardiac conditions, diabetes, and chronic respiratory diseases for a population of 10,000 for a three-month period, with medicines in line with the 2015 WHO Essential Medicines List and WHO package of essential noncommunicable disease (WHO PEN) interventions for primary care in low-resource settings. The effectiveness of the NCD kit is under evaluation. WHO PEN provides simplified clinical algorithms which can be used to reinforce staff training on NCD care.

Implementation and monitoring

In the post-acute or protracted phase of an emergency, NCD care should be expanded to include the management of sub-acute and chronic presentations of previously identified NCDs, providing ongoing care and palliation. Once the initial package of services is implemented, a more comprehensive assessment of needs should be undertaken, and services expanded to manage those treated before the emergency for conditions such as non-insulin dependent diabetes, coronary artery disease, hypertension, cancer or chronic respiratory disease. The decision to actively seek out previously undetected or asymptomatic cases will depend on the capacity of healthcare services.

The management of NCDs should be integrated into existing primary healthcare services from the start of the response or as soon as possible, with resources used to strengthen national systems. Where this is not possible, humanitarian agencies may provide services directly or support public services. Referral pathways should be rapidly established, but will depend on resources and context.[18] In countries where much of the day-to-day NCD care is delivered at the secondary/tertiary level, efforts should be made to reorient care to the more cost-effective primary care level, with rapid scale-up of staff training.

Several organizations (MSF, ICRC) have developed ready-to-use clinical guidance for NCD care in the context of humanitarian emergencies.[19] A package of essential NCD interventions for humanitarian settings (PEN-H)[20] has been adapted from the WHO PEN package for primary care.[21] PEN-H is primarily intended for medical officers, nurses, nurse practitioners and other clinical staff who provide NCD care in these settings. It covers NCD conditions, their risk factors and provides detailed flowcharts for the diagnosis and management of a range of cardiovascular diseases (including heart attacks, stroke, heart failure and hypertension), diabetes (including diabetic ketoacidosis) and chronic respiratory diseases (including asthma and chronic obstructive pulmonary disease). The London School of Hygiene and Tropical Medicine maintains a database of clinical and operational guidance and tools.[22]

Ensuring a regular supply of good quality generic medicines and equipment aligned with national or WHO or UNHCR Essential Medicines Lists, is recommended. It may not be possible to maintain patients' existing treatments and introducing new or expensive treatments may not be sustainable. Supply challenges, including physical interruptions due to insecurity, destruction of transport networks, overwhelming demand, poor management, insufficient storage capacity for medications, particularly insulin which requires a cold chain, often present immediate barriers to care in humanitarian crises.

People living with NCDs and their risk factors need regular follow-up at the primary care level to monitor disease control and prevent or manage long-term complications (e.g. using aspirin in those at high cardiovascular risk, ensuring good hypertension and diabetes control and screening for some complications, such as a diabetic foot). This involves regular access to clinical consultations, medicines, medical devices and laboratory tests. Promoting patient self-management and empowerment is likely to be beneficial but evidence for their use in humanitarian settings is lacking. Providing good quality care requires data collection and monitoring as well as functioning chronic care systems.

Patient education is particularly important in the case of mobile populations where patients often access different health services and providers. Adherence to treatment can be enhanced by staff following simplified protocols, with good communication skills. Health promotion is important and can be life-affirming. While people in humanitarian crises may have limited available or affordable food options and may be dependent on calorie-dense food aid, originally designed to address undernutrition, organizations such as the World Food Programme may be able to provide appropriate alternatives, e.g. low salt, low-fat food, food vouchers or cash-based system, including for those with specific NCDs such as hypertension, diabetes or high cholesterol.

Exercise advice should be context-adapted, taking into account security and cultural norms.

Primary prevention is not prioritized during emergency response but is important when emergencies become chronic. Community leaders (including displaced health professionals who may not be permitted to work in healthcare where they have settled), volunteers and self-help groups can lead health promotion activities, and encourage people to access healthcare services and to adhere to long-term treatment.

Evaluation and early recovery

The Sphere association has identified general indicators and targets for measuring performance for the prevention and management of NCDs but a set of joint, specific indicators spanning health system-, facility- and patient levels are being developed by the informal Inter-Agency Working Group on NCDs in Humanitarian Settings.

Internal operational reviews as well as post-response evaluations are critical to ensure ongoing learning and improvement of services for people with NCDs. Recovery planning should commence early in the post-acute/protracted (>6 months) phase of the crisis, with the aim of ensuring public health and healthcare systems are fully restored in time.[23]

Notes

1. UNHCR. Global trends: forced displacement in 2021. Geneva: UNHCR, 2022. https://www.unhcr.org/globaltrends.html.
2. Slama S et al. Care of non-communicable diseases in emergencies. *Lancet* 2017;389: 326–30.
3. Responding to the challenge of non-communicable diseases. UNHCR and UN Inter-Agency Task Force on the Prevention and Control of NCDs, 2018.
4. Hayman KG et al. Burden of cardiovascular morbidity and mortality following humanitarian emergencies: a systematic literature review. *Prehosp Disaster Med* 2015;30:80–8.
5. Jawad M et al. The impact of armed conflict on cardiovascular disease risk: a systematic review. *Heart* 2019;105:1388–94.
6. WHA74 Agenda Item 13.2: resolution on diabetes prevention and management, including access to insulin; WHA72 Agenda Item 12.4: Promoting the Health of Refugees and Migrants. WHO.
7. Health Cluster coordination guidance for heads of WHO country offices as cluster lead agency. WHO, 2019.
8. *Sphere Association. The Sphere Handbook: Humanitarian Charter and Minimum Standards in Humanitarian Response*, fourth edition, Geneva, Switzerland, 2018.
9. IASC Reference Module for the Implementation of the Humanitarian Programme Cycle. Inter-Agency Standing Committee, United Nations, 2015.
10. Political declaration of the third high-level meeting of the General Assembly on the prevention and control of noncommunicable diseases Report by the Director-General, Annex 4. WHO, EB 150/7, 2022.
11. WHO Guidance on preparing for national response to health emergencies and disasters. WHO, 2021.

12 IASC. Multi-Cluster/Sector Initial Rapid Assessment Guidance Revision July 2015.
13 Health Cluster 3/4W Tool. WHO, 2021.
14 Minimum Initial Services Package (MISP) for Sexual and Reproductive Health (SRH) in Crisis Situations. United Nations Population Fund, 2020 (web site).
15 Integration of NCD care in emergency response and preparedness. WHO, Regional Office for South-East Asia, 2018.
16 UN Interagency Task Force on NCDs. *Responding to non-communicable diseases during and beyond the COVID-19 pandemic.* WHO and UNDP, 2020.
17 Integrating non-communicable disease care in humanitarian settings – an operational guide. UNHCR, International Rescue Committee and the Informal Inter-Agency Group on NCDs in Humanitarian Settings, 2020.
18 UNHCR's principles and guidance for referral health care for refugees and other persons of concern. UNHCR, 2009.
19 Non-communicable diseases: programmatic and clinical guidelines. MSF, 2016.
20 Miller L, Mendis S et al. Package of essential non-communicable diseases interventions for humanitarian settings (PEN-H). International Rescue Committee and USAID, 2020.
21 Package of essential noncommunicable (PEN) disease interventions for primary health care. WHO, 2020.
22 Mortlock A et al. NCDs in humanitarian settings: resources and tools. London School Hygiene and Tropical Medicine, web site.
23 Disaster recovery guidance series: health sector recovery. PAHO/WHO/IRP/GFDRR, 2017.

52 The role of human rights in NCD prevention and control

Lynn Gentile, Maria Chiara Campisi, Nyasha Chingore

Human rights are rights everyone has simply by existing as human beings. These universal rights are inherent to every person in the world, regardless of nationality, sex, national or ethnic origin, colour, religion, language or any other status. They range from the most fundamental – the right to life – to those that make life worth living, such as the rights to food, education, work, health and liberty. They are not granted by any state, but are recognized in international, regional and national legal instruments that make them actionable entitlements. Human rights are part of the overarching principles of the WHO Global NCD Action Plan.

Human rights are important instruments for health, including the prevention and control of NCDs

Human rights provide binding standards

The right to health is recognized by numerous human rights instruments, such as the Universal Declaration of Human Rights, the International Covenant on Economic, Social and Cultural Rights and the Convention on the Rights of the Child. It is also acknowledged by the Constitution of the World Health Organization and the WHO Framework Convention on Tobacco Control. Unlike policy options, human rights are legally binding on States and must be implemented.

As human rights are interdependent and interrelated, the right to health can only be fully realized when other human rights are upheld. How much we enjoy the rights to social protection and work, for instance, will have a bearing on whether we can afford to access health services. Our access to adequate, healthy food and nutrition affects our health. Civil and political rights such as freedom of association and assembly enable people to organize and advocate for better health services, while the right to information empowers people to make informed decisions about their health and lifestyles.

A human rights-based approach to health aims to ensure that laws, policies, practices and processes with an impact on health further the realization of the right to health for all and are guided by human rights principles. As such, States

DOI: 10.4324/9781003306689-57

have an obligation to guarantee the availability, accessibility and acceptability of health goods, facilities and services for everyone on an equal footing. These should be of good quality, scientifically and medically appropriate, and respectful of confidentiality and medical ethics. A human rights-based approach also requires that government and those delivering services be held accountable for meeting their obligations under the right to health framework. Where the action is inadequate or where violations have occurred, effective remedies should be readily accessible.

Economic and social rights such as the right to health may be realized progressively. States should still, however, ensure the enjoyment of minimum essential levels of the right to health. These 'core obligations' include:

- Non-discriminatory access to health facilities, goods and services (including essential drugs), especially for vulnerable or marginalized groups.
- Ensuring access to minimum essential food which is nutritionally adequate and safe.
- Adopting and implementing a national public health strategy and plan of action which address the health concerns of the whole population.[1]
- More broadly, ensuring access to education, adequate housing and adequate water and sanitation.

Human rights provide special protection for vulnerable and marginalized groups

Human rights are especially concerned with people in situations of vulnerability and marginalization, such as those who are most likely to be affected by NCDs – and least likely to benefit from measures to address them. These groups are often discriminated against or subjected to stigma, which undermines their right to equal access to good quality health services. The human rights framework encourages the adoption of temporary special measures to achieve substantive equality, and these are a useful tool for achieving equal opportunities for healthy living, particularly when employed within a legal and policy environment where equality and non-discrimination are actively protected. With its emphasis on universal and equal access to quality health care, goods and facilities and the protection of marginalized groups, a human rights-based approach is essential for expanding access to preventative, curative and palliative care for those living with or at risk of developing an NCD.

Human rights require action on the underlying determinants

The right to health includes action on the underlying socio-economic, commercial, environmental and structural factors which determine or influence people's ability to live in the best health possible. These 'determinants' of health are mostly found outside of the health care system, in the conditions in which people are born, grow, live, work and age. Consequently, the health of individuals, communities and populations requires more than medical care.[2] Tackling NCD risk factors means, for instance, taking into account how socio-economic status, age, cultural norms, gender and other distinctions affect exposure for different populations, and addressing the root causes of such differences. NCDs are more prevalent among the socially and economically disadvantaged such as people living in poverty or those with relatively little education. Dealing with inequalities and discrimination, including where they intersect is, therefore, a key intervention for NCDs.

Human rights call for individual, community and broad stakeholder participation

Participating in decisions which affect our lives is a right and a core principle of a human-rights-based approach. Consequently, communities, civil society and those living with NCDs have a right to participate in developing, implementing and monitoring the NCD response. Facilitating community participation is also beneficial as health and related services are more likely to respond to the real needs of people living with NCDs. Community-led responses include advocacy, campaigning, service delivery and participatory research.

Human rights and health policy

The United Nations bodies responsible for monitoring how States meet their human rights obligations have provided guidance on measures needed to build human rights into health policy. The Committee on Economic, Social and Cultural Rights, for example, has worked on interpreting the content of the right to health protected under the International Covenant on Economic, Social and Cultural Rights. The following are particularly suitable for planning and programming to address NCDs:

Data collection

Collecting comprehensive data is part of a human rights-based approach to health.[1] Data should be disaggregated by age, gender, exposure to risk factors, prevalence of NCDs, geographic region, education, wealth categories and other distinctions as locally relevant. Disaggregated data helps to identify disparities and barriers to access to health care, patterns of discrimination, underserved areas, priority health problems, underlying determinants and vulnerable populations or groups. Relevant actions include:

- Allocating sufficient resources to expand and institutionalize data collection capacity.
- Analyzing, disseminating and using disaggregated data for policy formulation, impact evaluation, programming and information sharing, for instance, on cost-saving strategies such as the NCD best buys.

- Using disaggregated data to identify accountability gaps and to monitor and review health system performance, including the extent to which health systems are successfully implementing health-related human rights into the NCD response.

Prevention

It goes without saying that exposure to the risk factors for NCDs has a strong influence on the likelihood of developing an NCD. Other determinants of health in the context of NCDs include poverty, discrimination, access to education, adequate housing, food and nutrition, early childhood development and health in adolescence (Chapter 37 on the life-course). Given that NCDs are largely preventable, policy measures should be aimed at addressing both the determinants applicable to and known risk factors for NCDs, including tobacco use, harmful use of alcohol, physical inactivity and unhealthy diet (Chapter 17 on social determinants). As all health-impacting sectors, such as trade, agriculture, food systems, education, housing and finance are implicated, coordinated action is essential (Chapter 36 on population and high-risk strategies; Chapter 41, on fiscal measures; Chapter 53 on whole-of-government responses). Human rights-based approaches support, for example:

- An in-depth assessment, at the national and sub-national levels, of administrative, structural, social and other barriers to accessing treatment and care and how they affect various population groups.
- An in-depth assessment of the prevalence of risk factors for NCDs, including being overweight or obese, tobacco use, alcohol abuse, physical inactivity and unhealthy diets across population groups (see chapters on these risk factors).
- Cost-effective interventions to prevent occupational lung diseases, lifestyle interventions to prevent diabetes, whole-of-school programmes that include quality physical education, availability of adequate facilities and programmes to support physical activity for all children and access to clean energy for cooking in order to reduce indoor air pollution

Legal frameworks

Laws determine, to a great extent, how much everyone enjoys their health and health-related rights. Measures to ensure an enabling legal environment should have as a primary objective the repeal, rescission or amendment of laws and policies that restrict or hamper the realization of these rights, and the enactment of positive laws and policies to support them.[3] A holistic approach to creating an enabling legal environment looks beyond health-specific laws and examines what makes people vulnerable. For example, gender inequality is a major factor in women's vulnerability to cervical cancer. Legal frameworks to support the prevention and control of NCDs are important in:

- Reducing exposure to NCD risk factors.
- Regulating the private sector in order to tackle commercial determinants of health.
- Addressing stigma, discrimination and inequalities both within and outside of the health sector.
- Ensuring stakeholder participation in priority-setting, policy and programme design, implementation, monitoring and evaluation, and in accountability mechanisms.
- Enabling governments to assume full accountability for an effective NCD response and rights holders to claim their right to health.

A number of these issues are described in more detail in Chapter 46 on law and NCDs.

Planning and budgeting

Even in resource-constrained environments, the right to health means that States should allocate their maximum available resources for its optimal realization.[4] This implies the proportionate and rational allocation of resources for the NCD response, covering the health and health supporting sectors such as education, food and social protection. Examples of measures include:

- An assessment of the human rights measures required as part of the NCD response (e.g. protecting child health, promoting breastfeeding, regulating the food industry) in all relevant sectors, using disaggregated data to identify priorities.
- The development of comprehensive and time-bound plans of action providing for explicit action to ensure that these measures are implemented, together with related monitoring systems.
- Identifying, through the sharing of good practices and the provision of technical support, cost-effective interventions for the prevention and treatment of NCDs, adapted to the national context.
- The establishment of participatory budget formulation and review processes involving the representation of all stakeholders, particularly people living with NCDs.
- Human rights impact assessments of NCD policies and programmes – either as a standalone measure or integrated into broader impact assessments.
- The allocation of resources adequate to implement the areas above.

Availability, accessibility, acceptability and quality of health care

It has been estimated that more than 90% of people living in low-income countries have no legal right to health coverage and that, globally, about 39% lacks coverage.[5] Even where legal entitlements to health coverage are provided for, these are often inadequate or not implemented, with the result that they fail to meet the requirements of availability and affordability. Large parts of the population – particularly in rural areas – are also excluded from access to health services due, for instance, to insufficient numbers of skilled health workers, poor infrastructure, limited benefit packages and high co-payments.[6] From a human rights perspective, States (as principal duty bearers) are under an obligation to ensure the creation of conditions which would assure to every person all appropriate medical service and medical attention in the event of need.[1] This is an important objective of universal health coverage (Chapter 38).

Broadening health coverage for NCDs on an equitable basis requires identifying gaps in health coverage and access to services, taking into account populations whose health care costs are likely to expose them to financial hardship. Health coverage for all should then be integrated into the legislative and policy framework to ensure the formal recognition and protection of the right to health. The following are key elements to incorporate into the framework:

- The cost of the service should be met collectively by regular periodical payments which may take the form of social insurance contributions or of taxes, or of both.
- Health services should cover all members of the community, whether or not they are gainfully occupied.
- Complete preventive and curative care should be constantly available, rationally organized, provided by sufficient numbers of skilled health workers, and, so far as possible, coordinated with general health services.
- Complete preventive and curative care, available at any time and place to all members of the community covered by the service, on the basis of non-discrimination.
- The establishment or strengthening of social protection floors comprising basic social security guarantees and including, at a minimum, access to a nationally defined set of goods and services essential for NCDs, and meeting the criteria of availability, accessibility, acceptability and quality.
- Legal literacy programmes to enhance states' accountability and empower individuals and communities to access health services and claim their other health rights.

Accountability

Human rights-based accountability calls for promoting the accountability of multiple actors at various levels, within and beyond the health sector, while emphasizing that the ultimate responsibility for upholding human rights remains with governments. An important obligation is the duty to protect human rights from violations by third parties, such as private sector entities, which has a clear application in the NCD response. Accountability requires many forms of review and oversight, such as administrative, social, political and legal mechanisms and processes. Examples of actions include:

- Regular reviews, conducted in a participatory and inclusive manner, of whether, and the extent to which, health systems are delivering NCD services consistent with human rights norms.
- Establishing and/or strengthening transparent, inclusive and participatory processes and mechanisms, with jurisdiction to recommend remedial action, particularly at the national level, both within the health and the justice systems.[7]
- Ensuring that violations of the right to health and health-related rights can be effectively tackled, including through legislative measures to address criminal and civil liability, ensure access to justice and provide for compensation where appropriate. The WHO FCTC, for example, addresses liability and provides Parties with options for taking legislative action or promoting their existing laws, where necessary, to deal with criminal and civil liability.

Notes

1 CESCR general comment no. 14: the right to the highest attainable standard of health (Art. 12). Office of the High Commissioner for Human Rights, 2000.
2 Report of the special Rapporteur on the right of everyone to the enjoyment of the highest attainable standard of physical and mental health, Dainius Pùras. Office of the High Commissioner for Human Rights Council, United Nations, 2015.
3 Technical guidance on the application of a human rights-based approach to the implementation of policies and programmes to reduce preventable maternal morbidity and mortality: report of the office of the United Nations high commissioner for human rights. UN Office of the High Commissioner for Human Rights, 2012.
4 International covenant on economic, social and cultural rights. Office of the United Nations High Commissioner for Human Rights, 1966.
5 World social protection report 2014–15: building economic recovery, inclusive development and social justice. ILO, 2014.
6 Scheil-Adlung X (Ed.). *Global evidence on inequities in rural health protection: new data on rural deficits in health coverage for 174 countries*. ILO, Geneva, 2015.
7 Keeping promises, measuring results. Commission on information and accountability for women's and children's health, WHO, 2011.

Part 6
Stakeholder action for NCD prevention and control

53 Whole-of-government response for NCD prevention and control

Roy Small, Tamu Davidson, Conrad Shamlaye, Nick Banatvala

Whole-of-government action on NCDs is an example of the Health-in-All-Policies approach (HiAP), which promotes joint action across sectors to advance health and health equity. This approach systematically considers the health implications of public policy decisions and seeks synergies across health and development broadly.[1,2] Actors beyond the health sector have a large impact on the prevention and control of NCDs – and thus multisectoral action is a cornerstone of almost all national NCD action plans, as well as the WHO Global NCD Action Plan, and the political declarations and outcomes of high-level meetings. The importance of joint action across government sectors is highlighted throughout this compendium, including in chapters on the best buys and other recommended interventions, social determinants of health, commercial determinants of health and NCDs through the life-course.

A whole-of-government approach encourages sectors to collaborate, identify and act toward mutually beneficial gains (win-wins) whilst avoiding policies and actions that conflict. Too often sectors work in siloes, with incentives not always aligned with public health. It is important that different parts of government are clear on their respective responsibilities in delivering country action to address NCDs. This requires shared understanding and agreement on aims and objectives, sufficient incentives to act, quantifiable targets, and a commitment to monitor and account for progress. This chapter outlines actions that ministries beyond health can take to strengthen national responses to NCDs and the role of ministries of health in supporting this.[3]

Examples of actions by sector

Agriculture

- Implement import/export duties that make nutritious foods (such as fruits, vegetables) more affordable, and unhealthy foods and beverages less affordable.
- Develop and promote initiatives to improve access to healthy and nutritious foods such as promoting cottage farming, gardens in cities and direct farm-to-customer sales.

DOI: 10.4324/9781003306689-59

- Evaluate and monitor food policies and programmes to assess their impact on health and nutrition.
- Promote and support economically viable alternatives to tobacco growing and protect children from being used as labour for tobacco farming.
- Protect against industry interference in policymaking (e.g. farmers' and consumers' organizations that serve as tobacco or food industry front groups).

Education, sports, children and youth

- Include the risks associated with tobacco, alcohol, unhealthy diet and physical inactivity into the core curriculum.
- Include quality physical activity in sufficient amounts into the curriculum and promote extracurricular activities, as well as nutrition education initiatives (e.g. walk to school programmes and gardening activities).
- Ban the advertising, promotion and sponsorship of tobacco, alcohol and unhealthy foods and beverages in and around schools as well as other places where youth frequently gather, including by closing loopholes in corporate social responsibility initiatives, and ensure regulations concerning the marketing and sale of these products are enforced.
- Establish standards to ensure that foods and beverages provided or sold in schools are healthy and meet healthy nutrition guidelines.
- Work with ministries of health to ensure that vaccines for human papillomavirus infection (HPV) and hepatitis B (which protect against cervical and liver cancers, respectively) are included in routine childhood vaccination programmes.

Environment and energy

- Promote low-emission public transport and implement road-user charging schemes/urban road pricing to encourage active mobility.
- Phase out fossil fuel subsidies, and tax fuel and motor vehicles to reduce exposure to particulate matter.
- Map how the national NCD epidemic intersects with climate, environmental, energy and related policies and work across sectors to improve the health of people and the planet in line with the Compendium of WHO and other UN guidance on health and environment.[4]

Finance and planning

- Work with other parts of government to understand the full impact of NCDs on healthcare budgets and the economy, the return on investment from scaling up action to prevent and control NCDs, and how non-health sector budget contributions can be strategically allocated to address the determinants of NCDs, with accountability mechanisms for delivery in place.

- Work with ministries of health and other sectors to ensure that public sector finance for NCDs is adequate and being used on evidence-based and cost-effective interventions, including by promoting universal health coverage and being inclusive of marginalized populations.
- Support and where appropriate lead the development, implementation and effective administration of health taxes on tobacco, alcohol and sugar-sweetened beverages, reform fossil fuel subsidies and consider the potential for additional tax revenue to be invested in policies and programmes for NCDs and sustainable development broadly (see Chapter 3).
- Support government initiatives to disinvest in health-harming industries such as the tobacco industry.
- Invest in alternative livelihoods and healthier, more economically productive and environmentally sustainable crops for tobacco farmers.

Food and drugs

- Promote the use of clear, accurate and easily understandable food labelling (see Chapter 24).
- Regulate and ultimately eliminate the use of trans fats in the food chain.
- Test, measure and regulate the content of tobacco, alcohol and food products as appropriate.
- Adopt measures requiring public disclosure of toxic constituents in tobacco products and well-designed pictorial health warnings for tobacco products.

Foreign affairs

- Support the development (and monitoring) of bilateral and multilateral agreements that include, or establish strong protections to advance, effective NCD prevention and control measures, for example regulatory, fiscal and legislative measures on the price and regulation of unhealthy products.
- Promote and strengthen international cooperation for capacity-building, resource mobilization and use, and information exchange on best practices.
- Facilitate ratification of the WHO Framework Convention on Tobacco Control (FCTC) and the Protocol to Eliminate Illicit Trade in Tobacco Products.

Internal administration/home affairs

- Support implementation and enforcement of restrictions/bans and other public health measures to reduce population exposure to tobacco, alcohol and unhealthy foods and beverages, for example reduced hours of sales, and marketing restrictions, including to children.
- Promote legislation and support its implementation and enforcement to ensure all indoor workplaces, public places and public transport are smoke-free.

Justice and law

- Provide input and assistance in the development of legislation and regulations (e.g. nutrition labelling and advertising laws, regulations to control tobacco, harmful use of alcohol and air pollution).
- Provide support for enforcement of and/or compliance with NCD prevention and control laws and regulations.
- Identify and promote opportunities to advance NCD prevention and control in relevant laws of non-health sectors (e.g. environmental protection, labour and healthy workplace laws).
- Protect obligations under the WHO FCTC in bilateral and multilateral agreements.

Labour and employment

- Raise awareness among the public and employers about productivity losses due to NCDs and how these can be avoided.
- Ban tobacco use on work premises and provide employees with access to tobacco cessation services.
- Develop internal guidelines for alcohol consumption by staff, including restricting or banning consumption on work premises and during work hours.
- Establish standards, safeguards and regulations to protect workers from air pollutants and other hazardous conditions.
- Ensure the availability of healthy foods and beverages on work premises, including in vending machines.
- Unite key partners such as chambers of commerce employees and employers organizations to identify and incentivize collective NCD responses.

Media, information and communication

- Raise awareness of the NCD epidemic and what actions government, non-State actors, and the public can take to prevent NCDs and ensure early diagnosis and treatment are accessed by everyone.
- Work with policymakers, civil society and consumer groups to promote and implement restrictions/bans and international and national recommendations on advertising, promotion and sponsorship regarding tobacco, alcohol and unhealthy foods and beverages, and highlight issues around indoor and outdoor air pollution.
- Raise awareness of the tactics of tobacco, alcohol, food and beverage and fossil fuel companies to interfere with the implementation of effective NCD prevention and control measures.
- Monitor and hold the government, industry, and others to account in their response to NCDs.

Revenue authorities and customs

- Assist in adopting and implementing effective measures to collect tobacco, alcohol and sugar-sweetened beverage taxes and reduce evasion of taxes or duties.
- Support the development of tax policies that reduce the affordability of health-harming products and raise government revenue.
- Encourage healthier behaviours and healthier products through price and tax measures (e.g. subsidizing fruit and vegetable sales and vendors, decreasing import duties on fresh fish and implementing excise taxes on processed food producers to incentivize product reformulation).

Social and family welfare

- Ensure marginalized populations (for example women, children, indigenous peoples and the poor) have equitable access to essential NCD health services and benefit from health promotion programmes.
- Raise awareness of tobacco, alcohol and food and beverage industries' marketing to the above groups, and support efforts to combat this, as well as measures to reduce indoor air pollution.
- Ensure NCDs are considered in broader social protection policies.
- Promote the importance of collecting data on social determinants of NCDs, trends of NCDs and the impact of NCD programmes in marginalized populations.

Trade

- Be aware that unregulated trade liberalization and foreign direct investment as well as transnational advertising, marketing and promotion are increasing the availability of tobacco, alcohol and unhealthy food and beverage products.
- Use price and tax measures, import and export tariffs, and subsidies to reduce demand for tobacco and alcohol and promote a healthy diet.
- When establishing trade agreements, negotiate strong public health protections (e.g. protection of TRIPS flexibilities) and include language that clarifies the right to regulate unhealthy products.

Urban planning and transport

- Improve supportive infrastructure for, and the safety and accessibility of, walking and cycling, and public transport.
- Promote structural measures to reduce ambient and household air pollution (see Chapter 27).
- Promote safe access to green spaces, recreational facilities and pedestrian-friendly streets.

- Promote smoke-free public places including transportation, workplaces, housing and parks/green spaces; assist in the monitoring and enforcement of smoke-free policies.
- Raise awareness of the harms of second-hand smoke in public places, private vehicles and residences.
- Promote the concept and development of Healthy Cities (see below).

Working effectively across sectors

As the lead sector for the prevention and control of NCDs, the health sector needs to engage effectively with other ministries, and doing so can be challenging.[5] Working across sectors requires an understanding that:

- Ministries of health and other ministries respond to stakeholders with different interests and do not always share goals and objectives. Other ministries may require support to understand how NCDs impact their sector and the steps they can take to respond while advancing their core interests. NCD investment cases, described in Chapter 40, as well as advocacy across different parts of government by the UN system and other development partners, can be helpful in this regard.
- Ministries beyond health should be proactively involved in the development of national multisectoral action plans, and not expected to implement a plan that they have no ownership of. This requires the health sector to engage with non-health ministries early in the process of plan development, and to sustain meaningful engagement through drafting, finalization, launch, implementation and monitoring. Health ministries should similarly participate in and support the development of strategies and action plans of other ministries. Establishing or strengthening governance mechanisms dedicated to whole-of-government NCD action, and meeting regularly, is also important to ensure broad-based buy-in and ownership.
- Buy-in at a high level across all ministries is required to demonstrate leadership and commitment – with incentives (e.g. promotion or secondment) provided to staff engaged in the prevention and control of NCDs as a cross-government issue. Cross-government collaboration should be a clear objective in the annual work plans of relevant staff working on NCDs.
- Dedicated experts can also drive progress, and many countries strengthen their response by ensuring that cross-government engagement involves a mix of senior and technical staff.
- Efforts should be made to coalesce around a set of priority actions on NCD prevention and control, guided by the WHO best buys, costing action and assigning roles and responsibilities, along with timelines and specific, measurable, attainable, relevant and timebound targets.
- Ministries of finance, parliamentarians and others must be supported to make budgets available for different sectors to implement their areas of

responsibility. Accountability and monitoring mechanisms should be in place to track progress, celebrate and share success, and identify challenges.
- Inter-ministerial groups (which may cover NCDs as a whole or specific issues, for example nutrition or tobacco control) need to be established to agree on action, monitor progress and ensure partners are held accountable. The involvement of civil society partners will strengthen the effectiveness and impact of such groups.
- Informal networks are important in building trust and understanding across sectors.

Governments may consider that convening and coordinating functions for the government's multisectoral NCD response is more effective if undertaken by a central coordinating office, such as the head of state's office, cabinet office or a ministry of development planning.

The role and importance of Heads of State and Government

Heads of State and Government and their offices have a crucial role to play in driving forward action on NCDs. Their leadership helps to:

- Establish health as a core objective of national development.
- Provide sustained political commitment to promote public health as a government priority and, as part of this, keep NCD prevention and control on the national agenda, including convening different government agencies and promoting action beyond government.
- Fulfil obligations under the WHO FCTC (if the country is a Party; if not, promoting accession).
- Take action to prevent industry interference in government policymaking.
- Hold ministries accountable for the development and implementation of policies that support the prevention and control of NCDs.

The role and importance of legislative bodies

Legislative bodies such as parliament, congress and senates are also critical in supporting a whole-of-government response to NCDs. They should act to:

- Support the adoption and oversight of policies and legislation for the prevention and control of NCDs and ensure that government policies do no harm and protect health from undue commercial and other vested interests.
- Ensure that impacts on NCDs, especially on vulnerable populations, are considered in all new legislation and budgets and in strengthening the legal and policy environment for NCD prevention and control.
- Hold government and non-State actors accountable for their support (or lack of support) for delivering national NCD strategies and action plans.

- Take steps to reduce conflicts of interest between government officials/ civil servants and health-harming industries, and ensure that commercial interests do not adversely influence legislative processes for health.

The role and importance of cities and local councils

The increase in urban populations means that cities are an important setting for multisectoral action for responding to NCDs and the examples provided earlier apply equally to local and regional councils and bodies – and their elected officials, including mayors.[6] The Partnership for Healthy Cities is a global network of around 70 cities committed to preventing NCDs and injuries.[7] Examples of whole-of-government action across this network include: (i) clearing the air with new smoke-free areas in Bandung, Indonesia; (ii) reducing traffic, air and noise pollution in Barcelona, Spain; (iii) building healthier school and restaurant environments in Lima, Peru; (iv) tackling the dual challenge of tobacco use and COVID-19 in Ahmedabad, India; and (v) building a smoke-free and more equitable city in Kampala, Uganda.

Challenging public and political misperceptions

Persistent misperceptions around NCDs debilitate and undermine whole-of-government responses. Where countries do not account for the full costs of NCDs across sectors or prioritize the right to health, they may believe that any economic benefits provided by health-harming industries (e.g. tax revenue and employment opportunities from the tobacco industry) justify deregulation. Higher levels of NCDs are often considered to be an inevitable by-product of population aging and successes in combating communicable diseases; however, like many communicable diseases, NCDs cause substantial *premature* mortality and morbidity which can be prevented. Individuals are often held solely responsible for unhealthy behaviours by focusing on choice paradigms which fail to consider how the broader environment shapes choice. The negative effect of such examples of misperception is to absolve governments of responsibility and accountability for protecting populations from NCDs and their risk factors. Evidence-based policymaking, individual empowerment and community and civil society engagement, including media engagement, are important to address misperceptions.

The private sector

The interests of a number of private sector entities, most notably the tobacco industry, conflict with NCD prevention and control. Where private sector and public interests are misaligned, there is a big risk that such companies will interfere with government's efforts to develop and implement rights- and evidence-based policy and action to prevent and control NCDs. The WHO FCTC includes obligations for governments to protect against tobacco industry interference in policymaking (Chapter 33), and robust governance mechanisms across sectors are important to reduce industry interference more broadly. Efforts to better align private sector and public interests can advance NCD prevention and control (e.g. food product reformulation, collaboration with the sporting goods industry). Civil society, including the media, has roles to play in highlighting the impact of the private sector on NCDs. The roles of the private sector and public-private partnerships are described in Chapters 56 and 57.

Notes

1 Health in all policies (HiAP). *Framework for country action.* WHO, 2014.
2 Health in all policies: a guide for state and local governments. American Public Health Association, 2013.
3 Examples adapted from: (i) Secretariat of the WHO FCTC and UNDP. National Coordinating Mechanisms for Tobacco Control. Toolkit for Parties to implement Article 5.2(a) of the WHO FCTC. 2019; and (ii) What government ministries need to know about NCDs. WHO & UNDP, 2019.
4 Compendium of WHO and other UN guidance on health and environment - 2022 update. WHO, 2022.
5 Juma P. Multi-sectoral action in non-communicable disease prevention policy development in five African countries. *BMC Public Health* 2018;18:953.
6 The Power of Cities: Tackling Noncommunicable Diseases and Road Traffic Injuries. WHO 2020.
7 Partnership for healthy cities. https://cities4health.org/about-us.

54 Whole-of-society response for NCD prevention and control

Nick Banatvala, Roy Small, Pascal Bovet, Cristina Parsons Perez

A whole-of-society approach extends the whole-of-government approach by placing additional emphasis on the roles of the private sector, civil society, political decision-makers such as parliamentarians,[1] academic and research institutions, professional organizations and the media. It promotes institutional cooperation, coordination and coherence across sectors of government and society broadly for the prevention and control of NCDs.

This chapter describes the roles of parliamentarians and legislators, civil society, academic and research institutions and professional organizations in responding to NCDs. It also describes key issues in developing and sustaining partnerships. The roles of government, the private sector and the media in tackling NCDs are covered in other chapters and summarized in Table 54.1.

Parliamentarians and legislators

Parliamentarians and legislators are of critical importance for NCD prevention and control. Many of the WHO best buys (Chapter 34) require legislative and/or regulatory measures, for example: (i) increasing excise taxes and prices on tobacco products, alcohol, vehicles and fuel (Chapter 41); (ii) eliminating second-hand tobacco smoke in indoor workplaces, public places and public transport; (iii) eliminating industrially produced trans-fats from the food chain; and (iv) banning the use of asbestos and other toxicants in new construction and removing them where currently used.

Legislators are well-placed to facilitate a whole-of-government and whole-of-society response to NCDs – and to help ensure that governments and key stakeholders are held accountable for their actions (Box 54.1).

Table 54.1 The roles of government, the private sector and the media for prevention and control of NCDs

Sector	Examples of actions
Government (Chapter 53).	• Provide leadership, planning and coordination for effective multisectoral action. • Mainstream NCD prevention and control into the national development agenda and allocate adequate resources efficiently and sustainably. • Provide equitable access to NCD prevention and care through universal health coverage and action to address the determinants of NCDs. • Set and enforce standards for preventive, promotive, curative and rehabilitative health services. • Ensure legal, regulatory and fiscal environments that enable health and well-being for all. • Drive partnerships, ensuring safeguards for effective private-sector collaboration.
Private sector entities (Chapters 56 and 57).	• Work constructively with governments to create environments that reduce population exposure to NCD risk factors and enable access to health services. • Reformulate foods to eliminate trans fats and limit levels of saturated fats, sugar and salt. Increase the availability and affordability of healthy and nutritious foods and beverages. • Ensure responsible marketing practices, particularly for children and youth. • Ensure safe working conditions, including the elimination of second-hand smoke exposure, and implement workplace screening and wellness programmes. • Address environmental processes which cause NCDs and harm the planet.
Media (Chapter 50 on effective communication).	• Raise public awareness of NCDs and ways to reduce risk. • Advocate for legislative and regulatory action on the marketing of tobacco, alcohol and unhealthy foods and beverages, particularly to children and youth. • Consider impacts on NCDs in deciding what the media will/will not advertise/promote. • Keep NCDs on the public agenda through repeated coverage. Help sensitize and engage political leadership/policymakers on NCDs. • Publish high-quality scientific research on NCDs and present data in formats that suit the targeted audiences. • Hold others to account.

Whole-of-society response to address NCDs—what is the role of various stakeholders in society? WHO South-East Asia Regional Office, 2014.

> **BOX 54.1 EXAMPLES OF HOW LEGISLATORS CAN FACILITATE A WHOLE-OF-GOVERNMENT AND WHOLE-OF-SOCIETY RESPONSE TO NCD PREVENTION AND CONTROL[2]**
>
> - Raise awareness of the need for action, amongst fellow legislators, other branches of government and the general public.
> - Promote multisectoral action, including through strong multisectoral coordination mechanisms.
> - Ensure horizontal and vertical policy coherence, i.e. across and between government sectors at local, national, regional and global levels.
> - Press to incorporate NCDs into national development strategies, policies, programmes and financing frameworks.
> - Engage civil society and people living with NCDs in national NCD responses.
> - Support legal frameworks for social participation in health decision-making and for enabling civic space.
> - In budget allocations and expenditure reviews, consider the economic costs of not adequately addressing NCDs and the return on investment in scaled-up action.
> - Encourage the dissemination of accurate and trustworthy information and call out information that is inaccurate or misleading.
> - Support government to monitor public health, defend public health policies in litigation and strengthen enforcement, for example by ensuring action against those in violation of the law.
> - Ensure transparency and accountability in law-making and oversight processes, for example by supporting the development and dissemination of clear codes of conduct and disclosure mechanisms to safeguard against industry influence in policymaking, and by holding industry accountable for voluntary commitments.

It is important that legislators are aware of potential biases linked to the vested interests of industry and other stakeholders. Strong governance mechanisms must be in place to prevent legislators from being inappropriately influenced, including by ensuring that legislators declare conflicts of interest around the actions to prevent and control NCDs.

Civil society

Civil society refers to voluntary, non-governmental, not-for-profit organizations formed by people in the social sphere with commonly held values, beliefs or causes. It includes civil society coalitions and networks, protest and social movements, voluntary bodies, campaigning organizations, indigenous groups, professional associations, charities, faith-based groups, trade unions and philanthropic foundations. Civil society has been a powerful force in other global health and development responses, such as maternal and child health, HIV/AIDS and climate change. The political declarations of the high-level meetings on NCDs highlight the importance of civil society to an effective response as well as the need to foster partnerships between government and civil society (Chapter 31).

CSOs play a key role in four major areas in the prevention and control of NCDs (Box 54.2)

BOX 54.2 THE ROLE OF CIVIL SOCIETY IN THE PREVENTION AND CONTROL OF NCDs (FROM NCD ALLIANCE)[3]

- *Awareness:* Targeting the general public or specific populations with initiatives aimed at increasing knowledge and changing attitudes and behaviours (Chapter 47); raising public demand for improved rights and services (Chapter 52).
- *Advocacy:* Driving system change and influencing legislation, funding or policy for NCD prevention (e.g. Chapter 41) and/or control; mobilizing communities and people living with NCDs as agents of change (including contributing to the development, implementation and evaluation of policy and programmes) (Chapter 55).
- *Access:* Delivering health services, providing legal support, and providing practical assistance for accessing healthcare services (e.g. transportation and patient navigation) (Chapter 55), including in humanitarian situations (Chapter 51).
- *Accountability:* Tracking national progress and actions of the private and public sector against commitments and standards (Chapter 35).

In the NCD space, many CSOs focus on a single condition or risk factor. This can be advantageous since people do not have an 'NCD' – they have, for example, cardiovascular disease, cancer, diabetes or chronic respiratory disease, and the agendas for specific conditions or risks can be very different. However, many people have combinations of these diseases, and attention, investment and action for NCDs require bringing together the efforts and voices of NGOs working on disease-specific issues. The NCD Alliance was established to respond to this challenge by developing a network of organizational members, national and regional NCD alliances, over 1,000 member associations of its founding federations, global and national CSOs, scientific and professional associations, and academic and research institutions.[4] The growing network of over 66 national and regional NCD alliances across the world is evidence that coalition building is an integral part of NCD civil society. Given the linkages between NCDs and broader health and development, NCD alliances are increasingly engaging with other communities, such as those working on HIV and climate, to focus on win-win solutions.

Examples of action to maximize the potential of CSOs and communities to accelerate action towards the global NCD targets have been described.[5] They include:

- Establishing supportive legal, social and policy environments for civil society to thrive. In many countries, opportunities for flourishing civil society are repressed.[7] Governments need to be encouraged to foster and expand civic space for CSOs, and their development partners need to provide support in this process.
- Increasing investment in sustainable finance of CSOs and community systems to support CSOs and building capacity and skills in governance, advocacy, budget tracking, documenting best practices and holding others accountable.
- Encouraging the UN and governments to 'walk the talk' on their commitment to meaningful engagement of civil society, i.e. moving beyond tokenism by viewing CSOs and people living with NCDs as equal partners (Chapter 55) and experts in their own right, and creating fully inclusive processes at all levels of policy and programme design, governance, service delivery and accountability mechanisms.
- Emboldening the NCD community to hold governments and other development partners to account. As part of this, governments with the support of the UN and other development partners need to establish inclusive and transparent national accountability mechanisms that include CSOs and people living with NCDs, and to foster independent accountability efforts such as CSO shadow reporting.

Professional associations

Professional bodies are responsible for setting professional standards, accrediting professionals and providing ongoing training and professional development, including ensuring their members are fit to continue their duties. Professional bodies also have an important role in generating data, advocating for NCD prevention and control, providing technical support for the development of norms and standards and supporting their implementation. Professional bodies can influence policies around task-sharing or task-shifting (which can be particularly helpful for NCDs that require long-term treatment and care). While it is important for professional bodies to uphold standards for ensuring quality of care, they should also be open to supporting new and innovative ways of working effectively.

To support whole-of-society approaches, the WHO Global Coordination Mechanism on the Prevention and Control of NCDs (GCM/NCD) was established in 2014. GCM/NCD facilitates multistakeholder engagement and cross-sectoral collaboration and action across over 450 WHO Member States, UN organizations and non-State actors to support the delivery of the WHO Global NCD Action Plan. Examples of GCM/NCD activities are shown in Box 54.3.

BOX 54.3 EXAMPLES OF WHO GCM/NCD ACTIVITIES[6]

Working groups: (i) how to realize governments' commitments to engage with the private sector; (ii) how to realize governments' commitment to providing financing for NCDs; (iii) the inclusion of NCDs in other programmatic areas; (iv) alignment of international cooperation with national NCD plans; (v) health education; and (vi) health literacy for NCDs.

Communities of practice: including (i) meaningful involvement of people living with NCDs; (ii) NCDs, poverty and development; (iii) NCDs and health literacy; (iv) NCDs, health and law; and (v) women and NCDs.

Communication campaigns: e.g. Beat NCDs, NCDs & Me.

Knowledge Action Portal (KAP): an interactive online platform to enhance the understanding, interaction and engagement of its members on the prevention and control of NCDs.

Accountability: tracking commitments and contributions from civil society, philanthropic foundations and academic institutions on addressing NCDs.

Trade unions

Trade unions have an important role in promoting health, including the prevention of NCDs, in the work setting, working in partnership with employers and the workforce in the development, delivery and evaluation of a healthy workplace. The workplace can be an environment that protects workers' health and enables them to make healthy choices, without stigmatizing. Examples of workplace initiatives include cessation support for individuals who want to quit smoking, providing access to affordable, healthy food and beverage options for employees and implementing regular workplace screening for NCDs and their risk factors.[7]

Academic and research institutions

Although affordable, cost-effective interventions for NCDs exist, implementation is inadequate worldwide. Comparative, applied and operational research, integrating both social and biomedical sciences, is required to scale up and maximize the impact of existing interventions. Research and academic institutions, working in partnership with policymakers and funders, are key to:

- Assess, analyze and report on determinants of NCDs in various populations and subgroups.
- Assess, analyze and report on factors influencing the multisectoral, macroeconomic and social determinants of NCDs and risk factors in different settings.
- Develop and evaluate existing and new interventions, including practices and protocols, and the efficiency, availability, accessibility and cost-effectiveness of interventions within healthcare and other sectors, in different settings.
- Collate and disseminate epidemiological and socioeconomic data (e.g. surveys) to monitor progress and the impact of interventions (possibly in collaboration with local government).
- Develop monitoring frameworks (e.g. disease registries, databases of policies and practices, etc.) that can contribute to or be part of accountability mechanisms.
- Collaborate with government in the design, implementation and/or evaluation of policies and programmes.
- Ensure that knowledge and skills (including around NCDs) are continuously evaluated, strengthened, shared and taught at pre- and post-graduate levels.

More broadly, academic and research institutions are important for strengthening the scientific basis for decision-making and getting research into practice, providing technical advice to policymakers and practitioners working in government and other agencies (development of guidance and other tools), and contributing to building capacity through undergraduate and postgraduate training and professional development.

Developing and sustaining partnerships

An effective whole-of-society response is achieved both through individual actions of stakeholder groups and partnership across groups. Key to success is an appreciation of what each group brings to the table and an understanding of the power, influence and interest of each partner in moving the agenda forward. This is particularly important when developing multi-stakeholder plans and specific policies or programmes that require action beyond the health sector (e.g. taxes on tobacco products).

Institutional and context analysis (ICA) is a tool that analyzes the political and institutional factors in a given country or locality, and how these factors may impact NCD prevention and control positively or negatively. ICAs can uncover barriers to service access and delivery as well as to the implementation and enforcement of laws and policies for NCDs. They also inform how these barriers can be overcome, including through stronger leadership and alliances. The methodology for undertaking an ICA for NCDs is described elsewhere[8] along with examples of it in practice.[9,10]

An NCD stakeholder analysis in Bangladesh for example determined that: (i) policymakers, development partners, service providers, industry, research and academia, the media and civil societies are the main stakeholder categories; (ii) government, development partners and civil society had the highest levels of power and support for NCDs; (iii) tobacco and food industries had powerful positions in opposition of key NCD interventions; and (iv) non-health ministries had the lowest levels of interest.[11]

Examples of partnerships include those between the public and private sector (Chapter 57), and between governments and NGOs for health promotion and service delivery. A third example is a partnership between a range of civil society and development partners (academia, NGOs, international organizations and the media) to monitor progress and hold governments to account.[12] Guidance for developing and sustaining partnerships across sectors is widely available, including tools to: (i) identify organizations and individuals to engage or consider in a potential project: (ii) define elements of the partnership to be agreed upon by partners; (iii) assess the value, risks and implications of a partnership opportunity and inform a go/no-go decision; (iv) systematically assess what value might be created through partnership and at what cost.[13]

Strong and inclusive national and local governance mechanisms are essential for well-coordinated whole-of-society action on NCDs, including for planning, guiding, monitoring and evaluating the enactment of national policy with the effective involvement of sectors outside health. Effective governance mechanisms and structures ensure clear leadership, ongoing stakeholder engagement and effective implementation of a national multisectoral NCD strategy or action plan.[14]

Notes

1. Governance snapshot: whole-of-society approach: the coalition of partners for strengthening public health services in the European region. WHO, 2019.
2. What legislators need to know: noncommunicable diseases. WHO and UNDP, 2018.
3. Shoba J et al. Practical guide on how to build effective national and regional NCD alliances. NCD Alliance, 2016.
4. NCD Alliance. NCD Alliance Network. https://ncdalliance.org/who-we-are/ncd-alliance-network.
5. Dain K. A "whole of society" approach to non-communicable diseases must include civil society organisations. *BMJ Opinion*. December 6, 2019.
6. 2014–2019: 5 Years of the global coordination mechanism on NCDs. WHO, 2020.
7. *Work and well-being: a trade union resource*. London: Trade Union Congress, 2015.
8. Non-communicable disease prevention and control: a guidance note for investment cases. WHO and UNDP, 2019.
9. The investment case for noncommunicable disease prevention and control in the Kingdom of Saudi Arabia: return on investment analysis & institutional and context

analysis, August 2017. United Nations Interagency Task Force on the Prevention and Control of NCDs. WHO and UNDP, 2018.
10. Hutchinson B et al. The investment case as a mechanism for addressing the NCD burden: evaluating the NCD institutional context in Jamaica, and the return on investment of select interventions. *PLoS One* 2019;14:e0223412.
11. Elfarra RM. A stakeholder analysis of noncommunicable diseases' multisectoral action plan in Bangladesh. *WHO South-East Asia J Public Health* 2021;10:37–46.
12. NCD Countdown 2030 Collaborators. NCD countdown 2030: efficient pathways and strategic investments to accelerate progress towards the sustainable development goal target 3.4 in low-income and middle-income countries. *Lancet* 2022;399:1266–78.
13. Stibbe D et al. THE SDG PARTNERSHIP GUIDEBOOK: a practical guide to building high-impact multi-stakeholder partnerships for the sustainable development goals. The Partnership Initiative and UN DESA, 2020.
14. Toolkit for developing a multisectoral action plan for noncommunicable diseases. Module 2. Establishing stakeholder engagement and governance mechanisms. WHO, 2022.

55 The role of people living with NCDs in NCD prevention and control

Johanna Ralston, Cristina Parsons Perez, Charity Muturi, Catherine Karekezi

People living with NCDs have unique experiences of having lived with one and often several NCDs. They are experts in their own right and can provide first-hand insight into the challenges for the prevention, diagnosis, treatment, care and palliation of NCDs. This means they are essential stakeholders in designing and implementing policies and programmes for NCD prevention and control, including broader health system issues such as health care delivery, as well as shaping research design and delivery. With first-hand experience of the impact that NCDs have on how they live and work, people with NCDs can identify barriers and solutions that policymakers and health professionals may not readily see or cannot provide. People living with NCDs can also play a critical role in providing support to others in coming to terms with and managing their condition, either directly or through formal and informal disease-specific associations or self-help groups.

The Global Charter on Meaningful Involvement of People Living with NCDs (developed by the NCD Alliance in collaboration with those with NCDs) describes this population as 'a broad group of individuals who have or have had one or multiple NCDs as well as care partners'.[1] The Charter emphasises that people with NCDs bring a variety of perspectives, skills, and expertise from a range of professional, socio-economic and cultural backgrounds.

The voice of people and patients

In addition to being potential important partners among those who plan and provide health care, people living with NCDs can provide strong voices in the community about their diseases, helping to reduce stigma and discrimination, addressing modifiable risk factors as well as ensuring that their voice and that of their community is heard in advocating for resources and services for the prevention and control of NCDs, including universal health coverage and the reduction of out of pocket health expenditures.[2]

Unlike those with HIV/AIDS, the voices of people with NCDs were not an integral part of the original NCD narrative. In the early 21st century, the approach to NCDs was shaped by professionals representing the four main NCDs, in order to galvanize political action and resources to respond to the

DOI: 10.4324/9781003306689-61

lack of attention to these diseases, particularly in low- and middle-income countries. Because people with NCDs and communities were not initially systematically involved in this, their absence has been a major barrier to progress in NCD prevention and control. The use of 'people first' language, including the patient's voice and a narrative that defined the individuals beyond their diseases was instrumental in moving the AIDS narrative from AIDS patients to people living with HIV/AIDS. For example, the UNAIDS' Greater Involvement of People living with HIV Policy Brief (GIPA) specifically highlighted the importance of people with HIV participating in the development, implementation, as well as the monitoring and evaluation of policies and programmes. GIPA was instrumental in increasing and mobilizing resources, strengthening programmes and policies around HIV/AIDS and the setting and achievement of bold targets.[3] The NCD community has learnt from this experience, realising the power of first-hand knowledge and the importance of people-centred language, now referring for example to a woman with diabetes rather than a diabetic woman, or a person with obesity rather than an obese person.

Similarly, the responses to the recent COVID-19 pandemic have demonstrated the role of community engagement in fostering trust in government and public institutions and ensuring that health policies are responsive to local contexts and lived realities. The importance of people living with NCDs has been highlighted as critical in national responses to COVID-19 response and recovery.[4] Including individuals with lived experience is important in building the public's trust (which is often low) in responding to public health guidance – especially important to people living with NCDs, who are at high risk of complications from COVID-19.

While people living with NCDs should be involved in designing policies and programmes, as well as many aspects of health care delivery, this is not always straightforward as NCDs consist of a large number of conditions. Therefore getting consistent messages can be a challenge. Also, people living with NCDs may not wish to speak in public about their conditions for many reasons, including fear of being stigmatized or discriminated against. Nevertheless, there are a number of organizations that can help address these challenges, channelling and amplifying the voice of people living with NCDs, e.g. hospital and health care centres, including patient support groups; civil society groups (including national NCD alliances and disease- or risk-specific groups); and faith-based organizations and other community groups.

Ways of involving people living with NCDs in developing and implementing policies and services

The Global Charter described above sets out ways that those involved in developing policies and services should work with people living with NCDs. Adapted from the Charter, they are:

- Ensuring high-level commitment to the meaningful involvement of people living with NCDs in a way that recognizes the value of lived experiences and of community engagement, including embedding meaningful

involvement in organisational policies and processes, with the resources and internal capacities needed to sustain it.
- Identifying, creating and formalizing opportunities and mechanisms for meaningful involvement of people living with NCDs, including in governance and decision-making roles, policies, programmes, services and all aspects of the NCD response that affect them.
- Ensuring that meaningful involvement is contextually appropriate and spans across design and planning stages as well as implementation, monitoring and evaluation.
- Creating enabling environments and mechanisms for sustained and effective participation, particularly from marginalized groups, aimed at countering barriers and addressing power imbalances, inequalities and inequities. This includes sharing knowledge with people living with NCDs in culturally appropriate and accessible ways, such as adequate platforms for information exchange, using local languages and partnering with local services, enabling people living with NCDs to feel confident in participating, and sharing their views free of judgement, stigma or discrimination.
- Defining clearly and agreeing upfront on the purpose and terms for involvement, roles, responsibilities and expectations of all parties (including the identified groups of people living with NCDs) to build trust, commitment and mutual accountability. Provide feedback on the results of involvement and involve people living with NCDs in regular evaluation of such efforts.
- Develop transparent strategies to select and ensure the legitimacy of people living with NCDs as representatives and seek to engage a diverse range of constituencies/themes/experiences/ expertise/backgrounds.
- Strengthening the capacities of people living with NCDs through appropriate training, information, background, resources, technology, etc., to ensure their effective involvement.
- Providing support (such as logistics and financial support as feasible) to people living with NCDs in an equitable way to ensure that involvement is recognized, valued and accessible to all, leaving no-one behind.
- Using person-centred and inclusive language which respects the dignity and preferences of those being referred to.
- Ensuring sustained community engagement by supporting civil society organizations and connecting people living with NCDs with the communities they represent.

Table 55.1 provides examples of how the above can be translated into concrete activities. It is based on GIPA and adapted for people living with NCDs.

Examples of good practice

At the global level examples of good practices for the meaningful involvement of people living with NCDs in the prevention and control of NCDs, include The WHO Civil Society Working Group on NCDs, the WHO Global Compact on Diabetes and the WHO Global Coordination Mechanism on the

Table 55.1 Examples of how the engagement of people living with NCDs can be translated into concrete actions for NCD prevention and control

Policy-making process.	People living with NCDs participate in the development, monitoring and evaluation of NCD-related, as well as broader health and development policies and plans at all levels.
Programme development and implementation.	People living with NCDs provide knowledge and skills through participation in the governance of global and national organizations and in the choice, design, implementation, monitoring and evaluation of prevention, treatment, care and support programmes and research.
Leadership and support, group networking and sharing.	People living with NCDs take leadership of NCD support groups or networks, seek external resources, encourage the participation of new members or simply participate by sharing their experiences with others.
Advocacy.	People living with NCDs advocate for law reform (including rights); access to services; adequate health care delivery, including treatment, care and support; NCD prevention; resource mobilization to sustain NCD networks; and inclusion in research.
Campaigns and public speaking.	People living with NCDs are spokespersons in campaigns or speakers at public events and in other areas.
Personal.	People living with NCDs are actively involved in their own health and welfare. They take an active role in self-care and in decisions about the prevention and management of NCDs.
Treatment and management.	People living with NCDs support treatment through assisting and/or educating others on treatment options, including specific aspects of heath care not necessarily addressed by existing health care services, and share their experiences on side effects and adherence, coping with disease, and being involved as home-based and community health-care workers.

(Adapted from the GIPA framework for the NCD context)

Prevention and Control of NCDs.[5] Regional, country and local examples are provided below.

Developing policy

- In Kenya, people living with NCDs were included in the development and launch of the National Strategic Plan for Prevention and Control of NCDs

2020/21 to 2025/26. The plan was built on the expertise and legitimacy of people living with NCDs and they were involved in developing a country situational analysis. People living with NCDs raised issues around the need for greater availability and affordability of essential NCD medicines at primary health care; the disparity of cost of drugs; training and recruitment of specialist providers for NCD services; strengthening awareness around modifiable risk factors; and community mobilization to increase NCD awareness. People living with NCDs were also included in the Ministry of Health's NCD COVID-19 Sub Committee on Community Engagement, where they reported on challenges, including difficulties in accessing clinics and essential drugs, inability to pay for public health insurance premiums, barriers in accessing treatment and transport disruptions.
- The European Cancer Patient Coalition has mobilized a number of cancer patient groups on specific policy issues with a focus on health inequalities. In 2014, the Coalition launched the Cancer Patients' Bill of Rights with members of the European Parliament. People living with NCDs have been included in the development of national plans.
- Leaders and policymakers who have themselves been affected by, or seen the impact of NCDs, can be instrumental in promoting policies to tackle NCDs. Examples include a World Health Assembly resolution on rheumatic heart disease led by Australia and the establishment of a national strategy on obesity in the UK during COVID-19.

Governance and representation

- The NCD Alliance of Kenya is co-chair of the NCD Interagency Coordinating Committee (NCD ICC), which includes the promotion of and representation by people living with NCDs. The NCD-ICC spearheaded the development of the NCD Strategic Plan with technical working groups on cancer, diabetes, nutrition, essential drugs supply chain, as well as an advocacy group which included people living with NCDs.
- In the US, a group of physicians launched the Obesity Action Coalition to bring in the voices and perspectives of people with obesity. This led to changes in national legislation.
- Staff and governing bodies for Alcoholics Anonymous World Services include recovered alcoholics. Those providing support through Alcoholics Anonymous are those with lived experience of alcoholism.

Programmes, services and research

- The National Institute of Respiratory Disease's Bioethics Committee in Mexico explores complex challenges such as programmes for caring for those with a terminal illness. It includes people living with NCDs closely connected to the national NCD alliance.
- The OECD Patient-Reported Indicator Surveys (PaRis) initiative has been set up to assess the outcomes and experiences of patients managed

in primary care.[6] A Patient Advisory Panel advises on survey design and implementation and outreach activities.

Advocacy and public campaigns

- Our Views, Our Voices, an initiative of the NCD Alliance and people living with NCDs, promotes a people-centred lens in advocacy efforts of regional and national NCD alliances.
- People living with NCDs, supported by the NCD Alliance of Kenya, presented the Advocacy Agenda of people living with NCDs in Kenya[7] to the Cabinet Secretary of Health who subsequently committed to implementing the Agenda.
- The NCD Alliance of Kenya in partnership with the Ministry of Health created a platform for people living with NCDs to launch the National NCD Strategic Plan 2020/21–2025/26.

Supporting others with NCDs

People living with NCDs can play a critical role in providing support to others in coming to terms with and managing their condition, either directly or through disease-specific associations (e.g. diabetes, chronic respiratory diseases, various types of cancer, stroke) or self-help groups. Such patient-based associations or federations (which are distinct from professional associations) exist in most countries and are often led by people living with NCDs. They may be fully not-for-profit (with funding based on membership) or not-for-profit partnerships between individuals, the government and sometimes the private sector.

A number of patient-based associations and federations provide services that may not be provided by health care services and/or are best provided by those that have the unique experience of living with an NCD. They can provide practical knowledge and tips about solutions as only insiders can. Given that several hundreds of millions of patients across the world live with an NCD and many of them have a related disability that needs locally-tailored solutions, such associations bear a huge potential to help people living with NCDs to make day-to-day living with their conditions more productive. For example:

- Diabetes associations can advise those with diabetes on how to best manage repeat injections, where to find foot care and where to purchase shoes adapted for those that have diabetic foot complications.
- Associations for women with breast cancer can help fellow patients discuss concerns around their condition (e.g. issues around loss of hair associated with chemotherapy) and surgery (e.g. access to wigs, breast implants) and physical activity programmes (e.g. to improve upper limb functioning after breast surgery).
- Associations for stroke patients can assist in choosing and purchasing wheelchairs and other orthopaedic materials, or special equipment to be installed at home to facilitate mobility.

A way to go ...

The bottom line is that when individuals and communities are involved in shaping their own health and wellbeing, policies and interventions in both the public and private sectors are more likely to be successful ('nothing about us without us'). But all too often this does not happen sufficiently due to power dynamics, the absence of a culture in which this form of engagement is encouraged, and legal and structural barriers, e.g. (i) viewing those with NCDs with pity rather than as valued resource; (ii) promoting token engagement rather than encouraging leadership; (iii) those with NCDs being seen as a threat by professionals; and (iv) the expectation that inputs from those living with NCDs will be provided pro bono, including travel and subsistence.

Maximizing the value of the lived experience toward better prevention and health care, particularly in relation to disabling chronic diseases such as NCDs, will require greater efforts to systematically address power imbalances, and open up pathways for easier involvement and high-level commitment to include those with lived experience. Governments and their development partners have an important responsibility to work together alongside those with NCDs to develop the necessary legislative and policy frameworks to ensure that people with NCDs are fully included in decision-making and building capacity so that they can take on these roles.

Notes

1 Global charter on meaningful involvement of people living with NCDs. NCD Alliance (web site).
2 Voice, agency, empowerment - handbook on social participation for universal health coverage. WHO, 2021.
3 Policy brief: the greater involvement of people living with HIV (GIPA). UNAIDS, 2007.
4 COVID-19 omnibus resolution. UN General Assembly, 2020.
5 WHO civil society working group on NCDs, WHO 2018; WHO global diabetes compact, WHO 2021; and WHO global coordination mechanism on the prevention and control of NCDs.
6 Putting people at the centre of healthcare, PaRis survey of patients with chronic conditions. OECD, 2019.
7 The advocacy agenda of people living with NCDs in Kenya. NCD Alliance website, March 2018.

56 The role of the private sector in NCD prevention and control

*Nick Banatvala, Alan M Trager,
Mary Amuyunzu-Nyamongo, Téa Collins*

This chapter describes the role of the private sector in the prevention and control of NCDs. The importance of the private sector as part of a whole-of-society approach to tackling NCDs has been highlighted in the 2011 and 2018 UN political declarations of NCDs (Chapter 31) and the WHO Global NCD Action Plan (Chapter 32). The WHO Independent High-level Commission on NCDs also highlighted that relevant parts of the private sector can play an important role in making a meaningful and effective contribution to the implementation of national responses to NCDs.[1]

The term 'commercial determinants of health' is widely used to describe how private sector activities affect people's health positively or negatively (Box 56.1).

BOX 56.1 COMMERCIAL DETERMINANTS OF HEALTH

- Describe how corporate activities shape the physical and social environments in which people live, learn, work and play – both positively and negatively.
- Describe how the private sector influences the social, physical and cultural environments through business actions and societal engagements (e.g. supply chains, product design and packaging, lobbying, preference shaping).
- Impact a wide range of NCD outcomes (e.g. obesity, diabetes, cardiovascular health and cancer).
- Affect everyone, but particularly young people as lifestyle behaviour developed at an early age, as well as those with lower levels of health literacy.

Private-sector organizations (including transnational companies, micro, small and medium-sized enterprises, cooperatives, individual entrepreneurs, and farmers) can operate in the formal and informal sectors.[2] The private sector also includes corporate and commercial healthcare providers, which have a large and growing role in health systems worldwide – in some countries, private providers may be even responsible for a majority of healthcare services. While, in market economies, the private sector's first responsibility is to their shareholders and to their profitability, this does not preclude them from contributing to the prevention and control of NCDs, as profit is not in and of itself a conflict of interest.[3] A healthy workforce is essential for establishing and sustaining businesses, and employers in the private sector increasingly include the promotion of health and provision of healthcare for their employees as one of their core functions.

Private sector alignment with the prevention and control of NCDs

Private enterprises influence health through the distribution and sale of both harmful and health-promoting products, as well as through related lobbying and marketing activities.[4] This means that these industries directly and indirectly influence NCD outcomes positively and/or negatively. While some industries have values and core business models that are well aligned with global and national efforts to reduce NCDs, this is not always the case. And indeed some industries are misaligned entirely (Figure 56.1). The heterogeneous nature of the private sector makes engagement between the public and private sectors complex.

For well-aligned businesses, engagement is straightforward: the company's goals already result in a positive health outcome – and there are opportunities

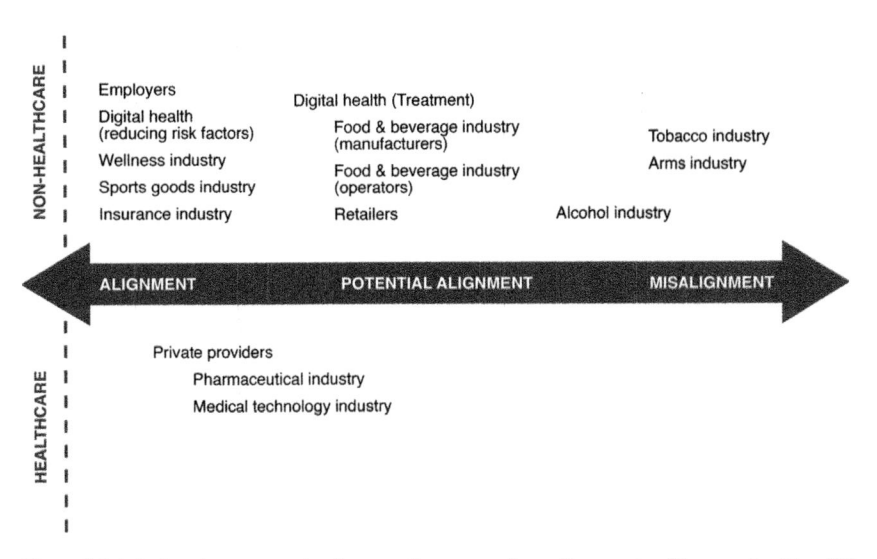

Figure 56.1 Industries categorized according to value alignment. (Trager A, Sim SY. Potential business models that involve private-sector support for national responses in preventing and controlling NCDs. PPT Initiative. 2019).

for dialogue and partnership. But things become more complex for those that are partly or imperfectly aligned. These businesses may sell a variety of products, including unhealthy ones. Efforts must be made to move these entities towards greater alignment.

Misaligned industries do not offer opportunities for engagement of any sort. The tobacco industry, for example, only causes harm to public health and wider socio-economic development. No efforts should be made to engage with this industry. The tobacco industry is not considered further in this chapter.

Well-aligned industries

The *sports and fitness industry* has an important role to play – both on its own and in partnership with governments – when it comes to increasing levels of physical activity in the population. These businesses should be encouraged to work with local and national authorities, local organizations, and other businesses to ensure that environments, programmes and opportunities for physical activity are widely available and tailored for people of all ages and abilities. Examples of collaboration might include developing knowledge to improve marketing and messaging of physical activity for different population subgroups; strengthening the capacity of healthcare professionals to help individuals improve levels of physical activity; developing applications of digital technologies that promote health and physical activity; contributing to education campaigns that promote physical activity; and being a partner to increase the availability and update of physical fitness facilities, for example through subsidized agreements.[5]

The *mobile technology industry* is increasingly being used to support governments in responding to NCDs. Mobile solutions for NCDs (including applications used in smartphones) can be used to help people quit tobacco use, monitor and increase physical activity levels, eat more healthily and better manage adherence to treatment. The mobile technology industry can also provide resources including technical expertise for issues such as communication infrastructure, interoperability between different data systems, diagnostic aids and capacity building at large (Chapter 49). However, it is also true that many of the mobile technology industry's products – like smartphones – can lead users to be more sedentary. The same industry needs to help find solutions to this.

Private sector employers have an important role to play in tackling NCDs in workplace settings. NCDs impose significant costs on businesses, such as economic losses due to absence from work (absenteeism), presence at work but not working at full capacity due to illness (presenteeism), and the loss of employees due to early retirement or death (Chapter 40). As such, employers are highly incentivized to provide healthy workplace settings. LEADERS is an example of a framework for employers for NCD workplace health programmes (Box 56.2).[6]

BOX 56.2 TACKLING NCDs IN THE WORKPLACE: THE LEADERS FRAMEWORK

- **L**ead from the top, with policies and pledges in place and leaders acting as role models.
- **E**ngage the cooperation, support and participation of employees (e.g. workplace health committees, formalizing engagement with employees, enlisting health champions), and encourage the active involvement of external partners.
- **A**ssess the needs of employees to establish workplace health priorities and design effective, evidence-based ways to tackle NCDs, with a clear plan of action.
- **D**o programmes that are based on the needs of employees with (or at high risk of) NCDs and that foster a broader health-promoting working environment. This includes ensuring relevant legislation is in place (e.g. health screening of employees, smoke-free regulations), developing and sustaining prevention and treatment programmes, and providing incentives for use of public transport, walk or cycle-to-work schemes.
- **E**valuate the impact of programmes.
- **R**ethink and adapt programmes in response to evaluations.
- **S**hare successes and challenges to encourage a culture of health within and beyond the organization.

Moderately well-aligned industries

These include the *pharmaceutical and medical industries*, which have an important role in scaling up access to essential medicines and preventive and treatment technologies (Chapters 44 and 45) and improving availability and affordability. Key areas for action should include:[7]

- Licensing and technology transfer (e.g. voluntary license through the Medicines Patent Pool).
- Broader and more rapid registration of medicines, vaccines and biologicals, especially in low- and middle-income countries.
- Transparency over the registration status of medicines, vaccines and biologicals, especially in low- and middle-income countries.
- More transparent, fair and equitable pricing (including differential prices according to country income).
- Adherence to recognized laws and regulations (e.g. around effectiveness, standards, safety, regulation).[8,9]
- Needs-based R&D, particularly for low- and middle-income countries.

- Equitable, publicly available access strategies to promote maximal coverage of medicines and health products.
- Promoting accountability and transparency.

Because NCD management often requires long-term treatment, there are potential conflicts of interest among industry, patient organizations, professional associations, health insurance companies, and public sector organizations which must be carefully identified and managed. This also applies to low- and middle-income countries where many locally produced 'branded generics' are aggressively marketed for the treatment of NCDs, that can lead to overtreatment. A number of pharmaceutical and medical industries are involved in corporate social responsibility (CSR) initiatives. However, the nature and impact of these activities on NCDs must be rigorously and transparently assessed.

When it comes to the private health and healthcare industries, it is important that they provide evidence-based prevention and treatment interventions at fair costs and, in the case of new treatments or extended indications of existing ones, full evidence of data on efficacy and side effects in a timely manner. Governments need to work with the private sector to ensure that these facilities are contributing to Targets 8 and 9 of the WHO Global NCD Action Plan (which call on providers to prioritize what works over newer, often more expensive technologies):

- At least 50% of eligible people receive drug therapy and counselling (including glycaemic control) to prevent heart attacks and strokes.
- An 80% availability of the affordable basic technologies and essential medicines, including generics, required to treat major NCDs in both public and private facilities.

It is also crucial that the healthcare industry does not exclude those with NCDs or at risk of developing NCDs – either directly or through charging higher premiums. Such policies are likely to increase inequalities and reduce the likelihood of preventive care, early diagnosis and treatment.

Skills and capacity within the private sector

Where there is good or reasonable alignment, the private sector should be incentivized to make their skills and capacity available to support broader efforts to combat NCDs. These can include:[10]

- Development of new and updated products that make a positive impact on NCDs.
- Supply infrastructure: in many countries, business controls the entire supply chain infrastructure – in the case of food, this can extend from farmers' fields to supermarkets.
- Reach and access: companies can significantly influence consumer behaviour – through marketing, the shopping process (e.g. placement, promotion of selected products, etc.) and, of course, the products themselves.

Such influence can be used productively to discourage NCD-associated behaviours and habits – for example, through a public awareness campaign.
- Brand: companies can use the social capital of their 'cool' brands to influence people's behaviour.
- Technical knowledge and capacity: companies bring technical knowledge/capacity in a range of relevant areas from product formulation to marketing know-how.
- Market-based approaches: companies are well-positioned to create sustainable long-term economic models (which in turn influence individuals' behaviour) by creating new products, new markets and new viable businesses.

The actions above can be undertaken either by private sector entities alone or in partnership with others, for example through: (i) platforms that allow for discussion, information sharing and/or collaborative action; (ii) informal alliances; or (iii) partnerships,[11] including more formal partnerships such as public-private partnerships that are described in Chapter 57. Full documentation and transparency in these mechanisms are required.

The private sector can also provide financial resources, including in-kind donations. However, agencies should be cautious in receiving such assistance, again ensuring that any such relationship with the industry is fully documented and transparent.

Industries where alignment is more problematic

Engaging with the food, and non-alcoholic beverage industries is complex. Healthy nutritious food is essential for life but ultra-processed energy-dense products (such as sugary drinks), if consumed to excess, constitute an unhealthy diet. The food industry uses a range of tactics to encourage consumers (particularly children) to buy unhealthy products, especially as many of them have low production costs, long shelf life, and thus high-profit margins. This is increasingly a problem among global conglomerates in low- and middle-income countries. Their tactics include using sophisticated marketing techniques, interfering in public policymaking processes, opposing evidence-based practices[12,13] and engaging in CSR activities of marginal public health gain rather than focusing on reducing the burden of NCDs by improving their core products (Box 56.3).

BOX 56.3 EXAMPLES OF ACTIONS FOR THE FOOD INDUSTRY, INCLUDING MANUFACTURED, RETAIL AND OUT-OF-HOME AND FOOD SERVICES

- Reformulate foods to lower sodium concentrations, saturated fats and sugar through the adoption of voluntary or mandatory standardized targets.

- Reformulate foods to eliminate or largely reduce (e.g. <1%) industrially-produced trans fats.
- Provide nutrition labelling on pre-packaged foods (total energy, sugar, saturated fats, salt, etc.), preferably using user-friendly interpretative labelling systems.
- Provide verifiable data for an independent accountability platform.

The food and non-alcoholic beverage industry retailers have an important influence in shaping markets. They should be encouraged to work with both manufacturers and national and local authorities to encourage people to have a healthy diet, through fiscal and other measures, such as marketing. Through legislation, retailers should be discouraged from promoting multi-buy or discounted offers of products associated with an unhealthy diet or placing such products at checkouts.[14]

Alcohol is associated with a range of health and social problems, and engaging with the *alcohol industry* is even more complex. Those working to promote public health across government and beyond the need to consider very carefully if and how they engage with this industry, and the impact of that, taking into account the following risks: (i) conflict of interest between the promotion of alcohol consumption and public health; (ii) the influence from the industry on those developing policies, norms and standards around alcohol; and (iii) conferring an endorsement of the alcohol industry's name, brand, product, views or activity. Funding (including sponsoring of events) and/or in-kind contributions from the alcohol industry are especially risky. Where there is a dialogue with the alcohol industry, it should be to encourage it to act in line with the global strategy to reduce the harmful use of alcohol including self-regulatory actions, adhere to the highest business standards by following existing rules and regulations and supporting public health initiatives to reduce alcohol-related harm, as well as making data available on sales and consumption of alcoholic beverages.

Incentives for better alignment

A variety of levers can be used to increase alignment among private sector entities that are moderately aligned or where alignment is problematic. Governments can use dialogue to highlight the importance they attach to public health (although not all parts of government attach the same level of priority to this. While some governments have promoted voluntary action to meet government-set targets[15] others consider regulatory and/or legislative action as the most (and in some cases the only) effective way of supporting individuals in making healthy choices. Those involved in developing policy can benefit from the increasing number of country case studies and reviews of experience to date.[16,17,18] Consumer and civil society pressure is also very important for driving action, making clear to private-sector stakeholders that improving public health is a core part of environmental, social, and corporate governance, and encouraging transparent monitoring and promoting accountability.

Transparency among government officials and their advisers

When public officers (both elected and unelected) involved in developing public policies have financial or other interests in industry, this information should be well documented, transparent and publicly available. Similarly, while it is helpful for governments to draw on experts outside industry, it can also be useful (and sometimes necessary) to draw on experts that have experience in the private sector and may have unique know-how on production processes of products (e.g. food or pharma). In all cases, it remains imperative that all interests and potential conflicts are well-documented and publicly available.

Notes

1 It's time to walk the talk: WHO independent high-level commission on noncommunicable diseases final report. WHO, 2019.
2 Private sector peer learning: peer inventory 1: private sector engagement terminology and typology. Understanding key terms and modalities for private sector engagement in development cooperation. OECD, 2016.
3 Hancock C et al. The private sector, international development and NCDs. *Glob Health* 2011;7:23.
4 Kickbusch I et al. Commercial determinants of health. *Lancet Glob Health* 2016;4:e895–96.
5 More active people for a healthier world. WHO dialogue with the sports industry on the implementation of the global action plan on physical activity (2018–2030). WHO, 2018.
6 Tackling NCDs in workplace settings in low- and middle-income countries. A call to action and practical guidance. NCDAlliance, 2017.
7 Roundtable on NCDs - strengthening the role and contribution of the pharmaceutical industry to respond to the 2011 political declaration of the high-level meeting of the general assembly on the prevention and control of NCDs. WHO.
8 Health product and policy standards. WHO. https://www.who.int/teams/health-product-and-policy-standards/standards-and-specifications/norms-and-standards-for-pharmaceuticals/guidelines.
9 Medical device regulations. Global overview and guiding principles. WHO, 2003.
10 Bauer K et al. An "all of society" approach involving business to tackle the rise in non-communicable diseases (NCDs). In *Commonwealth health ministers' update 2010* (pp. 137–48). London: Commonwealth Secretariat, 2010.
11 Collins et al. Interact, engage or partner? Working with the private sector for the prevention and control of noncommunicable diseases. *Cardiovasc Diagn Ther* 2019;9(2):158–64.
12 Lesser L et al. Relationship between funding source and conclusion among nutrition-related scientific articles. *PloS Med* 2007;4:e5.
13 Lauber K et al. Commercial use of evidence in public health policy: a critical assessment of food industry submissions to global-level consultations on noncommunicable disease prevention. *BMJ Glob Health* 2021;6:e006176.
14 Restricting promotions of food and drink that is high in fat, sugar and salt. UK Government. www.gov.uk/government/consultations/restricting-promotions-of-food-and-drink-that-is-high-in-fat-sugar-and-salt.

15 Salt targets 2017: Second progress report. A report on the food industry's progress towards meeting the 2017 salt targets. Public Health England, 2020.
16 Moodie R et al. Profits and pandemics: prevention of harmful effects of tobacco, alcohol, and ultra-processed food and drink industries. *Lancet* 2013;381:670–79.
17 Enhancing economic performance and well-being in Chile. Policy actions for healthier and more efficient food markets. OECD, 2021.
18 Public health and the food and drinks industry: the governance and ethics of interaction. Lessons from research, policy and practice. UK Health Forum, 2018.

57 The role of public–private partnerships in NCD prevention and control

Alan M Trager, Ethan Simon, So Yoon Sim, Nick Banatvala

NCDs represent a complex challenge for both governments and the private sector. These diseases are costly to treat and manage, they can negatively impact workplace productivity and they can jeopardize economic growth. By leveraging the strengths of the public and private sectors simultaneously, public–private partnerships (PPPs) can deliver results where governments or the private sector alone might fail. In the past, PPPs have been widely used for infrastructure projects, but are now increasingly being used to improve health and healthcare systems. There are opportunities to expand this approach to the prevention and control of NCDs.

Business models

A PPP is a collaborative organizational structure in which public, private, and/or nonprofit partners agree to share risks, resources and decision-making authority and responsibility. While PPPs can be modelled much like conventional businesses (with a set of structures and conditions that define revenue, financing, operational capacity, monitoring, etc.), they often require a more subtle and nuanced construction.

A successful PPP model will serve to maximize long-term value for both parties. For the public sector, this usually means better health outcomes, or lowered costs. For the private sector, it generally means some form of commercial gain, but note that immediate monetization is not a necessary prerequisite for long-term value. When structuring a PPP there are three key principles. The better these are met, the lower the risk, and the greater the opportunity a PPP presents.

Credibility of the partners, especially the public sector

For the private sector, making an impact on NCDs can be complex, expensive and laborious. Moreover, because reducing the impact of NCDs often involves significant and sustained lifestyle interventions, achieving results can often take years. Changing behaviours around diet and physical activity, for example, cannot be achieved overnight. For governments, this long-term outlook can

DOI: 10.4324/9781003306689-63

often run at odds with short-term political cycles, rapid changes in administrations and agendas and the need to control public expenses. For the private sector, it can conflict with shareholders' need to see quick returns on investment. It is crucial, therefore, that governments maintain a consistent commitment to their partnerships with the private sector regardless of short-term political winds, and that the private sector provides mechanisms to maintain long-term support for projects despite short-term risks.

Engaging the public as a partner

PPPs involving NCDs usually require significant engagement with the public. This is especially true when it comes to programmes that require behavioural change (e.g. promoting physical activity or healthy diets). PPPs that do not effectively engage the public as stakeholders in their own health (and ultimately their quality of life) will not be as successful. As voters also tend to have short-term views on how public money is used, PPPs that yield more immediate benefits to public health, or those that demonstrate benefits to revenue (e.g. taxes on cigarettes or sugar-sweetened beverages) are more likely to be welcomed by the public.

Recognizing that changing behaviours is hard

Habits can be difficult to change, and many of the behaviours that increase the risk of contracting NCDs are addictive and/or part of cultural norms – e.g. consuming tobacco, drinking alcohol and eating sugar and processed foods. It is crucial that successful PPPs address this reality by dedicating adequate resources to inducing and incentivizing behavioural changes and influencing social norms as required (e.g. by utilizing role models or influencers, etc.). PPPs that underestimate the scale of this challenge will be far less successful than those that do not.

Categorizing industries according to value alignment

Many private sector entities influence NCD outcomes – sometimes for better, sometimes for worse. Identifying whether a potential private-sector partner has 'aligned values' – that is, whether the pursuit of their vested interests leads to an improvement in public health – is the first step in building a successful PPP. Governments should work with private sector entities that have values that align with the overall goal of tackling NCDs. Well-aligned companies are those whose business model not only captures economic value but also positive health and social externalities. Examples of businesses that are likely to be well aligned include the digital health, wellness, sporting goods and health insurance industries.

Other industries are clearly misaligned, such as tobacco and arms. These industries should be excluded from PPPs.

Most industries, however, fall somewhere in the middle, and can be classified as 'potentially aligned'. This category includes the pharmaceutical industry, the medical technology industry, informal private healthcare providers and elements of the digital health industry focused on treatment. While these industries do engage in health-promoting activities, the viability of their products also relies on the presence of disease. Others may be only partly aligned, for example the food and beverage industry. While these industries may sell some unhealthy products, they can also benefit from reformulating less healthy products to meet healthier standards. Through a PPP, they may be incentivized to be more selective about the provision and advertisement of unhealthy products. Further details on classifying alignment across the private sector are included in Chapter 56 on the private sector.

PPPs can accelerate demand for healthier lifestyles and increased availability of goods and services that promote health. Using a well-designed incentive structure, the public sector could – for example – support the private sector in expanding the supply and availability of NCD prevention, screening and treatment options. Governments might also work with the private sector to bolster demand for healthy food and beverage options, using advertising and other public engagement strategies. PPPs can work to increase private competition in the markets for health-promoting products, which can stabilize prices and increase affordability. Even projects in non-health sectors can have an impact on NCDs – in the housing sector, PPPs can be used to ensure that new or renovated housing includes areas for play, access to public transport and allow the purchase of food to support a healthy diet. PPPs designed to create and maintain public parks can impact air pollution and encourage exercise. This is consistent with the 'health in all policies' approach (Chapter 53).

Business model types

PPPs can be divided into four types (Table 57.1).

As with all business models, stakeholders need to keep in mind contingencies around access to capital, stability of cash flow, commercial viability, customer base and retention rate, fair use of human resources, competitive landscape, marketing channels, infrastructure and macroeconomic conditions. In the case of NCDs, there is an inherent tension between long-term assets that require subsidies and multi-year agreements vs short-term political cycles that may result in subsidy reductions.

Key issues for building and sustaining public–private partnerships

Governance

While there are many different ways for the public and private sectors to engage with one another – from contracts to simple dialogues – it's the sharing of decision-making authority that makes PPPs unique. And while governments and corporations are often content to share this authority *in theory*, determining

Table 57.1 Business models of public–private partnerships

Business Model	Description	Application/example
Internalizing positive externalities.	Capturing the potential benefits of companies and industries that promote healthy behaviours: provides direct opportunities for partnership with 'perfectly aligned' industries.	• Partnership between city authorities, real estate agents and the local population to develop city parks or cycling lanes for exercise and relaxation.[a] • Partnership between government and private-sector employers to provide workplace wellness programmes such as workplace physical activity programmes, gym memberships, mobile apps to track employee fitness, biometric screenings, smoking cessation programmes and discounted insurance prices for employees.
Developing a market for healthy goods and services.	Markets for healthy goods and services provide opportunities for unlocking long-term value for 'potential alignment' industries as consumers become more attracted to healthy products. The profit motive can push existing food and beverage companies to reformulate their products to be healthier – less sugar, less fat, etc. Carefully designed PPP incentives can help encourage reformulation.	• Partnership between government and food and beverage businesses to provide healthier food and drink options. Businesses participating may be encouraged to apply for grants to develop and promote healthy menu options and accelerate timelines for reformulation.[b] • Partnership between government and employers to provide subsidies for employers to buy bikes for cycle to work or use public transport. • Companies pledge for each product sold (e.g. wellness products, sporting goods, digital health products), to donate the same or similar products to low- and middle-income countries or poor communities in their own country (buy-one, give-one model).[c]
Leveraging international organizations and the non-profit sector to reach consumers and patients in low-income countries or underprivileged persons in the same country.	Involves local and international organizations and the non-profit sector to assist in an operational and technical capacity, helping the public and private sectors come together more seamlessly. 'Imperfectly aligned' industries have relied on the non-profit sector to handle	• Gavi, the Vaccine Alliance, a partnership of funders (governments and donors) and the pharmaceutical industry (vaccine production including HPV vaccination) works with LICs to aggregate demand and create viable markets for immunizations. • The Defeat-NCDs online marketplace connects governments as buyers of medicines, diagnostics and equipment with private sector suppliers. By allowing multiple

(Continued)

Table 57.1 (Continued)

Business Model	Description	Application/example
	technical assistance for the coordination and distribution of goods and services in low-income countries or underprivileged persons in the same area, which has also enables them to secure new market shares while reducing transaction costs. These PPPs often rely not only on public subsidy, but also on donor support.	countries to pool their purchasing power, LICs get more for less, and suppliers are able to develop predictable markets. • Partnerships with local organizations (e.g. the local Red Cross or charitable organizations that provide food to those in need).
Traditional PPP models for healthcare infrastructure and services.	These can be elaborate arrangements or more simple government subsidies. Distinguished from privatization, private financing initiatives or the contracting of services. This model allows governments to take advantage of the agility and expertise of the private sector, while still maintaining responsibility and ensuring standards are in place for high-quality care.	• Private partners are enlisted by the government to co-finance, build and operate the facilities, but the facilities are ultimately owned by the government. Private partners are responsible for meeting agreed service quality benchmarks. • Partnerships to reduce waiting lists for routine procedures (e.g. laser therapy for diabetic retinopathy).

a Donahue J. Parks and Partnership in New York City: Adrian Benepe's Challenge (A). Harvard Kennedy School Case Program, 2004.
b Trager A, Lundberg C. Do the Elderly Have to Be Ailing? Singapore's Health Promotion Board. 2018.
c Marquis C, Park A. Inside the Buy-One Give-One Model. Stanford Social Innovation Review, 2014.

how exactly power will be shared and how it will be monitored and adjusted over time can be a challenge.

Negotiating a governance structure is one of the earliest challenges that partners will face. Partners must negotiate in a manner that develops trust and credibility. While the terms under which authority is shared can vary considerably, successful PPPs always emphasize accountability and transparency (including adequate monitoring of outcomes and finances) and ensure that both partners are acting in the best interests of the partnership. In order to minimize risk from external bodies and influences, PPPs are usually set up to be independent entities.

Aligning interests

While PPPs work best when the vested interests of both partners are well-aligned, governments and corporations often have divergent interests which can come into conflict. Partners should aim to move beyond framing conflicts of interest in a binary and reductive way, towards a more constructive and nuanced paradigm of a 'vested interest spectrum', which implies some flexibility around each party's intrinsic interests.[1] For example, while pharmaceutical companies do have an overall net positive impact on public health, the viability of their products still relies on the existence of disease. Similarly, while manufacturers of sugar-sweetened beverages are major contributors to obesity and diabetes, they may also profit from selling plain or sparkling water, which are healthy substitutes. Thus, it may make sense for governments to support certain aspects of a given industry's activity, but not others. By identifying private-sector entities whose market goals are reasonably aligned with services of the public sector, governments can use value alignment to identify suitable partners for a PPP.

The presence of conflicts of interest does not necessarily mean that a partnership is unviable. Managing conflicts of interest through careful incentive design is often more productive than avoiding them altogether. For example, ministries of health developing a PPP with the private sector to deliver healthcare services will need to ensure that the contractor does not cut corners to reduce costs, increase profits or make compromises on quality of care. To manage these challenges, payment schedules based on performance metrics can be agreed upon to determine how much the government will pay the contractor and establish mechanisms that discourage inappropriate use, including overconsumption of services. This means moving beyond broad, non-specific metrics such as number of patients served, to metrics around the quality of care (e.g. health-maintaining organizations where funding is allocated toward demonstrated and measurable health benefits). This way, the contractor is incentivized to work in the best interests of the public and the public purse, while still empowering the provider to find new efficiencies, innovations, streamline operations and reduce unnecessary costs.

Aligning interests also requires that both partners adopt a holistic understanding of agreed 'values'. While a private company is obligated to pursue a positive return on investment, this return does not need to come exclusively in the form of monetary profits. Returns can include strategic benefits, positive press and access to new markets (e.g. healthy products for the food industry). By accepting a broader range of returns, a PPP can better internalize positive externalities.

Recognizing externalities

Externalities can be negative or positive. Developing cycling lanes will increase the number of cyclists on city streets. This can increase bicycle accidents (negative externality) but also increase physical activity and reduce pollution and traffic (positive externalities). Strengthening education around health and NCDs not only benefits students but also positively impacts their families and the community at large. Improved screening and lifestyle interventions not only prevent NCDs for patients, but can also decrease healthcare expenditures, and increase economic productivity. The consumption of healthy foods can decrease healthcare costs, increase worker productivity and can also benefit local agriculture, reduce carbon footprint and create new jobs. Financing arrangements for PPPs should attempt to recognize and quantify these externalities in the PPP's business model. In doing so, governments and the private sector can identify and develop more win-win opportunities.

Engaging users as partners

Public engagement is crucial for PPPs, but 'the public' is not a single, monolithic entity. The 'general public' actually includes a complex fabric of overlapping cultural, social and economic groups, each with its own multivalent set of interests and norms. As such, an effective communication strategy is likely to require different approaches for different segments of the population. This is particularly important for PPPs where partnerships with the private sector may be viewed with concern or even hostility. Efforts to improve alignment typically involve engaging users as partners.

Capacity-building

Few professionals in the public or private sector possess the knowledge and skills for developing and managing PPPs – such as negotiation, political management, and stakeholder analysis. The number with experience in NCDs is even more limited. Building capacity, sharing best practices, and communicating lessons learnt are important if PPPs are to maximize their potential.

Performance measurement

As with any programme, defining success and regularly measuring performance is critical. This can be a special challenge in interventions run by PPPs as PPPs are structures that span many different institutions and sectors, with varying time horizons, priorities and values.

Note

1 Trager AM, Simon E. Public-private partnerships for health access: best practices. *World Economic Forum*, 2021.

58 Aid effectiveness and the role of multilateral and bilateral development agencies in NCD prevention and control

Nick Banatvala, Andrea Feigl, Nnenna Ezeigwe, Dudley Tarlton

This chapter describes the aid-effectiveness and financing-for-development agendas and their relevance for those working to prevent and control NCDs. The chapter also describes the contributions that multilateral and bilateral development agencies make to reducing the burden of NCDs.

Aid effectiveness

A series of high-level fora on aid effectiveness (Rome, 2003; Paris, 2005; Accra, 2008; and Busan, 2011) and conferences on financing for development (Monterrey, 2002; Doha, 2008; and Addis Ababa 2015) have developed and promoted a number of principles and areas for action for partners funding, implementing, and receiving development assistance (governments, multilateral and bilateral agencies, civil society, philanthropic organizations, and the private sector) to improve the impact of their investment on health and development outcomes along with setting targets to monitor progress (Box 58.1).

BOX 58.1 EXAMPLES OF PRINCIPLES AND BEST PRACTICE FOR DEVELOPMENT ASSISTANCE, WHICH SHOULD BE TAKEN INTO ACCOUNT BY THOSE WORKING ON NCD PREVENTION AND CONTROL.

- *Ownership*: Developing countries should set their own strategies for poverty reduction, improve their institutions and tackle corruption, play a more active role in designing development policies, and take a stronger leadership role in coordinating development assistance, including engaging fully with their parliaments and civil society.
- *Alignment*: Donor countries should align behind country priorities and objectives and use local systems.

DOI: 10.4324/9781003306689-64

- *Harmonisation*: Donor countries coordinate, simplify procedures and share information to avoid duplication.
- *Results*: Developing countries and donors shift focus to development results and results get measured.
- *Mutual accountability and transparency*: Donors and partners are accountable for development results.
- *Partnership*: Partnerships should move beyond traditional donors to include new governmental donors (including those from emerging economies), as well as foundations and civil society.
- *Financing*: Financing flows from development partners should align with the government.
- *Integration*: An approach that brings together economic, social and environmental priorities of countries, promoting trade and debt sustainability and addressing key governance issues.
- *Capacity building and absorptive capacity*: ensuring that development assistance builds capacity on the ground and that there is sufficient capacity to absorb the investment in a way that is sustainable.
- *Additionality*: development funds should not replace domestic funding and should ideally be adding to (or catalyzing) the quantity (and quality) of domestic investment.
- *Sustainability*: ensuring that support is provided in a way that allows activities to be continued after the investment. This requires social, economic and environmental dimensions are considered.

The aid and development effectiveness agenda has important implications for those working on the prevention and control of NCDs. Some examples are provided below.

- Countries (and where health is devolved, states or provinces) should have multisectoral NCD action plans in place that: (i) set out clear roles and responsibilities for government, international development agencies, civil society and the private sector; (ii) are aligned with broader health and development plans; (iii) have a prioritized set of actions that are evidence-based (WHO best buys and other recommended interventions – Chapter 34); (iv) have clear targets and indicators that are measured using monitoring and evaluation processes that contribute to building capacity in the country and which all partners are using.
- Prioritizing action from the demands and expectations of the many stakeholders that make up the NCD community and the myriad global and regional disease- and risk-specific strategies and action plans in addition to the WHO Global NCD Action Plan.[1] It is often more effective to focus on successfully delivering a small number of well-defined outcomes.

Multisectoral NCD plans need to be costed, resourced and include indicators that are sufficiently specific, time-bound and measurable, as well as meaningful and realistic for policymakers and practitioners on the ground.
- Prioritizing NCD action should take into account cost-effectiveness (described in Chapter 40 and elsewhere),[2] equality, equity and utility.
  - Equality: each individual or group of people has access to the same resources or opportunities.
  - Equity: recognizing that each person has different circumstances, with resource distribution based on the needs of recipients in order to reach an equal outcome.
  - Utility: allocation of resources according to their capacity to do the most good or minimize the most harm, for example, using available resources to save the most lives possible.
- Establishing multisectoral NCD coordination mechanisms (at national/federal and/or more local levels as required) that include partners across government and society (including those living with NCDs).[3] These mechanisms are important in ensuring that action plans are developed, implemented, monitored and evaluated in line with the principles and approaches described above. These mechanisms are most effective when led by senior political representatives, as this may encourage more effective participation of the non-health sectors.
- Countries and their development partners working together to scale up NCD financing: (i) low- and middle-income country governments (scaling up domestic investment for NCDs); (ii) high-income country governments and development agencies (catalytic financing and technical cooperation); (iii) multilateral agencies (global solidarity and cooperation); (iv) foundations and philanthropy (responsive and catalytic funding); (v) private sector (innovation, partnerships and social impact); and (vi) civil society (advocacy, technical expertise and accountability).[4]
- Countries using price and tax measures on tobacco, alcohol and other unhealthy commodities as part of a comprehensive strategy of NCD prevention and control and as a way of reducing healthcare costs, and providing a revenue stream for financing development, including for health activities and action on NCDs more specifically, although ministries of finance are often resistant to earmarking (hypothecating) funds in this way.
- Small standalone projects (for example, setting up smoking cessation services in one small part of the country or establishing services for screening of patients with cancer or cardiovascular disease without being part of a long-term sustainable government plan) may not be helpful. Listening to the NCD priorities of government rather than normative guidance is critical, not least to understand the politics of why a particular NCD intervention may or may not be right for the moment. Given especially the growing NCD burden, it is paramount that development partners recognize and align their support based on the disease burden in countries.

- Development partners should identify ways to encourage South-to-South and triangular cooperation. South–South cooperation refers to partnerships wherein two or more Southern countries pursue their individual or shared national or institutional capacity development objectives, while triangular cooperation refers to a South–South cooperation partnership with financial, technical or administrative assistance provided by an international development partner. Examples where these approaches have been used include action on tobacco control and action on nutrition and physical activity under the Association of Southeast Asian Nations.[5]

Multilateral agencies

United Nations agencies, development banks, other regional and international organizations, as well as bilateral government agencies are important in providing leadership and in supporting the prevention and control of NCDs at global, regional and country levels.

United Nations agencies

The political declarations of the 2011 and 2018 high-level meetings on NCDs (Chapter 31), highlight the leadership role of WHO as the UN's specialized agency for health, in supporting its Member States (taking into account that governments have the primary role and responsibility of responding to the challenge of NCDs) in their efforts to prevent and control NCDs, including through developing and promoting norms and standards (for example guidelines on screening for cervical cancer, management of NCDs in primary care, and guidelines on recommended intakes of nutrients, such as salt and sugar), providing technical assistance and policy advice, for example, around the implementation of WHO best buys and other recommended interventions described throughout this compendium, and monitoring and evaluating progress on preventing and controlling NCDs at country level (Chapters 4 and 5 on surveillance).

The WHO Director-General provides a report each year to the World Health Assembly on progress being made following the third high-level meeting on NCDs. The high-level meetings and resolutions on NCDs also recognize WHO leadership and coordination role in promoting and monitoring global action against NCDs in relation to the work of other relevant UN agencies, development banks and other regional and international organizations in addressing NCD diseases in a coordinated manner.

The UN has a presence in almost all low- and middle-income countries; however, the number of UN agencies in any one country varies considerably. The UN Country Team (UNCT) enables agencies to provide support to the government in a coherent and coordinated way, in line with each agency's mandate.

For NCDs, which require multisectoral action, this is particularly important as individual agencies have different entry points into government. A number of UN agencies have strategies that focus on (or emphasize) NCDs.[6,7] In addition, agencies have developed briefs and case studies that describe the contribution that they can make to support the delivery of the WHO Global NCD Action Plan,[8,9] for example the United Nations Development Programme (UNDP) on strengthening good governance and sustainable financing, the United Nations Children's Fund (UNICEF) on strengthening health literacy and health behaviours in children and adolescents,[10] the United Nations Population Fund (UNFPA) on cervical cancer, UNHCR – the UN Refugee Agency on actions to prevent and treat NCDs among refugee populations, and the Joint United Nations Programme on HIV and AIDS (UNAIDS) on NCD prevention and treatment among those with HIV and AIDS. A number of joint UN programmes exist to provide coordinated support to countries.

At the country level, a UN Sustainable Development Cooperation Framework (or equivalent) guides the planning, implementation, monitoring, reporting and evaluation of collective UN support to the 2030 Agenda implementation, and it is important that NCDs are considered for inclusion in these frameworks.[11,12]

As part of enhancing development effectiveness, the UN Inter-Agency Task Force on the Prevention and Control of NCDs was established in 2013 by the UN Secretary General to harness the collective efforts of the UN system to support Member States scale up action on NCDs. The Task Force reports to the UN Economic and Social Council each year. The Task Force consists of 45 UN system agencies with a WHO Secretariat. Activities are in line with its 2022–2025 strategy, i.e. (i) supporting countries to accelerate multisectoral action on the NCD- and mental health-related SDG targets – advocating for whole-of-government and whole-of-society action, and responding to the increasing demand for context-specific technical assistance from countries; (ii) mobilizing resources to support the development of country-led responses to meet the NCD- and mental health-related SDG targets; (iii) harmonizing action and forging cross-sectoral partnerships; and (iv) being an exemplar for an ever more effective UN system.

The Task Force has undertaken joint programming missions to more than 20 countries to support UNCTs in their efforts to provide technical assistance to governments in responding to NCDs. Mission reports with recommendations as well as progress reports are in the public domain.[13] These missions enable discussions to be held with ministers across government, parliamentarians and development partners in order to make recommendations on action that is required for consideration at cabinet level, e.g. establishing or strengthening governance mechanisms for NCDs, the need for multisectoral action on WHO best buys and other interventions and ways of making development assistance more effective (see below). The Task Force also develops policy and advocacy materials (e.g. sectoral briefs, agency briefs and issue specific briefs such as responding to NCDs during and beyond the COVID-19 pandemic and examples of action being undertaken by Task Force members). The Task Force also monitors how effectively UNCTs are including NCDs in their planning frameworks.[14]

The World Bank and regional development banks

The World Bank and regional development banks provide policy advice, technical support and financial assistance to strengthen the health system response and address key risk factors for NCDs. Investment lending is effective for scaling up domestic action on the prevention and control of NCDs. For example, the World Bank loan to Argentina focused on the prevention and control of NCDs among the poorest populations with three main components: (i) health services – training medical teams in early detection and effective control of NCDs, updating health care models and implementing electronic medical records; (ii) health promotion – promoting healthy behaviours and develop provincial NCD strategies; and (iii) institutional strengthening – targeting monitoring and surveillance capacities for NCDs and developing surveys and communication campaigns. The health services and health promotion components focused on implementation at the provincial, municipal and primary care levels, while the institutional strengthening work targets the central level and building an operational platform.[15]

The World Bank portfolio also includes a range of non-health investment operations that directly or indirectly contribute to NCD prevention, including: (i) promoting environmental health; (ii) expanding the use of safe and efficient cookstoves; and (iii) promoting fiscal and regulatory reforms.

Other multilateral agencies

Other multilateral agencies such as the Global Fund supports NCD prevention and control through their co-infections and co-morbidities policy (Chapter 28). Gavi, the Vaccine Alliance, a public–private global health partnership, provides support to a number of countries to scale up human papillomavirus (HPV) and hepatitis B vaccination to prevent cervical cancer and chronic liver disease, including hepatocellular cancer, respectively.

Other regional entities are also increasing their attention on NCDs. For example, the Africa Centres for Disease Control and Prevention has recently developed a new five-year strategic plan to support countries in Africa to scale up action on NCDs and mental health.

Bilateral development agencies

Overall, government development agencies have yet to prioritize action on NCD prevention and control.[16] Reasons for this include:

- An understandable desire to see NCD prevention and control being integrated into the broader health system or strengthening investments and broader governance frameworks, but also erroneous and dated claims that NCDs are not directly linked to poverty or development, and are attributable to affluence and Westernization. As a result, a number of NCDs

do not evoke the same feelings of empathy and social justice that result from diseases of childhood, HIV, TB and malaria infection and maternal mortality.
- Many governments put the onus of responsibility of acquiring NCDs on the individuals rather than on society, on personal choices rather than socio-economic circumstances, this misconception of the true nature of NCDs (the causes of which are deeply rooted in the society at large, i.e. social and commercial determinants) extends to development policy.
- There may be conflicts between policies to provide development assistance to support countries develop strong fiscal and legal action and policies that promote international trade.

The 2015 Addis Ababa Action Agenda on Financing for Development emphasized that while development (and therefore NCD prevention and control) should be financed primarily from domestic resources, it also recognized that development assistance was important in providing technical assistance to catalyze the scaling up of action. Further details on development assistance financing for NCDs is Chapter 39.

Nevertheless, there are a number of examples where bilateral development agencies have supported technical assistance projects related to NCDs, for example the FCTC 2030 project funded by Australia, Norway and the UK.[17] In 2020, Norway became the first country to publish a specific development assistance strategy for the prevention and control of NCDs.[18] The strategy explicitly aligns with the WHO Global NCD Action Plan, with a specific commitment to support action in a number of areas including taxing and regulating tobacco and alcohol; reducing deaths from air pollution; reducing harmful use of alcohol through the SAFER initiative (Chapter 26); and improving levels of healthy nutrition.

Notes

1 Wickramasinghe K. The development of national multisectoral action plans for the prevention and control of noncommunicable diseases: experiences of national-level stakeholders in four countries. *Global Health Action* 2018;11:1532632.
2 Jackson-Morris AM et al. 'Implementability' matters: using implementation research steps to guide and support non-communicable disease national planning in low-income and middle-income countries. *BMJ Global Health* 2022;7:e008275.
3 Toolkit for developing a multisectoral action plan for noncommunicable diseases. Module 2. Establishing stakeholder engagement and governance mechanisms. WHO, 2022.
4 Invest to protect NCD financing as the foundation for healthy societies and economies. NCD Alliance, 2022.
5 Collins TE. Time to align: development cooperation for the prevention and control of non-communicable diseases. *BMJ* 2019;366:l4499.
6 Programme guidance for early life prevention of non-communicable diseases. UNICEF, 2019.

7 Connecting the dots: towards a more equitable, healthier and sustainable future: UNDP HIV and Health Strategy 2022–2025, 2022.
8 UN Inter-Agency Task Force on the Prevention and Control of NCDs. United Nations Agency Briefs: responding to the challenge of non-communicable diseases. WHO, 2019.
9 UN Inter-Agency Task Force on the Prevention and Control of NCDs. Non-communicable diseases and mental health: case studies from across the United Nations system. WHO, 2019.
10 Programme guidance for early life prevention of non-communicable diseases. UNICEF, 2019.
11 Guidance note on the integration of noncommunicable diseases into the United Nations development assistance framework UNDP/WHO guidance note. WHO and UNDP, March 2015.
12 UN Inter-Agency Task Force on NCDs. Governments and United Nations Country Teams: Working together to deliver the NCD-related Sustainable Development Goals, 2021.
13 UN Inter-Agency Task Force on NCDs. Country missions and progress reports. https://www.who.int/groups/un-inter-agency-task-force-on-NCDs/country-missions.
14 United Nations Inter-Agency Task Force on the Prevention and Control of Noncommunicable Diseases. Integrating NCDs into United Nations Development Assistance Frameworks (UNDAFs): 2017 survey. WHO. 2017. https://apps.who.int/iris/handle/10665/259857.
15 International bank for reconstruction and development project appraisal document on a proposed loan in the amount of us$ 350 million to the Argentine Republic for a protecting vulnerable people against noncommunicable diseases project. World Bank, Report No: PAD535-AR, 2015.
16 Jailobaeva K et al. An analysis of policy and funding priorities of global actors regarding noncommunicable disease in low- and middle-income countries. *Global Health* 2021;17:68.
17 FCTC2030. https://fctc.who.int/who-fctc/development-assistance/fctc-2030.
18 Better Health, Better Lives. Combating Non-Communicable Diseases in the Context of Norwegian Development Policy (2020–2024). Norwegian Ministry of Foreign Affairs and Norwegian Ministry of Health and Care Services, 2020.

59 Leadership for NCD prevention and control

Pekka Puska, Nizal Sarrafzadegan, Bharathi Viswanathan, Nick Banatvala

Public health has been described as the art and science of preventing disease, prolonging life and promoting health through the organized efforts of society.[1] This definition certainly applies to the prevention and control of NCDs, where whole-of-government and whole-of-society action is essential.

The modern public health leader has been described as a 'transcendent, collaborative servant leader who knits and aligns disparate voices together behind a common mission', with skills that require the ability to 'pinpoint passion and compassion, promote servant leadership, acknowledge the unfamiliar, the ambiguous, and the paradoxical, communicate succinctly to reframe, and understand the "public" part of public health leadership'.[2] The modern public health leader also needs to strike the right balance between 'heroic' and 'unheroic' leadership and 'positional' and 'non-positional' leadership to achieve the above (Table 59.1). There is, however, no single or 'right' leadership theory, principle or style.[3]

Whole-of-government (Health in All Policies)[4] and whole-of-society approaches, along with the need for action across the whole of life (Chapter 37), as well as responding to the challenges of the social- determinants of health (Chapter 17), and indeed the full range of issues outlined in this compendium, means that public health leadership requires a broad and deep range of skills. This includes a sophisticated understanding of: (i) social justice and distribution of resources; (ii) making decisions when data are scarce; (iii) the roles and responsibilities of the state and the individual; and (iv) the balance between prevention and care.[2,5]

This chapter focuses on leadership in the context of implementing NCD prevention and control programmes, highlighting issues around *how to do*, as much of the rest of this compendium is on *what to do*. The inability to implement is a big challenge for leaders responsible for delivering the ever-increasing number of NCD policies, strategies, programmes and targets. Barriers that leaders face include inertia for change and a range of political, sociocultural, resource (human and financial) and commercial and professional interests.

Leadership for the development of successful NCD programmes

Experiences of large NCD prevention and control programmes have identified a range of issues that can guide leaders in designing and implementing such initiatives.[6,7,8] They are summarized below.

DOI: 10.4324/9781003306689-65

Table 59.1 Styles of leadership

	Heroic leadership	Unheroic leadership
Positional leadership: how decisions get made.	Calls the shots based on supposedly superior knowledge. Decides unilaterally.	Displays humility by drawing solutions out of others with judicious questions. Fosters joint ownership of decisions.
Non-positional leadership: using influence to persuade.	Shows courage, high risk, challenges status quo, rocks the boat.	Promotes a better way or sets an example in low-risk, everyday situations.

(Source: McCrimmon M. Is heroic leadership all bad? *Ivey Business Journal* Jan/Feb 2010.)

Ensure action is evidence-based. Population-based programmes should be based on solid evidence of NCD prevention and control measures with regard to impact.

In addition, it is necessary to have information, as much as possible, on the local NCD situation and feasibility, acceptability by users and stakeholders, existing capacity and overall costs of the planned programme. Many prevention programmes are based on population health information alone which, taken in isolation, is insufficient (Chapter 47 on scaling up behaviour change). Leaders must consider issues of persuasion, have a good understanding of social theory and how to deliver behaviour change at the population level and be able to spearhead social and environmental support and community organization.[9] Phrases for leaders to remember to include Kurt Lewin's 'nothing is as practical as a good theory' (i.e. good theory is practical precisely because it advances knowledge in a scientific discipline, guides research toward crucial questions, and enlightens the professional management) and 'the best way to understand something is to try to change it'.[10]

Leaders of national NCD programmes in the 2020s are in a more fortunate position than those championing early examples of comprehensive NCD programmes when it comes to the evidence and experience available in terms of the 'what to implement', although leaders still need to make difficult decisions around prioritising particular interventions where resources are scarce.[11] In addition, there will always be uncertainties and context-specific decisions to be made when it comes to the 'how to implement', including how best to engage with the population, and how best to promote behavioural change. Managing uncertainty and learning on the job remains an as important as ever for those leading NCD programmes.

Harness required resources. Leaders must remember that the success of a programme does not depend only on the proper theoretical framework and evidence available, but needs a comprehensive practical approach. It is important not only 'to do the right thing' but also 'to do enough of it', 'do it at the right time, when circumstances are ripe'. This requires sufficient financial and human resources from partners, stakeholders and non-health sectors. Decisions should also be made as to whether this is the right time for the intervention or whether it should be downsized. Robust plans with weak implementation are disheartening for all those involved and provide ammunition for those opposing the programme. The programme may be ineffective because the theoretical base was not correct, or the intervention was not intensive enough or not sustained over sufficient time.

Focus on outcomes. Long- and short-term outcomes should be identified, with progress charted and programmes adapted where required. The WHO Global Monitoring Framework (Chapter 35) provides a set of outcomes that can be used or adapted at the country level, depending on the context. Leadership must therefore be pragmatic and always emphasize the desired outcomes within the given period of time.

Limit targets. A challenge for NCD leaders is the overwhelming number of targets and indicators that have been developed at global and regional levels, in part because of the breadth of the NCD agenda, including diseases, risk factors and unifying determinants. In general, it is better to concentrate on a smaller number of key targets that everyone can focus on, recognizing that 'less is more' and a reduction in exposure to risk factors has a benefit across a number of NCDs, health and development.

Work through communities and their structures. The success of a programme ultimately depends on whether the community at large and stakeholders own and support the activities, participate in them and respond as planned. A programme should be serving the interest of the population and not the team driving it forward. Leaders should have personal interaction and presence in the community, and not only communication through media. Every community has a different structure and many informal networks, coalitions and NGOs. Leaders must be aware of the community capacity, acceptability of their interventions, and should think of equity too. Empowering the community towards demanding then performing NCD preventive actions is crucial.

Work with health services. While the task to influence the lifestyles of the population calls for intersectoral work far beyond the health sector, the role of the health sector remains central to NCD prevention and control efforts. NCD policies and programme leaders need to have the trust of health professionals and work closely with them.

Remain flexible. While a good theoretical framework and well-planned strategies are needed, a leader needs to be flexible in responding to any changing political, socioeconomic and epidemiological situation, as well as to new or emerging evidence on available interventions. Communication goes two ways: on one hand communicating the message and on the other hand listening to the views, issues, concerns and ideas of others, in order to modify the interventions and to respond to challenges, and to adjust the work towards successful outcomes, and respecting the ownership of the community.

Ensure positive messages. Communication around NCD prevention has traditionally used negative messaging ('what not to do' rather than 'what to do'). It is important that leaders are able to communicate information to policymakers and the public at large, in a positive and realistic way that emphasises changes that are incremental, feasible and attractive. Moving from 'do not smoke' to 'smoke-free' or from 'don't eat …' to 'enjoy heart healthy food' are some examples. Communities need to hear positive success stories and the results of programmes that they are part of.

Monitor and evaluate. Monitoring and evaluation (M&E) of process, impact and outcomes are essential, with resources in keeping with the size of the programme. All relevant stakeholders should be part of the evaluation process, from design to the dissemination of results and how the findings are to be used. Important lessons can be learnt from successes and failures.

National level programmes

Empowering local leaders. Leadership at the national level needs to work with and through those leading action at the regional/state or local levels. National leadership should always empower local leaders. National leaders should be committed and provide examples of best practices.

Delivering win–win solutions. Leaders will need to recognize that elected officials and communities have a range of competing priorities in addition to health. They should work to identify win–win actions that benefit health and areas important to others (e.g. increased revenue by taxing unhealthy products or improving public transport to meet environmental goals). Similarly, trust is best established by focusing on areas where there is political and community support for action. Once this trust is developed, there will be opportunities to expand a programme into more challenging areas and actions. Leaders need to be aware of private sector interests and work with those with aligned goals to their programme, and avoid being influenced by those that are not aligned.

Balancing carrots and sticks. NCD prevention requires a mix of 'carrot and stick', and leaders need to develop the right balance. Examples of carrots are increasing access to smoking-cessation services, subsidies for healthy food production, provision of opportunities for screening and health check-ups, prescriptions for accessing gym clubs and free and accessible health care. Examples of sticks include taxing unhealthy products, and implementing and enforcing a smoke-free environment. Elected officials and community people usually favour carrots, but sticks (which can involve regulatory, fiscal and legislative change) are often more effective, cheaper and cost-effective.

Translating evidence into practice. Overcoming the implementation gap between evidence and implementation requires an understanding of the political decision-making process and skills to influence personal networks. Intersectoral collaboration is important in bringing people around a common agenda and it helps ensure action and accountability. Strong evidence-based arguments and being able to respond to the counterarguments are therefore important. But the real power for change comes from the people: voters or consumers. This is crucial to mobilize public support for the needed actions.

Engaging with the private sector. A particular challenge for those working on NCDs is how and when to engage the private sector and how to maximize the positive and minimize the negative impact they can bring toward the goals of NCD programmes, Increasing corporatisation of public health can stifle the ability of leaders to act as independent advocates for the health of the population. This is a particular issue for those working on NCDs, with the significant influence of the commercial determinants of health (Chapters 56 and 57 on the private sector and public-private partnerships).

Building capacity for leadership

A number of public health competency frameworks exist for public health leaders. One example is the Leaders for European Public Health project. It describes 52 competencies across eight domains (Box 51.1).[12] This framework has also been used by countries outside Europe.[13] While the skills and attributes can be learnt and developed to a large extent, leadership comes more naturally to some.

BOX 59.1 EIGHT DOMAINS OF PUBLIC HEALTH LEADERSHIP, DEVELOPED AS PART OF THE LEADERS FOR EUROPEAN PUBLIC HEALTH PROJECT

1. Systems thinking.
2. Political leadership.
3. Collaborative leadership: building and leading interdisciplinary teams.
4. Leadership and communication.
5. Leading change.
6. Emotional intelligence and leadership in team-based organizations.
7. Leadership, organizational learning and development.
8. Ethics and professionalism.

The importance of public health leadership is too often neglected and insufficiently promoted in many countries. Three approaches have been described to better train and develop public health leaders.[14] First, leadership programmes should be targeted to individuals who are moving from narrower management positions to public health leadership positions. Second, public health training needs a greater focus on understanding constructs of power and authority, and appreciation of political and socioeconomic disciplines in order that leaders have the necessary skills to influence policy and mobilize the community.

Third, good practices, and how to adapt them to local situations, should be shared and evaluated regularly and widely, given that public health policy is increasingly global.

Those in leadership positions need to identify opportunities for developing and evaluating their leadership skills. This can be done through mentorship programmes, on-the-job training, and learning through 360-degree feedback. There are also a number of courses that support leaders develop knowledge and skills in the prevention and control of NCDs.[15,16,17]

Leading an NCD programme is hard work and challenging, but often very rewarding. Leadership requires commitment, dedication, networking and extensive collaboration with non-health sectors, with a recognition that without struggle there is often little or no progress. Scientists, public health practitioners, clinicians, politicians and laypeople can all make strong and effective leaders for NCD – by combining formal and personal skills.

Notes

1 Acheson ED. On the state of the public health [the fourth Duncan lecture]. *Public Health* 1988;102:431–37.
2 Koh HK. Leadership in public health. *J Canc Educ* 2009;24:S11–18.
3 Freys S. An overview of leadership principles and theories. In Applegate J et al. (eds.), *Leadership in healthcare and public health*. Athens, OH: Ohio University Press, 2018; 27–44.
4 Leppo K et al. *Health in all policies: seizing opportunities, implementing policies*. Ministry of Social Affairs and Health, Finland, Helsinki, 2013.
5 Turnock BJ. *Public health: what it is and how it works*, 3rd ed. Burlington, MA: Jones and Bartlett Learning, 2004.
6 Puska P. Why did North Karelia – Finland work? Is it transferable? *Global Heart* 2016;11:387–91.
7 Soltani S et al. Community-based cardiovascular disease prevention programmes and cardiovascular risk factors: a systematic review and metaanalysis. *Public Health* 2021;200: 59–70.
8 Sarrafzadegan N et al. "Isfahan healthy heart program": a practical model of implementation in a developing country. *Prog Prev Med* 2018;3:e0014.
9 Batras D et al. Organizational change theory: implications for health promotion practice. *Health Promot Int* 2016;31:231–41.
10 Yorks L. Nothing so practical as a good theory. *Hum Resour Manag Rev* 2005;4: 111–13.
11 Puska P et al. *The North Karelia project: from North Karelia to national action*. Helsinki: University Printing House, 2009.
12 Czabanowska K et al. In search for a public health leadership competency framework to support leadership curriculum-a consensus study. *Eur J Public Health* 2013;24: 850–56.
13 Mahajan P. European public health leadership competency framework: what does it say about Indian public health professionals? *Eur J Public Health* 2016;26(Suppl 1):79–80.
14 Day M et al. Time for heroes: public health leadership in the 21st century. *Lancet* 2012;380:1205–06.
15 Galaviz KI et al. The public health leadership and implementation academy (PH-LEADER) for non-communicable diseases. *Health Syst Reform* 2016;2:222–28.

16 Erzse A et al. Building leadership capacity to prevent and control noncommunicable diseases: evaluation of an international short-term training program for program managers from low- and middle-income countries. *Int J Public Health* 2017;62:747–53.

17 *Non-communicable diseases management course.* Imperial College, London. https://www.imperial.ac.uk/school-public-health/primary-care-and-public-health/teaching/whocc/courses/non-communicable-diseases-management-course/.

Index

access to medicines *see* medicines
accountability **253–259**, 286, 344, 365, 389–390, 399, 405, 407
Addis Ababa Action Agenda 2015 291, 440
Agenda for Sustainable Development 2030 23, 27, 132, 231, 244, 252, 259
aid effectiveness **434–440**
air pollution 26, 118, 120, **201–207**, 230, 234, 266, 341, 387, 396, 397, 429, 440; ambient air pollution 201; household air pollution 201, 203, 205; particulate matter 118, 120, 121, 201, 394
Air Quality Guidelines 202
alcohol 49, 50, 53, 60, 92, **194–200**, 214, 246, 271, 274, 298, 302, 305–306, 340, 343, 344, 355, 357, 358, 370, 377, 387, 396, 397, 440; harmful use 59, 63, **194–200**, 211, 212, 227, 230, 231, 234, 257, 424; risky use 197
ambient air pollution 201
approaches for NCD prevention and control *see* individual approaches and population approaches
asthma 118–119, 121, 122

bad cholesterol *see* LDL-cholesterol
bariatric surgery 70, 80
behaviour *see* health behaviour
behavioural support programmes 358
Be He@lthy Be Mobile programme 365
best buys and other effective and recommended interventions 54, 78–79, 99, 101, 107, 110, 120, 121, 146–147, 152, 197–198, 232, 236, **246–252**, 269, 296, 297, 324, 332, 340, 349–351
bilateral development agencies **434–440**
body mass index (BMI) 16, 35, 50, 67, 74–77, 91, 92, 107
breast cancer **91–96**, 318, 416

breastfeeding 78, 92, 130, 142, 146, 248, 272, 388
burden of disease *see* disease burden

cancer **83–90**, 210, 213, 318, 328, 330, 415; breast cancer **91–96**, 318, 416; cervical cancer **98–104**, 214, 438, 439; colorectal cancer **106–110**; endometrial 77, 83, kidney 77, liver 77, 83, 84, 86, 210, 213, 250, 394, 439, lung cancer 14, 15, 86, 118, 119, 203, 207, 322; oesophageal 77, 84, prostate cancer **112–116**, stomach 77, 83, 84
cancer control programmes 86–88
cancer registries 88–89, 96, 104, 110, 116
cardiovascular disease (CVD) **45–50, 52–56**, 58, 62, 77, 89, 118, 141, 149–150, 153–154, 158, 166, 186, 196, 213; alcohol use 196; best buys 54; dietary fats and cholesterol 149–150, 153–154; effective interventions 54; HEARTS technical package 63; recommended interventions 54; risk scores 54–55, 62, 153, 268; total risk approach 54–55
cerebrovascular disease *see* stroke
cervical cancer **98–104**, 214, 438, 439
CHOICE analysis 246
cholesterol **149–156**; HDL-cholesterol 151; LDL-cholesterol 150–155; total cholesterol 150, 152–155
chronic obstructive respiratory disease **118–123**
chronic respiratory disease (CRD) 119; asthma 118–119; chronic obstructive respiratory disease **118–123**; pneumoconiosis 119
civil society 69, 171, 176, 189, 207, 222, 233, 238, 240, 245, 279, 352, 353, 377, 386, 396, 399–401, **404–406**

450   Index

Clean Household Energy Solutions Toolkit (CHEST) 120
Climate and Clean Air Coalition 207
climate change 18, 201–202, 206
Codex Alimentarius Commission (Codex) 179–184, 342
Collaborative Action for Risk Factor Reduction and Effective Management of NCDs (CARMEN) network 228
colorectal cancer **106–110**
commercial determinants of NCDs/health 48, 69, 78, 340, 388, 393, **418**, 440, 446
communication 145, 161, 364, 367, **369–374**, 396, 444, 446
community-based programmes 190, 227, 273
Conference of the Parties (COP) *see* WHO Framework Convention on Tobacco Control
contestable buys 297
Convention on Long-Range Transboundary Air Pollution 206
COPD *see* chronic obstructive pulmonary disease
cost-effectiveness *see* economic analysis
Country Pharmaceutical Pricing Policy 2020 328
COVID-19 26–27, 120, 212, 231, 244, 309, 326, 345, 380, 400, 412, 415, 438
CRD *see* chronic respiratory disease
CVD *see* cardiovascular disease

demographic transition 17–19
developmental programming 271
development assistance 290–292, 434–435
diabetes **66–72**, 74, 141, 145, 154, 166, 186, 203, 218, 279, 283, 331, 333, 335, 336, 380, 381, 387, 412, 416, 432; gestational diabetes 67, 271; obesity/overweight 47, 63, 66, 69, 145; type-1 diabetes (T1D) 66, 68–70; type-2 diabetes (T2D) 66–70, 127, 131
diagnostic and monitoring tools 336–337
diet (healthy *vs.* unhealthy) 49, 59, 60, 79, 80, **141–147**, 149, 151, **157–162**, **164–169**, 171, 179, 218, 227, 229, 230, 248, 258, 266, 271, 272, 274, 302, 371, 372, 397, 423, 424, 429; fruit and vegetables 59, 60, 79, 142, 147, 152, 161, 348, 373; salt 56, 63, 131, 142, 144, 146, **157–162**, 171–176, 372; sugar 142, **164–169**, 171, 172, 175–176, 179
digital technologies **362–368**, 420; e-Health 364, 366, 367; interoperability 366; m-Health 365; telemedicine 364

direct tax 303
disability-adjusted years of life (DALYs) *see* disease burden
disease burden **3–12**, 83; air pollution 202–203; alcohol use 194; breast cancer 91; cardiovascular disease 46–48; cervical cancer 98–99; cholesterol and trans fat 151–152; chronic respiratory diseases 119; colorectal cancer 106; diabetes 67–68; dietary risks 141, 142; disability-adjusted life years lost (DALYS) 4–5, 194, 209, 246, 286, 291; hypertension 58–59; obesity/overweight 76; physical activity 188–189; prostate cancer 112; sodium intake 157; sugar intake 166; tobacco use 134; unhealthy diet 141
Disease Control Priorities (DCP) 53, 280
dyslipidaemia 151, 221, 330, 359

economic analysis 291, **294–300**; cost-effectiveness 108, 218, 246, 251, 252, 294, 296, 297, 318, 320, 329, 335, 336, 436; return on investment 297–298, 394, 432
effective interventions *see* best buys and other effective and recommended interventions
e-Health *see* digital technologies
electronic cigarettes (nicotine and non-nicotine delivery systems) 137–138
endometrial cancer 77, 83
environment and environmental risk factors 6, 21, 77, 119, 211, 212, 216, 218, 229, 235, 242, 266, 272, 274, 285, 300, 309, 347, 348, 369, 371, 394, 413, 420, 445
epidemiologic transition 14–18
epidemiology **3–12**, 15–18, 46–48, 58–59, 67–68, 76, 83, 91, 98–99, 106, 112, 119, 134, 141, 151–152, 157, 166, 188–189, 194, 202–203; risk factors *see* air pollution; alcohol; diet; hypertension; infectious agents; obesity/overweight; physical (in)activity; social determinants of health; tobacco; trends *see* disease burden; transition
epigenome 217
Essential health service package 281–282
European Cancer Patient Coalition 415
EU Tobacco Products Directive 2014 342
excise tax 136, 168–169, 198, 303

family history *see* genetics
fats: saturated fats 149; trans fats 150; unsaturated fats 149–150

financing 26, 259, 277, 278, 281, **285–292**, 326, 329, 433, 435, 436, 438; development assistance 290–292, 434–435; out-of-pocket expenditure 278, 286, 289, 327, 329
Fiscal policies 144, 298, 300, 301, **302–307**
fixed-dose medication combination (polypill) 55–56, 155
food *see* diet
Food and Agriculture Organization of the United Nations (FAO) 143
Food Drink and Taxation to Promote Healthy Diet (Manual on) 164
food reformulation 144, 159, 168, **171–177**
fortification 173–174
Framework Convention for Tobacco Control *see* WHO Framework Convention on Tobacco Control (WHO FCTC)
Front-of-pack labels 160, 167, 179–181, 183, 184

genetics 49, 77–78, **216–223**, 355
genomics 216, 219, 222
gestational diabetes 67, 271
Global Action Plan for the Prevention and Control of NCDs 2013–2030 12, 37, 38, 40, 45, 53, 56, 58, 63, 71, 74, 79, 80, 83, 93, 109, 110, 123, 127, 136, 159, 167, 189, 192, 196, 197, 201, 213, 228, **234–239**, 246, 253, 277, 326, 332, 335, 338, 353, 377, 384, 393, 407, 418, 422, 435, 438, 440
Global Action Plan on Physical Activity 2018–2030 189–191
Global AIDS Strategy 211
Global Alcohol Action Plan 196
Global Coordination Mechanism on the Prevention and Control of NCDs 407
Global Diabetes Compact 72
Global Disease Burden project (GBD) 5–11, 17, 46, 59, 68, 76, 91, 92, 99, 107, 113, 119, 135, 141, 142, 151, 152, 157, 166, 175, 188, 189, 194, 195, 203; *see also* individual chapters on risk factors and NCDs
global health databases: Global Disease Burden project (GBD) *see* Global Disease Burden project (GBD); Global Health Estimates (GHE) 6; Global Health Observatory (GHO) 5, 6, 11–12
Global Health Observatory (GHO) 5, 6, 11–12

Global Initiative For Asthma (GINA) 122
Global Monitoring Framework for NCDs 89–90, 155, 214, 253, 254, 444
Global NCD Action Plan *see* Global Action Plan for the Prevention and Control of NCDs 2013–2030
Global Physical Activity Questionnaire 191
Global School-based Student Health Survey 35
Global strategy for the Prevention and Control of NCDs 2000 196, **227–228**
Global Youth Tobacco Survey 35
good cholesterol *see* HDL-cholesterol
government response *see* whole-of-government response
Grading of Recommendations Assessment, Development and Evaluation (GRADE) 322

HDL-cholesterol 151
Heads of State and Government 229, 231, 238, 399
health behaviour 129, 438; at individual level **355–360**; at scale **347–353**
Health Behaviour in School-aged Children Survey 35–36
health checks **317–324**
health financing systems 259, 278, 282, 285, 287, 288, 290, 309
Health4Life fund *see* United Nations Health4Life Fund
Health-in-All-Policies approach (HiAP) 393
health insurance 88, 265, 278, 286, 287, 289, 329, 336, 365, 389, 415, 422, 428, 430
Health Service Availability and Readiness Assessment (SARA) 37, 64
health systems 26, 28, 32–33, 95–96, 102, 116, 120, 129, 214, 235, 287, **308–315**, 365, 367–368
health taxes 25, 290, 298, 302–304, 307, 343, 395
healthy diet *see* diet
heart attack *see* cardiovascular disease
HEARTS package 54, 56, 63, 312–314
heated tobacco products (HTPs) 242–243
high blood pressure *see* hypertension
high risk approaches (individual approaches) for NCD prevention and control **263–269**; *see also* individual chapters on risk factors and NCDs
hormone replacement therapy 92
hospital-based cancer registries *see* cancer registries

452   Index

household air pollution 201, 203
humanitarian programming cycle 378–379
humanitarian response 27, 212, 309, 328, **376–382**
human papillomavirus (HPV) 86, 98–100, 103, 213, 214, 394, 439
human rights 235, **384–390**
hypertension **58–64**; *see also* individual chapters on risk factors and NCDs
hypothecation 303

immunisation 23, 86, 99, 120, 121, 213, 214, 259, 309, 323, 394, 439; *see also* human papillomavirus (HPV)
immunotherapy 87, 116, 221
import duty 303
indirect tax 303
individual approaches for NCD prevention and control **263–269**; *see also* individual chapters on risk factors and NCDs
inequalities *see* commercial determinants of health; social determinants of health
infectious agents 14, 15, **209–215**, 227, 244, 283, 370; bacterial agents 210; fungi 210, protozoa 210, viral agents 209–210
innovation 307, 335
Institute for Health Metrics and Evaluation (IHME) Global Disease Burden project (GBD) *see* Global Disease Burden project (GBD)
Institutional and context analysis (ICA) 408, 409
insulin resistance 66, 70
Intellectual Property (IP) 333
Interagency Coordinating Committee 415
International Code of Marketing of Breast-milk Substitutes 258, 272
internet-based GBD Compare tool 6, 7
investment case **294–300**
ischaemic heart diseases (IHD) *see* cardiovascular disease

kidney cancer 77

labelling (food) 144, 147, 152, 160–161, 167, 169, **179–184**, 340, 344
law *see* legislation
LDL-cholesterol 150–155
LEADERS framework 421
leadership 191, 251, 311, 352, 399, 434, **442–447**

legislation (including international instruments and domestic implementation) 136, 152, 160, 171, 179, 180, **340–345**, 367, 387, 395, 396, 424
legislative bodies 399–400
life-course approach 100, 128–129, 235, **271–275**
liver cancer 77, 83, 84, 86, 210, 213, 250, 394, 439
lung cancer 14, 15, 86, 118, 119, 203, 207, 322

mammography 93
marketing 79, 131, 144–145, 168, 169, 172, 173, 272, 273, 333, 341–343, 394, 420
mass media campaigns 372–373
media *see* non-state actors
medical technologies **332–338**
medicines 64, 94, 116, 122, 211, 212, 222, 259, 279, **326–331**, 338, 379, 381, 415
mental health 234, 258, 294, 370, 438
m-Health *see* digital technologies
microbiota 78, 107, 210
mobile technologies *see* digital technologies
monitoring, diseases and risk factors *see* surveillance
monogenic diseases 217
MPOWER package 56, 135, 242, 304
multilateral development agencies **434–440**
Multinational MONItoring of Trends and Determinants in CArdiovascular Disease (MONICA) Project 227
multisectoral action *see* Global Action Plan for the Prevention and Control of NCDs 2013–2030; population approaches for NCD prevention and control; whole-of-government response; whole-of-society response; and individual chapters on risk factors and NCDs
myocardial infarction *see* cardiovascular disease

National cancer control programmes 88
National Food-Based Dietary Guidelines 143, 145
National labour policies 272
nicotine replacement therapy 137, 358
non-calorie sweeteners 167
non-government organisations *see* non-state actors
non-state actors: foundations 237, 405, 407, 435, 436; media 53, 79, 136, 138,

144, 146, 147, 152, 159, 161, 168, 198, 231, 257, 258, 267, 348, 363, 369–374, 396, 402, 403, 409, 444; nongovernmental organizations 176, 189, 237, 238, 282, 333, 405, 409, 444; private sector 78, 138, 189, 237, 282, 311, 327, 329, 352, 373, 388, 400–403, 407, 409, 416, **418–425**, 427–429, 432–436, 445, 446; *see also* civil society
nutrition 79, 80, 128, 143–147, 152, 160, 167, 173, 174, 176, **179–184**, 272, 273, 307, 378, 384, 387, 394, 424, 437
nutrition labelling 144, 152, 160–161, 179–184, 307

obesity/overweight **74–80**, 86, 127, 180, 271, 273, 357, 358, 432
obesogenic environments 77, 78
oesophageal cancer 77, 84
official development assistance (ODA) 290, 291
out-of-pocket expenditure *see* financing; universal health coverage (UHC)
overweight *see* obesity/overweight

Package of essential noncommunicable (PEN) disease interventions for primary health care 56, 122, 380, 381
palliative care 86, 95, 102, 103, 110, 116, 311, 312
Pan American Health Organization (PAHO) 160
pap smear 87, 101
parliamentarians and legislators 398, 402, 404
particulate matter 118, 120, 121, 201, 394
Patient-Reported Indicator Surveys (PaRis) 415
PEN package *see* Package of essential noncommunicable (PEN) disease interventions for primary health care
people living with NCDs **411–417**
perceptions and practicalities approach (PAPA) 359
pharmacogenes 218
physical activity 26, 34, 53, 56, 58, 70, 77–80, 107, 131, 153, **186–192**, 230, 258, 266, 267, 271, 273, 274, 285, 322, 348, 355, 358, 370, 372, 373, 377, 387, 394, 420, 427, 433, 437
pneumoconiosis 119, 121
Political Declarations *see* United Nations High-level meetings on NCD prevention and control; United Nations political declarations
polygenic diseases 217, 220
polygenic risk scores 49–50, 218; *see also* cardiovascular diseases; cholesterol; genetics
polypill *see* fixed-dose medication combination
population approaches for NCD prevention and control **263–269**; *see also* all chapters on risk factors and NCDs
population-based cancer registries *see* cancer registries
population-level screening programmes 318–320; *see also* screening
poverty 21, 22, 26, 128–130, 278, 279, 289, 291, 386, 407, 434, 439
pre-diabetes 67, 68
premature deaths 21, 204, 295, 298, 300
pricing policies 144, 198, 328
primary care 56, 102, 191, 196, 213, 273, 287, 288, 308, 312–314, 322–324, 330, 336, 337, 380, 381, 437, 439
PRIME theory of motivation 356
Priority Medical Device Project 332
private sector *see* non-state actors
Progress Monitor (WHO) 257
proportionate universalism 129
prostate cancer **112–116**
Protocol to Eliminate Illicit Trade in Tobacco Products (WHO) 241, 242, 395
public–private partnerships (PPP) **427–433**, 446

radiotherapy 102, 110, 115, 332, 334
REASSURED criteria 337
recommended interventions *see* best buys and other effective and recommended interventions
reformulation (food) 144, 159, 168, **171–177**
regulation 145, 159, 168, 182, 197, 340–341, 343–344, 396, 424
REPLACE package 153, 174–175
resource allocation 278, **285–292**
return on investment *see* economic analysis
risk factors *see* epidemiology

SAFER initiative 196, 198
sales tax 303
salt 56, 63, 131, 142, 144, 146, **157–162**, 171–176, 372
saturated fats *see* fats

screening 62, 69, 86, 87, 93, 101–102, 108–109, 113–114, 153, 198, 273, **317–324**; opportunistic screening 109, 321, 322; systematic screening 113–114, 320
Service Availability and Readiness Assessment (SARA) survey 37
service delivery 279, 286, 288, **308–315**, 360, 379, 380, 409
SHAKE technical package 161–162
Small island developing States 23, 76, 259
smoking *see* tobacco
social determinants of health **127–132**, 143, 190, 210, 277, 285, 393, 397, 408
social media 198, 369, 371–374
Sodium Country Score Card 162
STEPwise Approach to NCD Risk Factor Surveillance 34–35
stomach cancer 77, 83, 84
stroke 7, 45–49, 54, 55, 263, 309, 370
sugar (including sugar-sweetened beverages) 142, **164–169**, 171, 172, 175–176, 179
surveillance: monitoring, diseases and risk factors 56, 63–64, 72, 80, 89–90, 96, 103–104, 110, 122–123, 132, 138–139, 147, 155–156, 162, 169, 176–177, 191–192, 199, 207, 214–215; principles **28–33**; tools **37–40**, 336–337
sustainable development goals (SDGs) **21–27**, 147, 207, 230, 231, 243, 244, 253, 258–259, 282, 291, 438, 440
sustainable financing *see* financing

taxes, health 26, 290, 298, 302–304, 307, 343, 395; *see also* Fiscal policies
tobacco/tobacco control 4, 35, 56, 86, 113, 120, **134–139**, 227, 234, **240–245**, 257, 266, 271, 274, 283, 285, 298, 302, 304–305, 341, 343, 347, 394, 396, 420, 437
trade **240–245**, 333, **393–409**
Trade unions 405, 407
trans fats *see* fats
transition 204, 274, 379; demographic transition 11, 17–19; epidemiologic transition 14–17; public health transition 18, 20
triglycerides 150
type-1 diabetes (T1D) 66, 68–70
type-2 diabetes (T2D) 66–70, 127, 131, 268

UHC Compendium 191
UHC2030 International Health Partnership 282

unhealthy diet *see* diet
United Nations Children's Fund (UNICEF) 292, 438
United Nations Department of Economic and Social Affairs (UNDESA) 259
United Nations Development Programme (UNDP) 292, 298–299, 438
United Nations Economic and Social Council (ECOSOC) 231, 235, 244, 259, 377, 438
United Nations General Assembly (UNGA) 229
United Nations Health4Life Fund 292
United Nations High-level meetings on NCD prevention and control 229–233, 302, 342
United Nations High-level Political Forum on Sustainable Development (HLPF) 231, 235, 259
United Nations Inter-Agency Taskforce on the Prevention and Control of NCDs (UNIATF) 243–244, 438
United Nations Outcome Document 2014 257
United Nations political declarations 2011, 2018, 2025 **229–233**, 257, 302, 342
Universal health coverage (UHC) 231, **277–283**, 329
unsaturated fats 149–150

vaccination *see* immunisation
value-added tax (VAT) 303

waist circumference *see* obesity/overweight
wasted buys 297
WHO Framework Convention on Tobacco Control (WHO FCTC) 135–138, **240–245**, 257, 341, 342, 390, 395, 396, 399, 400
whole-of-government response 27, 69, 147, 229, 352, **393–401**, 402, 438, 442
whole-of-society response 69, 229, 352, **402–409**, 419, 438, 442, 443
win–win actions/interventions/opportunities/solutions/strategies 23–25, 206, 266–267, 393, 406, 433, 445
World Bank 5–8, 46, 187, 188, 194, 240, 283, 365, 439
World Health Assembly (WHA) 102, 227, 235–237, 252, 253, 331, 377, 415, 437
World Trade Organization (WTO) 342, 343